The Development of
Modern Surgery

D1327427

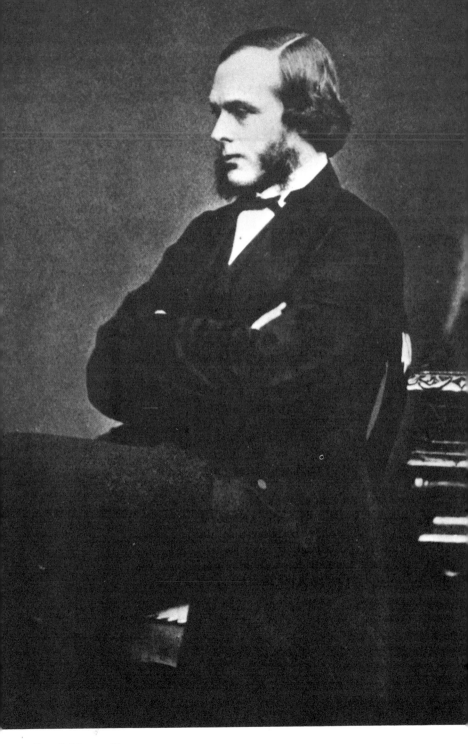

Joseph Lister, 1867.

The Development of Modern Surgery

FREDERICK F. CARTWRIGHT

THOMAS Y. CROWELL COMPANY

Established 1834 • New York

First published in the United States of America in 1968

Copyright © 1967 by Frederick F. Cartwright

All rights reserved. Except for use in a review, the reproduction or utiliza-
tion of this work in any form or by any electronic, mechanical, or other
means, now known or hereafter invented, including photocopying and
recording, and in any information storage and retrieval system is forbidden
without the written permission of the publisher.

Printed in the United States of America
L.C. Card 68-11287

THE CHICAGO PUBLIC LIBRARY

APR 1 1968 M

Contents

Illustrations

Preface

The history of surgery is so vast a subject that a full, detailed survey cannot be confined within the limits of a medium-sized book. For this reason, I have here tried to describe the development, rather than the history, of modern surgery. The modern science depends essentially upon basic principles evolved as the result of discoveries during the nineteenth century; I have therefore concentrated on the progress made in the last hundred and fifty years. This must not be taken to imply that no important work was done before 1800; there is a continuing story of real, although slow, progress which can be traced back into the misty times when the doctor was a priest or a magician or both. This earlier part of the tale may be found in one of the excellent histories of medicine listed in the bibliography.

Even with this limitation, it has been found necessary to select and, regretfully, to leave undescribed much that is of interest and importance. I have made this selection myself and the choice is entirely mine; I cannot expect unanimous agreement that I have chosen wisely. On the whole I have not introduced controversial matter, but in two instances, the chapters on anaesthesia and on Lister – subjects which have been my special study for a number of years – I have given a version of the story somewhat different from that commonly accepted; it seems dishonest to perpetuate legends, which I consider to be false, just for the sake of orthodoxy. On the other hand, limitation of space has not permitted discussion and there will be some, no doubt, who consider that I have been too didactic.

As this book is written primarily for the non-medical reader, a certain amount of explanation and simplification has been thought desirable. I hope that this will not deter the medical student or serious historian, for whose benefit a number of references have been provided. These are taken from British or American journals; having myself little French and no German, it would for me be little short of cheating to list references in a foreign tongue.

Examination of the bibliography will show that I owe a large debt to many who have written on the history of medicine and surgery in past years. Their work, and that of the medical authors who preface their chapters or articles with a short historical note, has been quite invaluable to me. I would here take the opportunity of most strongly commending the latter practice. The modern student is far too prone to think that there is no background to his subject; his mind is so fixed upon the present that he forgets that the past is the only map to the future.

I owe, too, a debt of gratitude to my colleagues who have so willingly answered my innumerable questions. Admittedly their replies have often been preceded by the remark that a first year medical student should have known the answer – but the opportunity offered was too good to be missed. I am particularly grateful to the following colleagues who have read and advised me on chapters; it is disappointing that so much of the valuable material which they gave me has had to be omitted: Mr H. C. Edwards (Wars and Wounds); Mr J. G. Yates Bell (Urology); Mr R. C. F. Catterall (Orthopaedic Surgery); Mr F. T. Moore (Surgery of Repair); Mr A. J. Heriot (Abdominal Surgery); Mr J. J. MacCabe (Surgery of the Brain); Mr L. T. Cotton (Surgery of the Lungs and Heart and the section on the thyroid); Mr S. R. Mawson (the ear); Mr P. Wright (the eye). I am also most grateful to my friends in the anaesthetic department for their generous help and understanding.

Almost the whole of the necessary research has been done in the library of King's College Hospital Medical School. Librarians in general are renowned for their helpfulness, but I think that we must be particularly fortunate at King's. So it gives me very real pleasure to have this opportunity of thanking Mrs Sargeant and her staff for their unfailing kindness and patience.

The Development of
Modern Surgery

CHAPTER I

The Surgeon in the Early Nineteenth Century

Although operative surgery can boast a very long history, the surgeon did not emerge as a specialist or even as a respectable practitioner until the nineteenth century. Professionally he was regarded as inferior to his associates, the physician and apothecary; a man of little education, he learned his trade by apprenticeship alone; he was compromised by a long standing association with the barber. The nature of his calling, the pain which he inevitably caused, the aura of death that surrounded him, these made him a figure from the thought of whom the patient shrank in horror – and not altogether without reason. Three essential needs had to be met before surgery could take its rightful place in medical science; these were a regular system of education, a means of destroying the pain of operation, and a lowered mortality. Our first chapters will therefore deal with the fulfilment of these primary needs.

Association with the encumbering barber was first ended by the surgeons of Paris in 1743; their example was followed by the London surgeons in 1745, largely through the initiative of William Cheselden of St Thomas' Hospital. The old Company of Barber-Surgeons gave place to the Company of Surgeons, at first little better than a trade guild, the function of which was to protect the interests of its members. Gradually this function widened to include the regulation of training. By 1800, when the Company became the Royal College of Surgeons of London, education had assumed a very important place in its undertakings.

But in 1800 the surgeon still acquired his professional education by apprenticeship only, and the value of apprenticeship depends upon the master's ability. Apprenticeship, although it has practical advantages as a method of training, can and does result in the handing down of bad tradition and obsolete methods from one generation to the next, unless supported by scientific teaching. It was not until after 1815 that anything in the nature of systematic education began to appear. This important advance followed the Apothecaries Act of 1815, when the Society of Apothecaries secured for themselves powers which placed in their hands the control of medical practice throughout England and Wales. Thereupon the Apothecaries insisted on a certain standard of general education and a set curriculum of study before a candidate might sit their qualifying examination. An apprentice, articled for a minimum term of five years, must have also attended two courses of lectures in anatomy and physiology and two courses in the theory and practice of medicine; almost of more importance in the future development of medical education, he must have walked the wards of a recognized hospital for a period of at least six months.

An apothecary was entitled to practise surgery.[1] For this reason, membership of the Royal College of Surgeons was not an essential qualification; the Surgeons, limited by their charter to the control of surgical practice in London and for seven miles around, found themselves in danger of losing their influence. They tried to obtain for themselves privileges similar to those of the Apothecaries but failed in their attempt. In order to maintain the prestige of their diploma they were forced to demand from their candidates certificates of having attended courses of lectures and of having walked the wards of a hospital, a curriculum similar to that of the Apothecaries, but with the emphasis upon surgery. The three or six months' medical and surgical 'firm' of the present day student is a relic of the two periods of six months' 'walking the wards' demanded for the licence of the Society of Apothecaries and membership of the Royal College of Surgeons. During the first half of the nineteenth century this, the 'college and hall', became the most popular double qualification.

These educational demands ultimately proved a death-blow

to the system of apprenticeship. In the early years the student-apprentice arranged his curriculum very much as he and his master pleased; he might go straight from a morning's work in the dissecting room to an afternoon session in operating theatre or ward, a system which had the obvious advantage over our own of allowing the student to correlate theory with practice. Lectures were arranged early in the morning or late in the evening so that the apprentice was free to attend to his master's business. The regulations imposed by Apothecaries and Surgeons resulted in an increased burden, for the apprentice, serving a term of five or seven years, could not attend hospital without prolonging his training for an additional year, unless he had the good fortune to be working in a town which possessed a recognized hospital. The burden became intolerable in 1824 when the Surgeons, anxious to raise the teaching standard, refused to recognize any school or hospital but those of London, Edinburgh, Dublin, and Aberdeen. Their action was followed by a storm of protest; for the apprentice working in the provinces could not possibly attend a hospital in London, the only recognized English centre, except at considerable expense and by lengthening his period of training. In 1832 the Surgeons were forced to relent and to recognize schools of anatomy in provincial towns possessing properly regulated hospitals. The result was the emergence of a number of provincial teaching centres, still very active today. But the difficulty remained; although the apprenticeship system lingered on for thirty more years, the school and hospital part of the student's training rapidly took precedence over his duties as an apprentice.

The physician was able to acquire a mark of distinction by obtaining a doctorate in medicine offered by the universities; no such mark of distinction existed for the English surgeon at the beginning of the nineteenth century. A higher surgical qualification, the fellowship, was originally mooted in 1832, purely as a means of securing a slightly more democratic method of election to the governing body of the Royal College of Surgeons of London, but the proposal was not accepted. The matter was again raised in 1836 when Astley Paston Cooper, president of the College, induced his colleagues to institute an examination which would entitle the successful candidate to be recognized as a teacher in anatomy, physiology, pathology, and surgery. But the new qualification did not prove popular; during the next two years only six candidates presented themselves, and the scheme came to an end in 1840.[2]

Three years later the College prayed a new charter, which was granted. The Royal College of Surgeons of London now became the Royal College of Surgeons of England, an extension of title, it is interesting to note, that was suggested not by the College but by the law officers of the Crown. The terms of the charter allowed for the election of a number of distinguished Members, three hundred in the first instance, to be Fellows of the College. Although the primary purpose of the new order of fellows was to form an electoral body, and the council of the College retained the right to confer fellowship by election, regulations for fellowship by examination were soon instituted. The original regulations demanded that the candidate must be at least twenty-five years of age and of certified good character. He must have spent six years in professional study, at least three in a recognized London hospital and one as a house surgeon or surgical dresser in a recognized hospital, not necessarily in London but in the United Kingdom. Every candidate was required to submit a written account of at least six clinical cases. The examination, to be held in two parts with a day's interval between, consisted of written papers on anatomy and physiology, surgery, pathology, and therapeutics. The papers were to be written from ten to five each day; the candidate might be questioned orally by the examiners and be required to perform dissections and operations upon the cadaver. At the first examination, held on 3 and 5 December 1844, twenty-four candidates successfully passed and were admitted as fellows.[3] The history of the modern surgical specialist starts with that first examination.

Thus the status of the surgeon in England underwent a radical change between the years 1815 and 1845; during this time he developed from an ill-educated technician, trained by apprenticeship alone, into a highly qualified member of the medical profession. In Europe and in America the change, although following similar lines, was somewhat slower. It is largely for this reason that London attained its importance as a world centre of surgery during the middle years of the nineteenth century.

Other factors contributed to the increased importance of London. In order to understand what happened it is necessary to go back for a few years. During nearly the whole of the eighteenth century Paris held pride of place as the centre of medical teaching and practice. The ambitious American or English doctor regarded a visit to Paris as an essential part of his training; French medicine and French surgery in particular exerted a profound effect upon the development of ideas in both countries. This French predominance, already waning by 1789, received a mortal blow in the Revolution when the extremists, bent upon destroying all real or imagined privilege, threw the professions open to anyone, qualified or not. But the French teaching persisted through the pupils of the original school and may certainly be regarded as one of the parents of American medicine. In France itself the old tradition was brilliantly carried on by a small number of men, predominantly interested in military surgery. Among these was Baron D. J. Larrey, Napoleon's chief surgeon and the idol of his troops. Larrey and others continued their work throughout the Napoleonic era and into the Restoration; they secured continuity of the pre-revolutionary tradition with the revived French school of the late nineteenth century.

Before the fame of Paris had started to wane, Edinburgh was already rising to the high place which it held at the end of the eighteenth century. The Edinburgh school derived from that of Leyden in Holland and depended for its excellence upon a far higher standard of teaching than was to be found in any other centre. The Monro dynasty of anatomists, grandfather, father, and son, all named Alexander Monro, made the Edinburgh teaching of anatomy famous, and anatomy is the basis of surgery. The third of the Monros did not share his forebears' brilliance – he is said to have contented himself with reading his grandfather's lectures, not omitting the words 'When I was a student at Leyden' – but an even more spectacular teacher was forthcoming in the person of Robert Knox. His classes were enormous; in 1828 five hundred and four students regularly attended his lectures; as the room would hold a maximum of two hundred, each lecture had to be repeated

5

three times a day, and Knox's assistants often spent as much as sixteen hours on end in the dissecting room. Not all of these students were reading medicine; besides physicians, apothecaries, and surgeons' apprentices there were 'English barristers, Scottish advocates and divines, scions of the nobility, artists, and men of letters.'[4] It is understandable that an artist should seek a knowledge of anatomy, but the reason which prompted a Scottish divine to do the same is less obvious.

At this time a knowledge of practical anatomy could only be obtained by leave of a resurrectionist, a ruffian who watched for funerals by day and who disinterred the body under cover of night. Teachers could acquire the subjects which they used for their demonstrations only by illegal trafficking with a ghastly crew who were certainly not above blackmail, and there are well-authenticated stories that some renowned anatomists tried to solve the difficulty by engaging in resur- rection on their own account. The high prices paid for fresh bodies in good condition and the fact that no questions could be asked by the purchaser tempted the more villainous type of resurrectionist to provide subjects by an easier method than that of rifling a grave. In 1829 the series of murders committed by Burke and Hare of Edinburgh and the tracing of at least one body to Knox's anatomy rooms provided a sensation which resulted in the ruin of Knox, the tarnishing of Edinburgh's good name and, after a similar murder in London, the passing of the Anatomy Act of 1832. This act permitted authorized medical schools to acquire bodies for the purpose of dissection. The Anatomy Act and the Apothecaries Act did more to advance the standard of education and respectability of the medical profession than any legislation before or since.

London had already started to rise before Edinburgh was passing into eclipse. An educational centre demands teachers, and the greatest of the London teachers were Scots by birth or education. First of these is John Hunter who did much to raise surgery from an empirical art to a science. Born at Long Calderwood, near Glasgow, in 1728, John Hunter set out for London at the age of twenty to study under the well-known surgeons William Cheselden of St Thomas' and Percival (or Percivall) Pott of St Bartholomew's. He then joined the army and served in Portugal for four years. On his return to

England he was appointed to the surgical staff of St George's Hospital and founded a school of anatomy and surgery in Leicester Square. Hunter was nothing of a scholar but he possessed an enquiring mind which urged him to undertake a great research into the wide field of physiology and comparative anatomy. A stumbling, tongue-tied lecturer, he successfully taught by demonstration and example; his outlook can best be summed up in his often quoted dictum (contained in a letter to Edward Jenner who introduced vaccination) 'Why think? Why not try the experiment?' He made no great advances or discoveries in surgery but, by correlating practice with comparative anatomy and physiological experiment, he placed surgery on a scientific basis.

John Hunter died at a meeting of the governors of St George's Hospital in 1793, but his teaching lived on. His pupils carried his methods into the nineteenth century. John Abernethy, who advised his rich patients 'to live on sixpence a day and earn it', became surgeon to St Bartholomew's; Astley Paston Cooper, a brilliantly daring operator who was the first man to amputate a leg through the hip joint, made the surgical name of Guy's Hospital. Another of Hunter's pupils, Philip Syng Physick, sometimes called the Father of American Surgery, spread the fame of John Hunter across the Atlantic.

The major Scottish invasion of surgical London came about as the result of the foundation of new London hospitals. For over five hundred years the two medieval hospitals of St Thomas' and St Bartholomew's were the only institutions which could possibly be given the name of teaching centres, but during the eighteenth century the rapid expansion of London made the provision of free treatment for the sick poor an urgent necessity. Thus came into being, often as out-patient dispensaries in origin, the Westminster (1715), Guy's founded as a kind of annex for the chronic sick of St Thomas' in 1721, St George's (1733), the London (1740), and the Middlesex founded in 1745. In all cases the medical schools attached to these hospitals are of later date, the earliest being that of the Middlesex, where an organized course of lectures commenced in 1785. The year 1821 saw the foundation of the first 'teaching hospital', when Dr Benjamin Golding opened Charing Cross 'to supply the want of a University, so far as Medical Education is concerned'. University College Hospital, first known as the North London, and King's College Hospital were founded respectively in 1834 and 1839 for the express purpose of providing clinical instruction for the students of University College in Gower Street and King's College in the Strand.

Appointments to the medical and surgical staff in the older hospitals were usually filled by the election of a favoured apprentice of the retiring member – a son, son-in-law, or nephew stood a particularly good chance. The increase in the number of posts and the lack of tradition in the newer hospitals made such nepotism less common; what had been almost a closed shop became more open to the outsider. In 1804 Charles Bell, youngest son of the large family of a Scottish Episcopalian clergyman who supported existence on £25 a year, decided to remove from Edinburgh to London. After a hard struggle he established himself as a teacher, served at the Battle of Waterloo, and in the same year was appointed surgeon to the Middlesex Hospital. He brought great renown to the Middlesex but, having declared that London was a good place to live in and no place to die in, he returned in 1835 to Edinburgh as professor of surgery. In 1835 Robert Liston, the most famous operating surgeon of his time, left Edinburgh for University College, London, and, four years later, the almost greater William Fergusson travelled the same road to the newly founded King's College Hospital, thereby making that small institution behind Lincoln's Inn Fields for a short time into the surgical centre of the world.

As these brilliant young men moved south – and there were others, physicians and surgeons both, who made the same journey – the centre of gravity moved with them from Edinburgh to London. The outcome was inevitable: the rise of London's influence at the expense of that of Edinburgh. This supremacy was maintained for some forty years, from the eighteen thirties until shortly after the Franco-Prussian war of 1870 when, for reasons which will be considered in their due place, initiative passed to the Germanic nations. At the end of the nineteenth century the United States of America began to move up to the leading place which they now hold. From the eighteen thirties onward, increasing ease of communication made interchange of ideas and personal demonstration more

8

widespread; medicine shared the tendency of other arts and sciences to become international rather than national. It is, however, true that the reputation of London stood higher than that of any other centre during the years 1840–70, which is the formative period of modern surgery. For this reason, and not because of the author's pride in his country's undoubted achievement, the story of these early years will be told with special emphasis upon the hospitals of London.

For it was in the hospitals that surgery developed. At first sight they had nothing to offer the ambitious surgeon; until 1848 he was a member of the 'honorary staff', unpaid, often expected to make donations from his own pocket in times of special financial stress, at all times required to put in time-consuming attendance at wards, out-patient department, and operating theatre. He could expect no private practice, for not a single London hospital possessed a pay-bed in which the surgeon might treat his fee-paying patients. The attraction of an honorary post lay in its prestige value; a tradition had grown up that the physician or surgeon to one of these institutions was reaching up to the heights of his profession; the coveted honours, membership of the councils of the Royal Colleges, fellowships of the Royal Society, court appointments, examinerships, all of these were awarded, almost without exception, to members of the honorary staffs of London hospitals.

It followed that the ambitious and more wealthy pupil desired apprenticeship to the hospital surgeon who, in his turn, charged far higher indenture fees than did his provincial or suburban colleague. Success bred success. The apprentice, having set up in practice on his own, recommended obscure or difficult cases to his old master; new apprentices, anxious to share the master's growing fame and perhaps to secure the reversion of part of his practice, were willing to pay still larger indenture fees. Some of these successful surgeons made enormous incomes; Astley Cooper earned as much as £15,000 a year, a sum quite impossible to express in terms of present day values, and the bulk of his income came from indenture or pupillage fees and from consultations – his butler is said to have made a steady £600 a year from showing patients in out of turn! There was, too, always the opportunity of 'placing' a favoured apprentice or relation; Astley Cooper succeeded his uncle,

William Cooper, on the staff of Guy's; two of Astley's nephews, Bransby Cooper and Aston Key, were in due course elected to surgeoncies on the Guy's staff.

The hospitals which these surgeons attended were quite different from the hospitals of today. They existed to treat 'the sick poor' and the sick poor only. Their patients were drawn from the slums of a Britain which was passing from a predominantly agricultural economy into the Industrial Revolution. We can read of these people in the pages of Dickens and see them in the illustrations of Hablot Browne. In London they were all-pervasive, for the slum areas were not confined to the East End or the districts around Drury Lane and Seven Dials. They infiltrated everywhere; great houses in Belgravia might face on to wide tree-planted squares but their back windows overlooked poverty stricken hovels lacking in elementary sanitation and water supply.

Thus there was little or no difference between the patients of a West End hospital, such as St George's, and those of St Thomas' in the Borough and the London in Whitechapel. They were of a type far removed from the occupant of a present-day ward. A clergyman, a comfortable small shop-keeper, the clerk occupying a safe stool, would no more have thought of entering a hospital than of entering the workhouse. We do not find members of 'respectable callings' among the patients until the late eighteen-sixties, when the influence of St John's House (the first Anglican Nursing Sisterhood) and of Florence Nightingale had done something to raise the standard of discipline and cleanliness in the wards. It is not surprising that a person with any pretensions to respectability should have preferred the expense and inconvenience of home nursing to the hospital, for the ordinary occupant of a hospital bed was indescribably filthy and infested with vermin, bugs, fleas, and lice. In this somewhat unsavoury connection it should be remembered that the nurse's cap, now worn as an adornment or badge of rank, has its origin as a full head covering to protect the hair from invading lice. Miss Emma Durham, one of the more notable nineteenth-century nurses, has left it on record that, during her time of hospital training in the eighteen seventies, it was customary to turn the gas full on when the nurses went to their dormitories at night so that a minute examination might be made of their persons and clothing. She tells, too, of a particularly filthy old woman who, after being given a cleansing bath, pressed a few halfpence into the nurse's hand with the remark that she must need 'a good drop o' gin' after the ordeal. And another woman refused the bath on the ground that she had never had such a thing in the forty years of her life.

Disease assumed a pattern very different from nowadays in these conditions of dirt and poverty. Sewage contaminated water supply brought epidemics of Asiatic cholera, which did not wholly disappear until well into the latter half of the nineteenth century. Typhoid and the other enteric fevers were so universally prevalent at all times as to be endemic, and, being nursed in the open wards of general hospitals without special precautions, placed medical and nursing staff at continual risk. The dreaded typhus fever, which from time to time devastated whole areas of Russia and the eastern countries, was by no means unknown in London. Shephard Taylor, in his *Diary of a Medical Student* records the deaths of two fellow students and a St John's Sister from typhus during the years 1863–7.[5] Occasional cases of true plague, the bubonic plague of the Black Death in 1348 and of the Great Plague in 1665, are still to be found in the hospital case-notes, although the black rat, by which the causative organism of bubonic plague is carried, was by then almost extinct in Britain. Gross malnutrition, even frank starvation at a time when it was possible to exist on less than half a crown a week, produced the diseases of vitamin deficiency, rickets and scurvy and the terrible infantile disorder known as cancrum oris, a spreading gangrene of the lips and mouth. Alcoholism, the bedfellow of misery and want, commonly united with malnutrition in its most distressing manifestation, delirium tremens. In some years alcoholism accounted for 10 per cent of all admissions to King's College Hospital, and alcoholism is the second commonest complaint to be noted in the past history of the patient.

Throughout the whole of the nineteenth century and well into the twentieth, tuberculosis was the commonest and most lethal disease of the town-dwelling population. The figures, as revealed in the case-notes, are quite staggering. In many years tuberculosis accounted for over a quarter of all in-patient admissions. Still more sinister and suggestive is the fact that tuberculosis receives bare mention in the past history of the patient. The disease was incurable; once diagnosed as tuberculous, the patient would not be readmitted to hospital except in the acute emergency of accident or of intercurrent illness. The surgery of tuberculosis accounted for over 20 per cent of all operations; removal of glands, the drainage of an abscess (the typical 'cold' abscess or the 'psoas abscess' derived from tuberculous infection of the spine) and the amputation of limbs for the classical 'white swelling' of scrofula which, although regarded as a separate entity, was caused by tuberculous infection of the joint.

The number of surgical operations was small. Even a man of the stature of Astley Cooper operated but rarely – although when he did operate his fees were very high. It was uncommon for a large teaching hospital to be able to boast of more than two hundred operations in a year; the comparable figure today would be in the region of ten thousand. In 1832 the *Lancet* reported as an item of interest that two operations were performed at St George's Hospital on 25 April and another three on 2 May.[6] Every hospital had its weekly operating day when the surgeons, in order of seniority, performed such operations as they deemed advisable. Horrible to relate, these regular sessions were a kind of free show; they were attended not only by surgeons and medical students but by members of the general public. A *Times* account of 1842 records that William Fergusson removed the whole of one side of the upper jaw from a twelve-year-old child, without any form of anaesthesia whatsoever, in the presence of over two hundred spectators.[7] In 1830 Aston Key of Guy's, by the advice of his uncle Astley Cooper, excised an enormous tumour, weighing fifty-six pounds, from a Chinaman who had travelled to London from Canton for the operation. The operation took two hours and was witnessed by a crowd of six hundred and eighty people; in fact the death of the unfortunate patient was attributed to prolonged exposure in an atmosphere so poisoned by human exhalations that many onlookers fainted.[8]

This operation is of interest for other reasons. The fact that the patient had travelled from Canton to London rather than to Paris or Edinburgh suggests that London was already becoming a renowned centre of surgery by 1830. Secondly, an attempt was made to revive the patient by means of six ounces of blood taken from the vein of a student in the audience, a very early example of human blood transfusion. Thirdly, the operation was regarded by many as quite unjustifiable and provoked a correspondence in the *Lancet*. A certain Dr J. M. Titley wrote that he had particulars of thirteen similar operations performed by various surgeons. Of these thirteen patients, only one had died; in this case, he said, the operation had lasted eight hours and the tumour weighed one hundred and fifty-six pounds.

The comparative rarity of operations was not due to any lack of skill on the part of the surgeon, but was on account of the agony which he caused to his patient and to the high death rate. Of the so aptly named 'capital' or major operations, amputation was that most commonly performed and carried a mortality in the region of 40 per cent. Tuberculosis supplied the reason for many of these amputations and, despite the high death rate, amputation was the most hopeful treatment in the acute infection now called osteomyelitis but known to our forefathers as necrosis of bone. Road accidents accounted for a quite surprisingly high proportion of amputations. There is a modern tendency to think that 'the toll of the road' is a problem entirely caused by the motor car; it should be remembered that an average of four to five persons were killed each week in the streets of London alone during the eighteen sixties.[9] Many of these road accident victims would not have died today. Heavy drays and carts caused crushing injury of the limbs, the compound fracture or broken bone combined with an open wound, which almost inevitably resulted in death if amputation were not performed at once. Death was caused by generalized infection; the filthy dung-strewn streets teemed with bacteria and, since the surgeon did not know of their existence, there was no means of combating their attack.

The second reason for the small amount of operative surgery was the agonizing pain. The old time surgeon had necessarily to be a man of tough fibre but he was no sadist. He did not operate unless he judged operation to be entirely necessary. Because of this, disabilities which we should consider crippling went untreated; procedures which we should regard as essential to save life were not attempted. Men, women, and children died from disorders, appendicitis for instance, which could now be cured by a simple operation. But sometimes these early surgeons were tempted into feats which we should consider to be unjustifiable in a world that knew neither anaesthesia nor any means of combating infection. It is hard to blame them, for they were wonderful craftsmen. Many of these brilliant technicians must have suffered from frustration; the limits imposed upon his manual dexterity and inventive prowess by the agony which he inflicted on his patient must surely have exasperated the ambitious surgeon.

In a situation such as this, with a fully conscious and perceptive patient, speed of operating was the primary attribute of the successful surgeon and the quality most loudly demanded by the writhing victim. Their speed of operating is fantastic. The eighteenth-century surgeon William Cheselden removed stones from the urinary bladder by the open operation of lithotomy in less than a minute; S. F. Morand, a surgeon of Paris, wrote that he had seen the same procedure completed in twenty-four seconds. Astley Cooper, amputating a leg through the hip joint for the first time in history, finished his operation in twenty minutes. This was in 1824; some ten years later, when the technique was better understood, James Syme of Edinburgh is reported to have done it in just over the minute.[10] It must, however, be acknowledged that these 'speed records' have been something exaggerated by modern authors. The minute-and-a-half amputation, the one minute removal of a stone, do not include the staunching of bleeding or suturing of the wound. Cooper, having removed the leg in twenty minutes, spent another quarter of an hour in securing the bleeding vessels and stitching up. The *Lancet*, reporting an unusual operation in 1833, remarks that 'the operation occupied a half an hour and the subsequent act of tying arteries, dressing, etc., was completed in a quarter of an hour more.' These 'subsequent acts' were not counted part of the operation; to our own minds they must have been excruciatingly painful, but the patient was probably too shocked by the pain of the actual operation to have much appreciation of them.

Nor could speed always be maintained. We have already seen that as much as two to eight hours might be taken over an unusual operation, and the opening years of the nineteenth century are notable for the number of new, daring operations introduced. Strangely enough, advance was chiefly in arterial surgery, generally regarded as one of the more recent branches to be developed. It was not, of course, the arterial surgery of today, but consisted of the comparatively simple and very dangerous manoeuvre of tying the artery with a silk ligature in order to occlude it. This was done to bypass an aneurysm, the weakening and ballooning of an arterial wall caused by injury or, more often in those days, by untreated syphilis. The surgeon tied the artery in order to force the smaller, collateral vessels to take up an increased blood flow; thus the circulation was adequately maintained but the large vessel no longer functioned and the weakened wall of the aneurysm no longer stood in the grave danger of rupturing through the accident of a blow or as the result of being unable to stand up to the arterial blood pressure.

There were other new operations as well; removal of tumours of the kind mentioned above; attempts to relieve the bowel by incision when a child was born with the congenital defect of imperforate anus. The great French surgeon Dupuytren reported that he once took over ten hours to repair the grossly distorted jaw of a Russian officer who had been wounded in 1814. The operation included extraction of teeth, the removal of a three-inch length of bone, and fixation of the fragmented jaw by a number of wires. The patient had to keep absolute silence for sixty days after operation, could take no solid food for three months, and, at the end of that time, it was discovered that his tongue had been cut almost in two by the wires which crossed his mouth. Despite all this he made a perfect recovery which, wrote Dupuytren, was 'considerably favoured by the docility, courage, and confidence of the patient, which did not desert him for a moment during the course of the long and painful treatment.'[11]

The surgeon possessed no map to these heroic procedures – whether they were justified or not. He could follow the classical plan of amputation, or Cheselden's method of extracting a urinary stone, and a few other operations described in the text books of surgery; for the rest he was entering entirely new ground, with only his exact knowledge of anatomy to guide him and his superb technical skill to smooth the way. Because speed was all important, the surgeon had no time to pause and

consider his next step when improvising a new procedure; unexpected difficulties, the urgent emergency that can face any
surgeon when embarking on the unknown, demanded lightning
decision and immediate action.

It follows, then, that the successful surgeon of the pre-
anaesthesia era must have been a man possessing a combination
of remarkable and unusual qualities. He needed a wide and
exact knowledge of anatomy, outstanding manual dexterity,
and the capability of acting upon an immediate decision. While
showing outward sympathy, he must have been able to develop
a case-hardened insensibility to the signs of acute suffering;
only thus could he have retained calm judgement when operating upon the conscious patient. The weakling could not undertake surgery, for the resistance of the muscles to pain demanded
strength above the average on the part of the operator who
reduced a fractured bone or a dislocated joint. Nor was mere
physical strength enough; with strength there must go perfect
muscular co-ordination if the surgeon were to perform deft and
delicate work. This controlled strength is remarked by contemporary biographers: Robert Liston is said to have had the arms
and hands of a Hercules, yet he was renowned for the artistic
delicacy of his operating. Some of them became so completely
ambidexterous that they could use their knife with either hand
at will; others are reported to have grasped the spurting end of
an artery with the fingers of one hand, to have thrown a ligature
around it with the other, and to have tied the knot of the ligature with the teeth. Usually adduced as evidence of their dirty
habits, it is more just to place this latter to the credit of their
dexterity.

The practice of these surgeons was at once more circumscribed and more catholic than that of their modern descendants.
It was more circumscribed because pain and death imposed a
limit upon surgery proper; it was more catholic because the
surgeon undertook a type of work that he would not do today.
The reason was an economic one. 'Was not a large part of
Mr Abernethy's practice of a medical kind?' a member of a
Select Commission asked G. J. Guthrie in 1834. 'So is my own,'
replied Guthrie – who had the distinction of qualifying as a
member of the Royal College of Surgeons at the tender age of
sixteen – 'and so is every surgeon's in London.' His reply,

although too sweeping to be entirely true, correctly described the state of surgical practice at the time. The average man just could not make a living only from surgery.

The apothecary functioned as a kind of general practitioner who dispensed his own medicines. The proud physician, a man of education and learned in the classics, was primarily interested in diagnosis. He therefore tended to deal with the type of disease which cannot be detected by superficial examination; overt disease he regarded as the province of the surgeon. Thus the surgeon undertook the duties of the present day dermatologist; he treated diseases of the skin and venereal disease in particular; as late as the second half of the nineteenth century we find recent advances in the treatment of syphilis and gonorrhea classified under the heading of 'surgery'.[12] Sir Jonathan Hutchinson, a well-known and very competent surgeon of the London Hospital, was a skin-doctor first and foremost, remembered today for his description of the signs of congenital syphilis rather than for any great advance in operative technique.

The surgeon tackled every kind of operation in the limited field of surgery. There was no such thing as the modern specialist, interesting himself solely in surgery of a particular part of the body or of a selected group of disabilities. As we shall see in later chapters, this type of work had fallen into the hands of untrained men who, if not wholly deserving the name of 'quacks', were by no means bound by ethical rules or orthodox methods. It is of interest that the Royal College of Surgeons of England, in their original regulations for the fellowship, refused to countenance any member who practised exclusively as a dentist, aurist, oculist, chiropodist, or orthopaedic surgeon. The College did not so much disapprove of specialization as of the odour of charlatanry which surrounded these specialities. They were, to use a modern popular term, the 'fringe medicine' of yesterday; many of them have now entered orthodox medicine, just as some 'fringe' practices will no doubt enter the orthodox medicine of tomorrow.

Some idea of the ordinary work of a young, ambitious surgeon can be gained by studying the case-book of William Fergusson. Between 1829 when he was twenty-one years old and 1839 when he was appointed to the staff of the newly founded King's College Hospital in London, Fergusson worked first at the Royal Dispensary and then at the Royal Infirmary in Edinburgh. His case-book covers a period of seven years, 1830–7. Thirty-nine operations are recorded. Of these, eight were immediate life-saving procedures, attempts to relieve acutely obstructed bowel resulting from untreated hernia, the 'strangulated hernia'. This was one of the emergencies which more commonly presented itself to the surgeon; he attempted to push the bowel back through the constricting ring of the hernial sac into the abdominal cavity, a method which he called taxis, but if he failed the only hope was open operation. That such operations were extremely dangerous is shown by the fact that three of Fergusson's eight patients died, a mortality of nearly 40 per cent. Fergusson notes that one of the survivors became his servant a month later. Next there are six amputations, one through the thigh in a child of only nine years old, and one of the arm when Fergusson remarks 'the arm was off in fifty-four seconds'. Three of these six amputations were on account of tuberculosis. One amputation was for necrosis or osteomyelitis, which has already been mentioned as a common reason and four more operations were for the same disease. Thus eighteen of the thirty-nine cases would nowadays be classed as 'emergency' surgery.

The remainder were operations of election; they were not essential in that the patient would not have certainly died without speedy surgical intervention. Four of these are border-line; the patient would not have died within a matter of days but could not have survived for long, all four being for cancer of the breast. One died of pneumonia soon after operation, but there is no mention of how long the remaining three lived. There are twelve operations which certainly cannot be considered essential; two circumcisions, the treatment of a birth mark on a child's face, an attempt to reconstruct a congenital deficiency of the vagina in a child of twenty months old, and no less than eight operations for the congenital deformity of hare-lip. All of these patients survived operation, and Fergusson states that the eight repairs of hare-lip were all successful.

Of the five so far unmentioned, no less than three operations have entered medical literature. In one of these Fergusson tied the subclavian artery, for the first time in history, to relieve an aneurysm in the upper part of the arm. He was successful but the patient, a farm worker given to drink, died some four years later from exposure, having spent all night in the open fields during a snowstorm. The second case is a remarkable one; a girl of nine inhaled a plum-stone which became lodged in the trachea. Several doctors made repeated but unsuccessful attempts to dislodge it and, after some hesitation, Fergusson decided that the only possible way to remove the stone was by open operation. He cut through the rings of the trachea in the neck and, after considerable difficulty, managed to remove the stone with a hook and a pair of forceps. Fergusson records that the patient thereupon leaped from the grasp of her friends and danced round the room, clapping her hands with joy. Unfortunately the girl did not survive for long; her parents made her into a fairground exhibit and she died a few weeks later from, in Fergusson's words, 'her continual gadding about'.

It is tempting to record the last of these remarkable operations in full, but the details are of medical interest only. A much shortened version will serve to present a picture of the surgical methods of those days. On 3 March 1831 Fergusson was asked to see a twelve-hour old baby who had been born in one of the tenement houses 'in the north back of the Canongate' in Edinburgh. The child had passed no motion since birth and, on examination, Fergusson found that no opening was present in the normal position of the anus; death must very soon take place for the child was already vomiting dark-coloured matter.

Fergusson told the mother that only an operation could save her baby's life and she asked him to make the attempt. He consulted with his colleagues, among them the great Robert Knox, as to whether it would be better to try to reach the bowel by cutting into the abdomen itself or to open up the normal site of the anus, through the perineum, in the hope that the blind bowel end might be easily found. The former of these procedures, known as Littre's operation or colostomy, had been attempted on several occasions; in a later chapter we shall see that it is one of the parent operations of modern abdominal surgery. But grave danger was well-known to attend opening the abdomen; Fergusson, rather against the opinion of his colleagues, decided to try the perineal approach. He therefore cut into the perineum but, although he carried his incision to a depth of an inch and a half, he failed to find the bowel. 'It was therefore evident' he wrote 'that nothing further could be done for the child in this direction.'

Fergusson was not the type of man to abandon a case as hopeless. He had reason to believe that a communication existed between the blind end of the bowel and the urinary bladder. Next morning at half past six he visited his small patient again, determined to try cutting into the bladder itself in the hope of finding the bowel that way. He introduced a metal guide or director into the bladder, so that he could feel the point at which to make his incision. Then he cut from below upwards on to the director. 'To my great satisfaction,' wrote Fergusson 'the meconium (a term for a new born child's first motion) flowed out after making the incision. I allowed as much to flow as would, and then introduced a small clyster pipe (enema syringe) with a bag of water attached to it and, by injecting the fluid, I washed out the cavity that had been opened. As there was no danger at this point of the wound healing, I left the parts undressed.'

Fergusson had saved the child's life. Recovery was slow; at one time he suspected the onset of erysipelas – the nature of which was not then understood but is now known to be due to wound infection – and he ordered poultices wrung out of a solution of lead acetate. There is a letter, found loose in Fergusson's case-book, which tells the rest of the story. The boy – his name was David Collison – lived for six years; then, in the letter writer's own words and spelling, he died from 'a deceased lung occasioned, I suppose, by the dregs of the measalls' on 29 July 1837.

Six of these thirty-nine patients died as the result of operation, which can be expressed as a mortality of 15 per cent. High though this is, it is not so great as some writers would have us believe to be the rule in the early part of the nineteenth century. We must remember, too, that these were special operations, regarded by Fergusson as of particular interest. His day-book, the record of his visits, reveals the more ordinary work of a surgeon, the passing of bougies to dilate a stricture of the urethra (one unfortunate patient received this treatment on more than fifty occasions), the setting of bones and the reduction of dislocations, opening of abscesses, dressing of cuts and sprains, attendance at a 'duello' in the Braid Hills when, it seems, neither contestant required his services.

Fergusson's work is typical of his period; it reveals that surgery was limited but wider in scope than one would have thought probable in the absence of anaesthesia. There are no abdominal operations; with this important exception, a selection from his thirty-nine cases would often appear as a present day operating list by a general surgeon. In some respects his scope is actually wider than that of a modern general surgeon; for instance, the removal of a foreign body from the trachea would nowadays be undertaken by a specialist in laryngology and the repair of a hare-lip would more commonly be the province of a plastic surgeon. We shall find, as the story unfolds, that there is a steady tendency for the bounds of surgery to enlarge while the field of the individual surgeon becomes more restricted.

Such, in brief outline, was the state of surgery in the years which immediately preceded the introduction of anaesthesia. The men who practised this surgery were often ill-educated and, with very few exceptions, of little culture or refinement. Sometimes they were quite uncouth, rude and rough with their patients to the point of brutality, men of the stamp of Liston and Abernethy. They possessed no effective means of allaying the pain which they inevitably inflicted, knew nothing of the cause of the infections that killed so many of their patients. The treatment and nature of shock was a closed book; blood transfusion was nothing but a dangerous experiment; the science of pathology, upon which the surgeon now leans so heavily, was not yet a science. They worked in conditions which we should consider impossible, with instruments that, although well made, were primitive in design and few in number; even their means of lighting would be regarded by a modern surgeon as hopelessly inadequate.

But they were craftsmen, probably technically more skilful than the majority of their descendants. Not only their work but their hobbies testify to their manual ability; Liston, an enthusiastic yachtsman, rigged his own boats; Fergusson built his own furniture besides designing and making the prototypes of his intruments, some of which have not been bettered and are in use today. It was this manual skill combined with their daring and ingenuity that enabled them to overcome all the difficulties imposed by their lack of knowledge. They laid a worthy foundation for the great advances made possible by the discoveries of the next thirty years.

CHAPTER 2

Anaesthesia

There is an eighteenth-century word, bottom, which implied the ability to meet all the pains and injustices and discomforts of life with cheerful unconcern. Bottom and bottom only supported the patient who was submitted to surgery until little more than a century ago. The fortitude of these patients is amazing. In 1830 Scott of the London Hospital removed the whole of one side of the upper jaw, the first occasion on which the operation was done in England. When preparations were made to carry the victim back to his bed, he indignantly protested and insisted on walking to the ward unaided. On 31 December 1811 Henry Cline of Guy's extracted a stone from the bladder of a gentleman described as 'about forty years of age, who, to the advantages of a liberal education, unites an uncommon share of cheerfulness, and a firmness of mind which does not forsake him under the most trying circumstances'. This stout-hearted gentleman wrote an account of his ordeal, from which the following extract is taken.

'My habit and constitution being good, it required little preparation of body, and my mind was made up. When all parties had arrived, I retired to my room for a minute, and bent my knee in silent adoration and submission, and returning to the surgeons, conducted them to the apartment in which the preparations had been made. I was prepared to receive a shock of pain of extreme violence, and so much had I overrated it, that the first incisions did not even make me wince, although I had declared that it was not my intention to restrain such impulse, convinced that such effort of restraint could only lead to additional exhaustion. At subsequent moments, therefore, I did cry out under the pain, but was allowed to have gone through the operation with great firmness.

'The forcing up of the staff, prior to the introduction of the gorget, gave me the first real pain. (The staff was a curved director upon which the surgeon made his incision, and the gorget a sharp tubular instrument.) But this instantly subsided after the incision of the bladder was made, the rush of urine appearing to relieve it, and soothe the wound.

'When the forceps was introduced, the pain was again very considerable, and every movement of the instrument, in endeavouring to find the stone, increased it. After several ineffectual attempts to grasp the stone, I heard the operator say, in the lowest whisper, "it is a little awkward, it lies under my hand. Give me the curved forceps:" upon which he withdrew the others. When the other forceps was introduced, I had again to undergo the searching for the stone, and heard Mr Cline say, "I have got it." I had probably by this time conceived that the worst was over; but when the necessary force was applied to withdraw the stone, the sensation was such as I cannot find words to describe. In addition to the positive pain, there was something most peculiar in the feel. The duration, however, of this really trying part of the operation was short; and when the words "now, sir, it is all over!" struck my ear, the ejaculation of "thank God! thank God!" was uttered with a fervency and fulness of heart which can only be conceived. I am quite unable to describe my feelings at the moment. The most captivating vision to the sight, the most enchanting harmony to the ear, or a combination of everything that is calculated to delight the senses, must fall far short of the perfect blessedness of my situation. With respect to the pain, I am persuaded that if it were possible to concentrate what I have often suffered in one night, into the same space of time, it would have been less endurable. Upon the whole, should I be again similarly afflicted, I should not hesitate in again submitting to the same mode of relief, provided I could place myself in equally able hands.'[1]

This philosophy of bottom, this unquestioning acceptance of the pain of surgery, did more to delay the introduction of anaesthesia than anything else. In a world which regarded fortitude as a desirable virtue and which counted suffering of small importance, the pain of rarely performed surgical operations aroused little interest and no protest. A change in Man's attitude towards suffering in general was necessary before his attention would be directed towards the pain of surgery in particular. Thus the introduction of anaesthesia is a dramatic outward expression of Man's inner change from eighteenth-century brutality to our own more humane pattern of behaviour. It is worth remembering that anaesthesia is roughly coeval with Arnold of Rugby, with the Mines Act of 1842 and the Factories Act of 1833, with the disappearance of duelling and the attempted suppression of the prize ring, with reforms in service discipline and of the penal code.

Means of anaesthesia had existed for many years. Alcohol and opium, both capable of destroying pain, have been known and used in medicine since time immemorial. Sulphuric ether, one of the more popular anaesthetics, had certainly been prepared by Valerius Cordus about 1540, and was purified to a degree probably capable of producing anaesthesia by Godefroy von Froben in the early eighteenth century. Nitrous oxide, the dentist's 'gas' of today, first prepared in an impure form by Joseph Priestley in 1772, was manufactured as a reasonably pure gas from ammonium nitrate, the process now used, by the French chemist Berthollet in 1797.

In 1800 that remarkable young man, Humphry Davy, who lived to discover sodium and potassium and to invent the miner's safety lamp, published the results of a three years' research into the properties of nitrous oxide. At the end of this book he made the first direct suggestion of a practicable means of anaesthesia in the words 'As nitrous oxide in its extensive operation appears capable of destroying physical pain, it may probably be used in surgical operations in which no great effusion of blood takes place.' In 1824 Henry Hill Hickman, a young surgeon of Shifnal in Shropshire, set out to find a means of anaesthesia by animal experiment, using his own exhaled breath, carbon dioxide gas, and simple deprivation of air. Hickman succeeded in producing unconsciousness for a sufficient length of time to allow a minor operation, with recovery of the animal. Suggestion or hypnosis, a possible but unreliable means of anaesthesia, entered medicine at the end of the eighteenth century, largely through the work of the Frenchman

Anton Mesmer, from whose name the popular term 'mesmerism' is derived.

The knowledge was there but the will to use that knowledge was not. None of the many and lengthy reviews of Davy's important book so much as mention his suggestion of anaesthesia. His friend Samuel Taylor Coleridge showed some interest; William Allen, lecturer in chemistry at Guy's Hospital, certainly lectured his class on nitrous oxide, probably forecast the use of the gas in surgery, and possibly demonstrated its pain-allaying property to the surgeon Astley Cooper. But that was all; nitrous oxide became a scientific plaything, the 'exhilarting' or 'laughing' gas much favoured for demonstration at popular lectures.

Hickman's work fared no better. He published a pamphlet (only one copy is known to exist now) which was laughed to scorn in the two periodicals which troubled to review it.[2] A young man of some persistence, he visited Paris in 1828 to lay his findings before the Academy, but he met with little or no encouragement. Bitterly disappointed, he returned to practise in Ludlow, whither he had removed from Shifnal, performed no more experiments, and died in 1830 at the age of thirty years.

Ether entered medicine as one of the group of drugs known as antispasmodics, often prescribed for asthma and even in cases of pulmonary tuberculosis. It became a 'popular' remedy. The author possesses his great-grandmother's manuscript book of household management, dating from 1830; here, sandwiched between a method of making brimstone and treacle and a recipe for lobster cutlets, are directions for administering ether by inhalation during an attack of croup. The inhalation or actual drinking of commercial ether as a substitute for alcohol became a social scourge in the nineteenth century. Though never widely prevalent in England, the habit spread throughout Ireland, Russia, and parts of America with disastrous results.

It is noteworthy that the first anaesthetics to be given in America came as a direct result of the so-called 'ether frolics'. It has already been mentioned that alcohol and opium can be used to dull pain. To be effective, the dose of opium would have to be dangerously large. Alcohol, the obvious pain-killer, was little used by the well-trained surgeon in a good type of practice.

Classed as a stimulant drug, it was supposed to increase blood loss and was therefore contraindicated in surgery, except in the form of 'sips of wine' to support the patient's strength. The less orthodox practitioner, the ship's surgeon or the jack-of-all-trades in a backwoods village of America, paid little attention to medical theories. He knew that a drunken man is more or less insensible to pain and so he made his patient drunk with rum or whisky before operation. Thus, when ether drinking or inhalation became a popular habit, a surgeon who had witnessed the effect of ether would naturally substitute that more powerful intoxicant for the usual dram of spirits. Into this category of practitioners falls Crawford Long of Jefferson, Georgia, who first administered ether to James Venables on 30 March 1842, before removing a small tumour from his neck. Long, himself an addict, had both purveyed ether and led the frolics.

Mesmerism, hypnosis, or animal magnetism came into very limited use as a means of allaying the pain of surgery during the late eighteen thirties. It was considered successful, although we now know that surgical anaesthesia, even for minor operations, cannot be attained by hypnosis alone in more than ten per cent of subjects. John Elliotson, professor of medicine at University College, London, tried his hand at it in 1837, but was forced to resign his chair in 1838 as a result of his colleagues' adverse criticism. James Esdaile of the East India Company achieved considerable success among Hindu convicts but failed to produce convincing results when he tried his method in Scotland. Perhaps the Scots are more hard-headed than the Hindus. James Braid of Manchester, to whom we owe the term 'hypnosis', was another advocate of mesmerism who met with some success. Mesmerism as a means of dulling surgical pain also became fairly popular in France and in America, where one of the leading exponents was a surgeon named John Collins Warren, whom we shall meet again in the course of the next few pages.

These early experiments did not form part of the chain of events which led to the discovery or, more correctly, the introduction of anaesthesia. They did, however, help to condition the minds of the medical profession to the idea that painless surgery might one day be feasible. The continuing tale starts with the discovery of the exciting effect of small doses of nitrous oxide by Humphry Davy in 1798–1800. Davy worked in Bristol with the physician Thomas Beddoes. This eccentric genius was surrounded by a quite outstanding circle of men and women; indeed, it is tempting to describe them as the 'most remarkable' collection of people ever to gather in one place. They included the poets Southey, Coleridge, and Wordsworth, James Watt the engineer, Roget of Roget's *Thesaurus*, Maria Edgeworth the novelist, the great potters Thomas and Josiah Wedgwood. It was Southey who forged the first link in the chain by writing that 'the atmosphere of the highest of all possible heavens must be composed of this gas', his poetic description of the exhilarating effect of a small dose or inhalation of nitrous oxide.[3]

These words appear in a lecture advertisement distributed in America by Gardner Quincey Colton. Little is known of Colton. Despite his American-sounding conjunction of names, he appears to have been an Englishman who emigrated to America after a short career as a student of science at University College, London. By legend he was in the employ of Phineas Barnum, the great showman.

In early December, 1844, Colton arrived in the small town of Hartford, Connecticut, advertising a grand demonstration of the effects produced by inhalation of nitrous oxide. His demonstration duly took place at seven o'clock in the evening of Tuesday, 10 December. A man named Sam Cooley and his friend, Horace Wells, a dentist of the town, formed two of the audience. Cooley inhaled the gas, became wildly excited, and tripped over a seat, cutting his shin. He continued to roar with laughter despite his injury. When questioned by Wells, Cooley denied any knowledge of the accident and seemed surprised to find that he was bleeding from a quite severe cut on the leg.

Wells had the wit to see that nitrous oxide might be of some use in his dental practice. He was still young, twenty-nine years of age, and his portrait suggests that he was a kindly, intelligent, civilized type of man. He certainly had an inventive brain but, as we shall see, he must have been of unstable mind. He consulted with his partner, J. M. Riggs, and between them they persuaded Colton to administer nitrous oxide to Wells 'to a point hitherto unknown' while Riggs extracted one of his molar teeth. The experiment was performed at about ten o'clock in

the morning of Wednesday, 11 December, and proved successful. Wells is credited with saying on recovery 'It did not hurt
so much as the prick of a pin. This is a new era in tooth-
pulling.'

In fact he was wrong; nitrous oxide did not introduce
anaesthesia. Wells used the gas on some fifteen occasions in his
dental practice with sufficiently good results to satisfy him.
Foolishly optimistic, he prematurely asked permission to give a
lecture-demonstration at the Massachussets General Hospital.
His lecture took place before a large audience early in January
1845. At the end, Wells called for a volunteer; a medical
student who had an aching tooth offered himself as a subject.
Wells applied the skin bag of home-made nitrous oxide, allowed
the student to inhale for a minute or so and proceeded to extract
the tooth, whereupon his patient leapt from the chair with a
scream. The audience hissed Wells out of the theatre as an
imposter and, when the student afterwards denied that he had
felt any pain, it was suspected that there had been collusion to
defraud. We now know that patients under the influence of
nitrous oxide may react quite violently and noisily to the pain
stimulus, yet be unable to perceive the pain or to remember
anything afterwards.

It is convenient to finish the story of Horace Wells and
nitrous oxide before considering the events that led to the
successful introduction of anaesthesia. Wells' life became pure
tragedy. He persisted with experiments in anaesthesia and
laid claim to the discovery. His brain started to fail until, from
being eccentric, he lapsed into frank insanity. Wells committed
suicide on 24 January 1848, while held in the Tombs Prison,
New York, on a charge of throwing acid over a prostitute. But
Colton never lost faith in nitrous oxide; a man of generous
nature, he claimed no recognition for himself and assigned full
credit to Wells. He formed the Colton Painless Extraction
Company and, by 1873, had administered gas to 67,455 patients
without a fatality. Colton visited Paris in 1867 in order to
demonstrate nitrous oxide; although the French practitioners
showed little enthusiasm, he aroused the interest of a resident
American dentist, Dr Evans, who is perhaps better known for
his feat of smuggling the Empress Eugenie out of Paris during
the riots preceding the Commune. Evans demonstrated nitrous

oxide at the National Dental Hospital, London (now the dental school of University College Hospital), where it was used for a short time but temporarily abandoned. However, Coleman of the London (now Royal) Dental Hospital became an enthusiastic advocate and it is largely through his efforts that nitrous oxide came into general use as a dental anaesthetic.

Meanwhile William Thomas Green Morton, a friend and one-time partner of Wells, had also been experimenting with nitrous oxide but he soon came to the conclusion that the gas, by no means pure and stored in skin bags which allowed contamination with air, was too uncertain for practical use. The story of what now happened is obscure. Morton had attended the chemistry classes of Professor Charles Jackson in Boston; it would seem that he now put his problem to Jackson, who drew his attention to the similarity in action of nitrous oxide and sulphuric ether. This similarity had already been the subject of a short paper, written either by Davy or by Michael Faraday, in the last number of the *Journal of Science and the Arts* for 1818.

Morton tried ether without success. He returned to Jackson who told him that he had been using commercial ether, heavily contaminated with water and spirit. This was the type of ether commonly used in 'ether frolics', so weak that it could be drunk without immediate harm. Jackson advised a trial of pure rectified ether and gave Morton the address of a chemist, Burnett, from whom it might be obtained. This is the basis of Jackson's later claim to the discovery of anaesthesia. Morton may or may not have then performed a number of experiments of a semi-scientific kind, using as his subjects goldfish, insects, a pet dog, and himself. His account must be viewed with suspicion but one of his experiments is beyond doubt; on or about 30 September 1846 Morton administered ether to a patient named Eben Frost for the extraction of some broken-down teeth. This trial was successful.

Morton was a very different type of man from Wells. One can feel some kind of affection for Wells, but Morton must have been a thoroughly unpleasant character. He was an unprincipled self-seeker who tried to patent anaesthesia and to extract a royalty for every anaesthetic administered; he was a charlatan who, from the start, attempted to hide the fact that he was using ether by colouring it with a red dye and adding a scented oil; he was a reckless ignoramus who once held a lighted candle before the mouth of an anaesthetized patient when warned that ether was too inflammable for safety. But he was also brave, pushing, and forceful, the type of man who will fight for recognition of his discovery. His bravery is shown by the choice of place for his first public demonstration. He asked permission to show his method at the Massachussetts General Hospital where Wells had met with so disastrous a failure. On 14 October 1846 Morton received a note from the house surgeon that John Collins Warren, the senior surgeon, had invited him to be present on the following Friday morning at ten o'clock to administer 'the preparation which you have invented to diminish the sensibility to pain'.

Shortly before ten o'clock on Friday, 16 October 1846, a large crowd assembled in the operating theatre of the Massachussetts General Hospital. There were doctors, medical students, members of the public. Some of them had come to try and detect any trickery, perhaps to run Morton out of town if he failed. Some had come out of mere curiosity, perhaps hoping to see something new or at least to join in the boos and hisses if there was nothing new to see. A few, probably á very few, would be bitterly disappointed if Morton did not justify his claim.

The patient, Gilbert Abbott, aged twenty-three and a painter by trade, was brought to the theatre and seated upright in the red plush covered operating chair, furnished with the necessary straps. John Collins Warren entered with his house surgeon and dressers. He waited for a few moments, glanced at his watch, and turned to the audience with the words 'Dr Morton is not here. I presume he is otherwise engaged.' There came a laugh from those who thought that Morton's courage – or his impudence – had failed him.

At this moment Morton hurried into the theatre, carrying in his hands a glass globe containing a red fluid, and accompanied by Eben Frost. He had been delayed by a last-minute difficulty with his inhaler. Warren rounded on him with that remark which must make the whole of this story ring true in the ears of any anaesthetist who has been late for an operation 'Well, Dr Morton, your patient is ready for you.' Morton asked the patient if he would like Frost to describe his experience, but Abbott refused. Then he told Abbott to close his lips round the wooden vent of the glass globe and to breathe backwards and forwards over the surface of the liquid. At first the patient coughed, then his breathing became quieter and more regular and his lips relaxed from their tight hold upon the vent. Satisfied that Abbott was unconscious, Morton repeated Warren's words 'Well, Dr Warren, your patient is ready for you.'

Warren made a cut in the skin of the neck, three inches long, and dissected out a tuberculous gland. Abbot neither moved nor cried out during the three minutes of this operation. He stirred uneasily as Warren put in the few stitches and Warren bent down to him. 'Did you feel anything?' he asked. 'I thought,' answered Abbott sleepily 'I thought I felt someone scratching at my neck.' Once again Warren turned to the hushed, astounded audience, 'Gentlemen,' he said, 'this is no humbug. We have seen something today that will go round the whole world.'

This is the classical story – there are several versions which vary in minor detail – of the first successful demonstration of anaesthesia. The news did indeed go round the world. It reached England on 16 December and London on 17 or 18 December. The first British anaesthetics were given at the house of Dr Boott in Gower Street, London, and at the Dumfries and Galloway Royal Infirmary.[4] Which of these two can claim priority is of little importance; the important date is 21 December 1846 when Robert Liston of University College Hospital amputated a leg and removed an ingrowing toenail, both patients being under the influence of ether. Liston was the most renowned of London surgeons, possessing, it is said, a technical skill in operating that has probably never been equalled and certainly never been surpassed. 'This Yankee dodge beats mesmerism hollow,' said Liston. 'It is a fine thing for operating surgeons,' he wrote to Boott. The acceptance of ether by the leading surgeon of London did more to introduce anaesthesia into England than any 'first' administration.

Other London hospitals followed suit. Reports of success came from Glasgow and from Edinburgh, where the surgeon

James Syme and his hated colleague James Young Simpson were among the first to introduce ether into their practices. In France Joseph Malgaigne and Alfred Velpeau, who had stated in 1837 that the dream of painless surgery was nothing but a chimera, used ether with success. Later they both condemned it as unreliable. Far away primitive Russia of the Tsars was not slow to follow; by April 1847 Professor N. I. Pirogoff of St Petersburg had evolved a method of reinforcing, or even substituting, the inhalation of ether by rectal injection of the vapour. So great was his success that modern Russians have claimed Pirogoff as the 'discoverer' of anaesthesia. It has been said that, within a year of Morton's demonstration, hardly a single major operation was performed in the civilized world without ether. In fact this is too sweeping to be true; James Syme, for instance, preferred not to use ether for certain operations, and there are many reports of patients who themselves refused the unknown hazards of painless surgery in the early years. Bottom was not yet dead.

Nor was ether by any means a perfect or even a reliable agent. Too irritating for comfortable inhalation, causing profuse salivation and sickness, often impure and so not sufficiently potent; reports of failure became not uncommon as the months of 1847 passed, although such failures were less numerous than reports of success. Just a year after the introduction of ether, James Young Simpson suggested the substitution of chloroform, which had been first prepared in 1831. Simpson's original experiment can hardly be called scientific. According to a contemporary account, he and two other doctors named Keith and Duncan wrapped table napkins around their heads and inhaled chloroform from their wine glasses after a dinner at Simpson's house. Swift loss of consciousness led Simpson to observe that this was 'better and far stronger than ether'.

Without more ado he arranged to administer his new drug to a young woman who was to have a small tumour removed from her breast. Simpson, an obstetrician, was at the last moment prevented from attending by a call to one of his patients. As the operation was only a very small one, the girl consented to have it done without any anaesthetic. When the first cut in her skin was made she fainted and died. This is usually presented as a narrow escape for chloroform; had the first patient to inhale chloroform died at once, the drug would have been abandoned. But this death is a clear case of the accident known as 'vagal inhibition', the sudden cessation of the heart's action which may occur for some quite trivial reason. The author knows of an exactly parallel case; a girl of eighteen was washing a milk bottle which broke in her hand and inflicted a small cut on one finger; the girl 'fainted and died'. We find similar deaths when searching the records of pre-anaesthesia operations. It is very unlikely that Simpson's patient would have died had chloroform been administered; this should serve to remind us that anaesthesia has not only given freedom from pain to the patient and increased operating time to the surgeon but has also lessened the risk of death from shock. This fact is often forgotten.

Simpson waged a great fight on behalf of anaesthesia. Opposition to painless surgery was trivial but, when Simpson first introduced ether and then chloroform into his midwifery practice, there came cries of protest from the Church and from godly laymen. Simpson, a sturdy fighter, a ripe liar on occasion, not above shamming illness when cornered, possessed just the type of character to do scornful battle against reactionary ignorance. The stories are legion but here we must content ourselves with only one which, with its sequel, sheds a light on the kind of man he was.

To the argument that it is both unnatural and sinful to allay the pain of childbirth, Simpson replied that the Almighty was the first obstetric anaesthetist, for He had caused a deep sleep to fall upon Adam who slept at the birth of Eve. The churchmen replied that Adam's painless labour had occurred before the Fall; the Curse of Eve reads 'in sorrow shalt thou bring forth children'. Simpson then claimed to have consulted the Hebrew script; the Hebrew word had been mistranslated, for the true meaning is not 'sorrow' but 'effort'. Apparently the agument was taken no further but the present writer felt he would like to know the truth and asked the opinion of a learned professor of Hebrew. His reply is uncompromising. The Hebrew word means 'sorrow' or 'suffering' and nothing else. Simpson won his fight with the aid of Queen Victoria, who decreed the use of chloroform at the birth of Prince Leopold in 1853, the chloroform being administered by the first specialist anaesthetist, John Snow. Queen Victoria is worthy of a high place among the pioneers of humane midwifery, for there is no doubt that her example led to the collapse of opposition.

Chloroform, introduced at the end of 1847, became the most widely used anaesthetic agent for the next sixty years. More pleasant to inhale than ether, far more powerful and, as a consequence, far more easy to administer successfully, chloroform would be the perfect anaesthetic agent did it not suffer from one fault, and that fault soon became all too obvious. More reliable than ether, chloroform is also more dangerous; this is the reason why it has now been replaced by other drugs. There can, however, be little doubt that chloroform, despite its relative danger, was the only feasible agent for general use in those days. John Snow answered his critics with the argument that he used chloroform in preference to ether for the same reason that he used phosphorus matches in place of a tinder box. The comparison is exact.

Anaesthesia at first directly affected only the surgeon and his patient; it brought no immediate advance in the scope or techniques of surgery. The affect upon the patient must be obvious to anyone; the affect upon surgeons was profound. Warren, after Morton's first demonstration, spoke to the audience in a voice broken with emotion; the steel-nerved Liston ended his first painless operation with tears in his eyes. Let us try to share the feelings of these basically kindly men who had been accustomed to inflict torturing pain and who now found themselves faced, almost unprepared, with an unconscious subject in place of an agonized creature, screaming and writhing against his restraining bonds. It must have been a deeply emotional experience.

There is no reason to wonder that anaesthesia brought in its train no dramatic change in surgical technique. When we look beyond the suffering individual, we see that the greatest gift of anaesthesia is not freedom from pain but prolonged operating time. The priceless boon of Time was not given to the surgeon at once. These primitive anaesthetics, administered from a variety of ingenious but ill-designed apparatus, consisted of inhalation for a period of two or three minutes only. The patient was not 'kept under'. The surgeon operated with his accustomed speed during the short minute or two before his patient regained consciousness. So, if we glance through the pages of a journal such as the *Lancet* for the years 1848 and 1849, we find little change in the pattern of surgery. There are endless references to painless operations, to ether and to chloroform – the latter would nowadays be described as 'a major break-through' for it is supposed to give excellent results in the treatment of typhus fever and delirium tremens.[5] But operations are no more frequent and the scope of operative surgery has not been extended.

Ten years later the medical journals reveal a very different picture. In 1858, after eleven years experience of anaesthesia, the surgeon is found to be operating far more often and to be covering a much wider field. The fact that the number has increased is shown by the tendency to report a series of operations rather than to give an account of a single operation. But the great change is in the type of surgery performed.

In the first chapter we saw that the surgeon was often faced with the urgent need to deal with a strangulated hernia. He rarely attempted to repair the ordinary hernia or rupture. The average man suffering from this disability lived a life of discomfort and impaired efficiency, only partially relieved by the support of a truss, until he either strangulated or died from some other cause. In 1858 the editor of the *Lancet* wrote that 'the radical cure of ... hernia is attracting considerable attention among surgeons.'[6] There are descriptions of several different methods by which the deficiency in the abdominal wall can either be plugged or oversewn and strengthened. Another report deals with plastic surgery, the repair of that type of injury which sometimes occurs as the result of difficult childbirth; here we read of operations devised to close a fistula between the vagina and the rectum, or between the vagina and the urinary bladder.

Then there are improvements in the method of treating fractures. The French surgeon Chassaignac had introduced a new technique of immediate splinting with a strong plaster which immobilized the broken ends of the bone so that they could not cause greater damage by piercing a large vein or artery. This having been done as an emergency treatment, the patient was put safely to bed and anaesthetized. Then the plaster was cut away over the site of fracture, the broken bone ends brought into apposition, the necessary traction or extension apparatus applied, and the limb replastered.[7] Such a method of dealing with a fracture would have been unthinkable before the days of anaesthesia.

The greatest change is seen in the technique of treating diseased joints. We saw in the first chapter that the white swelling of scrofula or tuberculosis was one of the commoner reasons for amputation of a limb. Before anaesthesia this was the only method, amputation of the limb above the joint infected by tuberculosis. In 1831 James Syme of Edinburgh had advocated excision of the diseased surfaces of the joint, leaving the bone ends and the surrounding tissues, but this was rarely practised because such an operation could not be performed speedily. Anaesthesia made the method possible and, in the *Lancet* of 1858, we find a number of references to excision of the knee and even of the hip joint. This type of operation had the advantage that the patient was left with a fairly useful limb although it was, of course, rigid because the joint had been removed and the cut bone surfaces united together to form a solid mass. Another operation that became popular at this time was Syme's amputation of the heel, instead of the whole foot. One paper in the *Lancet* reports a series of twelve Syme's amputations, and mentions that the operation had been modified by Pirogoff of Russia and by Busk of the Seamen's Dreadnought Hospital.[8]

During these years there had been a steady advance in surgery throughout the world. We may call this the transition period for, as we shall see in the next chapter, another and equally important advance had to be made before operations could be performed with reasonable safety. Among the more notable surgeons of this transition period are N. I. Pirogoff of St Petersburgh, who has already been mentioned. Pirogoff held the post of professor of surgery for forty-five years and was an excellent teacher. Besides the advances that he made in anaesthesia and in operative techniques, he organized the Russian nursing service in the Crimean War and may be described as the Russian counterpart of Florence Nightingale.

In Germany Bernhard von Langenbeck of Berlin devised many new operations, among them a method of repairing cleft palate, for which he is remembered today. Langenbeck's retractor, an instrument for holding skin and muscle away from the operation wound, is still in common use. He also founded the *Archives of Clinical Surgery* which held pride of place as the most influential continental journal of surgery during the nineteenth century. Contemporary with Langenbeck was Georg Friedrich Stromeyer of Hanover, primarily a military surgeon, who made great advances in what would nowadays be called orthopaedic surgery.

Antoine Lembert of France invented a special kind of stitch for sewing together the edges of a wound in the intestine so as to ensure no leakage. This 'sero-muscular suture' is used today in operations which involve joining one part of the alimentary tract to another. Joseph Malgaigne was another surgeon who made new advances in orthopaedics. Auguste Nélaton, a urologist, invented the flexible rubber catheter by which the bladder could be more easily emptied; before this catheters had been made of metal. He also devised a porcelain tipped probe to investigate bullet wounds, the porcelain becoming marked by lead when rubbed against the bullet. This probe was first used on the Italian patriot Garibaldi to detect the bullet which entered his ankle at the 'battle' of Aspromonte in 1862.

America, too, was rapidly gaining an important place in surgery. Samuel David Gross of Philadelphia, an able surgeon and writer, published his *Practical Treatise on Foreign Bodies in the Air Passages* in 1854; his book influenced the development of laryngology in Britain as well as in America. Better remembered today is James Marion Sims, world famous for his work on the diseases of women. He was specially successful in his operations for the repair of fistulae between the vagina and urinary bladder. Sims was the first man to attempt removal of gall-stones, but his patient died a week later.

There were many fine surgeons in Britain. Edinburgh could boast James Syme, perhaps the greatest surgical teacher of any age, known as the surgical miser who 'never wasted a word nor a drop of ink nor a drop of blood'. In London, now the centre of surgical practice, three men dominated the scene during the twenty years which followed the introduction of anaesthesia. Brodie, Fergusson, and Paget; between them they span the whole nineteenth century, for Benjamin Collins Brodie was born in the year 1783 and James Paget died in 1899 at the age of eighty-five.

Neither Brodie nor Paget can be said to have shone as an outstandingly brilliant operating surgeon, although Brodie was on the staff of St George's and Paget on the staff of St Bartholomew's and both made enormous incomes. Men of very similar qualities, they are of importance in the history of surgery for reasons other than technical ability. Both brought a new intellectual approach to their subject; both managed to combine a cultured, even aesthetic, mode of life with the active practice of what had so recently been little better than skilful butchery. Brodie became well known not only as a surgeon but as a physiologist and, in his later years, as a philosopher. A good administrator, he was chosen to be the first president of the General Medical Council when that august body was founded by the Medical Act of 1858. Joseph Lister was the first surgeon to be created a peer; Brodie was offered that honour but declined on the ground that his fortune was insufficient to support a hereditary title.[9] Paget we shall meet in a later chapter. Both of these men, in their outlook and their approach, were far more akin to the learned eighteenth-century physician than to the eighteenth-century surgeon. They did much to raise the status of the surgeon in England.

A quite different type was William Fergusson whom we met, as a young man, in the first chapter. By now he had settled in London and, after Robert Liston's death in 1847, became recognized as the finest operating surgeon in England. Born of very humble parents at Prestonpans in 1808, he achieved every honour open to a surgeon before his death in 1877; a baronetcy, surgeon to Queen Victoria and her Prince Consort, president of the Royal College of Surgeons, president of the British Medical Association among others. He had a hard struggle for many years, first at Edinburgh and then in London, where he was appointed to the newly founded King's College Hospital in 1839 on the recommendation of Astley Cooper. His daring, the speed of his operating, his coolness in emergency, are part of medical history. It is said that a student was in danger of missing the whole operation if he blinked an eyelid. More factual is the story that a knife once broke in Fergusson's hand at a moment when delay would have been agonising to the patient. He threw the useless handle on the floor and unconcernedly completed the operation with the broken blade held between his fingers.

A medical historian, the late Sir Gordon Gordon Taylor, described Fergusson as 'a flamingo of a man' and this unusual comparison gives a good idea of his colourful personality. Tall, powerful, handsome, of magnificent presence, he lived life to the full with uninhibited enjoyment. It is characteristic of him that he drove from his home in George Street, Hanover Square, through the mean slums surrounding King's College Hospital in a yellow coach with postillions and two Dalmatian dogs, specially trained to run beneath the rear axle. The latter detail is no evidence of eccentricity; Dalmatians were much in demand as guard dogs for carriages. He loved to be a convivial host at the Albion Tavern in the City, where he supped with journalists, writers, minor poets and artists, actors and, no doubt, actresses. A famous editor of *Punch* is said to have written 'Look out for me at seven, look after me at eleven. Lemon' in reply to one of Fergusson's invitations.

Fergusson belonged to the old school and he retained his remarkable speed of operating into the age of anaesthesia. He was no deep-thinking scientist but a practical man of his hands 'the greatest practical surgeon of our time' wrote James Paget of him. He made his fame in no narrow, specialized field; cutting for the stone, surgery of bones and joints, operations for hare-lip and cleft palate, resection of the upper jaw, these are some of the procedures attached to his name. After the coming of anaesthesia he turned his special attention to resection of the diseased joint in place of amputation of the limb, a type of operation which he described as 'conservative surgery'.

He remained in active practice until only a few weeks before his death at the age of sixty-nine. He lived into the years when, as we shall see, the surgeon began to depend upon other departments of medical science, but Fergusson, a man of his hands, would have little to do with these new aids. The story is told that he was once lecturing to a class on the diseases of bone when a daring student asked him if the views that he was putting forward were not at variance with those of a German scientist named Niemeyer. 'Why, man,' shouted Fergusson, 'Nehemiah was a minor prophet of the Old Testament. He wrote nothing on necrosis or caries.'

Fergusson was the last and perhaps the greatest of that early nineteenth-century school of surgeons who relied for their success solely upon their own technical skill and a knowledge of anatomy. Saluting his memory, we salute the passing of an epoch.

CHAPTER 3

Lister

Lister. The two short, close-bitten syllables of that name signal the point at which ancient surgery gives place to modern. Anaesthesia gave freedom from pain; the work of Lister, antisepsis, made surgery safe. The two are complementary; without anaesthesia 'the endless fiddle-faddle' of antisepsis would have been impossible; without antisepsis, anaesthesia alone could have brought little advance in surgery.

So in the year 1865, with anaesthesia established and antisepsis awaiting, a new age is about to open. Before telling the story of this new age we must first consider how true are the legends of the old. Legend tells us of the dirty pre-Listerian surgeon and his special operating frock-coat, stiff with blood and pus. He is supposed never to have washed his hands before operation – but he must have been well aware of the risk he ran for he always washed them afterwards. He performed a limited amount of comparatively minor surgery; incision of abscesses, the occasional amputation, a rare and invariably fatal attempt to remove a cyst of the ovary. Somewhere between twenty and forty per cent of his patients died after operation and all his wounds became infected. He was happy so long as these wounds drained the cream-coloured discharge which he called 'laudable pus'; faced with more malignant infection, he did nothing but clap on another bread poultice and cheerfully proceed with his next operation. When Lister showed him that wound infection might be easily prevented, he paid not the slightest attention.

Such is the legend as it has been told in endless biographies of Lister and histories of medicine. We must admit that, at bottom, there lies a solid core of truth. But that core of truth has been overlaid by a mass of distortion and fabrication. Take, for instance, the very minor legend of the blood-stained frock-coat. A surgeon named St Clair Thomson relates that when he was a house surgeon 'he himself put on an old blue frock-coat for operations, which he had previously worn in the dissecting-room. It was stiff and glazed with dry blood.'[1] St Clair Thomson was writing of the time when he was Lister's own house surgeon in 1883. If Lister, who made surgery safe by his antisepsis, allowed his house surgeon to wear a blood-stained frock-coat at operation, how can we blame the pre-Listerian surgeon for doing the same thing? This is an example of present day distortion of fact; the modern surgeon wears special clothing, so the old-time surgeon who wore no special clothing must have been criminally dirty.

Here, then, is the first indication that something is wrong with the classical story and, as we search through the records of the pre-Listerian age, we find ourselves questioning whether that story, as commonly told and accepted, comes near to the truth. Mortality, particularly mortality from sepsis, was undoubtedly high, but nothing like so high as is suggested by many modern writers. And it was not dirty operative technique so much as the generally dirty conditions of nineteenth-century life which caused the danger.

Clear evidence of this is provided by a *Lancet* report of 1865.[2] Fifteen cases of amputation through the hip joint, all previously published in the *Lancet*, are analysed. In the whole series of fifteen there are nine deaths, which may be expressed as a mortality of sixty per cent. This is very high but, of course, amputation through the hip joint was a far more dangerous operation than a simple amputation through the thigh or shin. Eleven of the fifteen cases were operations of election; these were operations rendered necessary by disease; the surgeon could operate at the most suitable time and in the best possible conditions. Five of these patients died, a mortality expressed as just over forty per cent. The remaining four of these fifteen amputations were emergency operations for a compound fracture. All four died from sepsis. It is also noteworthy that sepsis caused the death of only two of the five patients who died after amputation of election. Thus, it was the filthy, dung-strewn streets, the fact that the wound became infected before ever the patient reached hospital, that accounted for the appalling mortality of emergency amputation.

Amputation may be said, in general, to have carried a mortality of about forty-five per cent. It was notoriously the most dangerous of all commonly performed operations, but this forty-five per cent mortality must not be taken as a standard when assessing the death rate of pre-Listerian surgery. We can gain some idea of the overall surgical mortality by searching the case notes and extracting the relevant detail. For this purpose we will take at random two books of notes, one for the year immediately following the introduction of anaesthesia, the other some twenty years later and just before surgeons started to practise antisepsis.

The first book shows that, of 126 patients, 34 were treated by open operation. The remaining 92 were treated by other means and did not undergo operation. Of the 34 operation cases four died, which may be expressed as an operative death rate of 11·8 per cent. Of the patients who were treated by means other than operation (poulticing, dressings, splinting and so forth) twelve died, which again is a mortality of just under 12 per cent. The effect of adding these two figures together is to leave the result unaltered; the overall surgical mortality for patients treated by any means, or judged to be unsuitable for operation, is a fraction under 12 per cent.

The second book deals with 160 patients; of these 135 were treated by open operation and 25 by other means. Twelve of the 135 operation cases died, and three of the 25 patients treated by other means; this can be expressed as a 9 per cent mortality for the first class and a 12 per cent mortality for the second. The effect of adding the two figures together is to give an overall surgical mortality of just over 9 per cent.

These figures are interesting. It is now often stated that anaesthesia, by widening the scope of operation, increased the surgical mortality.[3] We see that it had the reverse effect. Not only did the mortality of operation fall, probably because the surgeon had more time at his disposal, but also the overall surgical death rate was lowered by nearly 3 per cent. It is the overall surgical mortality that matters; a patient is just as dead whether death is caused by operation or by failure to operate; anaesthesia, by making operation possible, reduced the death rate.

An operative mortality of between nine and twelve per cent is very high, but not nearly so high as the twenty to forty per cent which many writers would have us believe was the rule in the days before antisepsis. We must be fair to the pre-Listerian surgeon; he was doing his best in general hygienic conditions which made cleanliness very difficult; he was fully aware of the risks that his patients ran and he made valiant, if unavailing, attempts to combat the dangers.

Sepsis was the primary cause of death. Of this there can be no shadow of doubt. Eight of the twelve operative deaths in the second of our case-books were directly due to sepsis. In 1859 Thomas Bryant of Guy's Hospital published a study of deaths following amputation, based upon three hundred cases.[4] He stated that 10 per cent of all amputations died from the one form of generalized sepsis called pyaemia, and pyaemia was the cause of death in 42 per cent of fatalities. Thus nearly half of all amputation deaths were attributable to only one of the recognized forms of sepsis.

Generalized sepsis or blood-borne infection was commonly known as hospital disease, subdivided into erysipelas, pyaemia, septicaemia, and gangrene. Hospital gangrene, the most feared, may have been gas-gangrene but there is some evidence to suggest that it was an entirely different infection, first appearing at the end of the eighteen forties, rising to a peak during the eighteen sixties, and now unknown. Septicaemia is a general invasion of the blood stream by bacteria; in pyaemia, abscesses form in all parts of the body; erysipelas is much like septi-caemia but is accompanied by a fiery rash. Save for pyaemia, infection occurred in the form of epidemics; a hospital might be free of septicaemia or gangrene for a year and then the wards would be devastated by a virulent outbreak.

Little could be done when an epidemic occurred. Treatment consisted of supporting the patient's strength with vast quanti-ties of alcohol and strong beef tea. Chloride of zinc or Condy's fluid was applied to the wounds. In the eighteen sixties the surgeon often used carbolic acid empirically, bedding and floors being soaked with carbolic lotion. Some hospital authori-ties tried passing a slow stream of chlorine gas through their

THE DEVELOPMENT OF MODERN SURGERY

wards.[5] Huge fires were kept burning even in the heat of summer in order to increase ventilation. The wise surgeon – and most of them were wise – ceased to operate and closed his wards. The wards were then fumigated with sulphur candles or a mixture of saltpetre and sulphuric acid, and the walls were scrubbed with chloride of lime.

In these times of epidemic the whole hospital population was placed at risk. The man admitted with a cut on his head, the student who pricked his finger when threading the needle to stitch the cut, were equally prone to infection as the patient on the operating table. Many doctors who performed autopsies and many porters who cleaned and sharpened the operating instruments lost their lives. Nurses, working long hours in the crowded wards, were particularly vulnerable to 'hospital throat', now known to have been a streptococcal infection which was at once the result and the cause of septicaemia.

Pyaemia was endemic, although outbreaks reached epidemic proportions from time to time. This is understandable, for the multiple internal abscesses of pyaemia derived from local infection by an organism now known as a staphylococcus. Practically speaking, all wounds became locally infected with these organisms, commonly found on the skin. Hence the term 'laudable pus' which has become the shibboleth of pre-Listerian surgery. So long as the thick, creamy staphylococcal pus drained freely from the wound, the patient's life was not considered to be in danger. But if the skin edges united and the wound healed too soon, a loculated abscess might be formed and so bring in train the grave risk of blood-borne infection and the generalized abscesses of pyaemia. For this reason students were often advised to prevent the premature healing of amputation wounds.[6]

The high mortality of amputation wounds resulted chiefly from the very large area of underlying tissue exposed during operation. But the necessity of securing blood vessels entailed another grave danger. Thread ligatures, unlike the modern catgut, are not absorbed by the body tissues. The only method of removing a ligature was to leave the long end dangling outside the wound and to pull on the same when the ligature was judged to be free. Sloughing of the tied vessel end, which freed the ligature, occurred between the seventh and fourteenth day after operation. Thus, for a week or a fortnight, the wound contained a number of foreign bodies, of a kind that, even today, are particularly liable to form an abscess. The surgeon clung to the use of these ligatures because he had found that they formed useful drains to lead away the pus from the interior of the wound; in the case books we often come across the one mysterious word 'Through'; this simply meant that pus, draining through the dressings, had appeared at the end of the ligatures.

The majority of surgeons were fully conscious of danger and recognized the limitations which the ever-present risk of fatal sepsis imposed upon their practice. They made heroic and not altogether unsuccessful attempts to combat putrefaction, the term which they used to differentiate generalized from local infection or suppuration. They had certain drugs classed as antiseptics, a heterogenous collection of more or less useless remedies such as bitters, ethereal oils, carbon dioxide, and metallic salts. Myrrh, the age old antiseptic of the Bible, was in common use as late as the eighteen fifties. In the first chapter we noted that William Fergusson, suspecting the onset of erysipelas, ordered the wound to be poulticed with a solution of lead acetate. Diluted zinc chloride, sulphate of zinc, boracic acid, Condy's fluid (a solution of zinc permanganate), these and many other salts were tried out as wound dressings. Nor should we sneer too superciliously at the much maligned bread poultice, for folk medicine not infrequently has some basis of reason. Foxglove tea has given us the useful drug digitalis; poppy juice, an ancient anodyne, has given us first opium, then laudanum, and lastly morphia and its derivatives. Bread, unadulterated by preservative chemicals, quickly grows a penicillium mould and may have been of some value in inhibiting local staphylococcal infection.

We find many suggestions of preventive measures in the literature. The first of these were concerned with the terribly prevalent infection, puerperal fever. Charles White of Manchester insisted on strict cleanliness and ventilation of the lying-in room as early as 1773. In 1843 Oliver Wendell Holmes of Boston, better known as author of *Autocrat of the Breakfast Table* than as a doctor, rightly advised that students or obstetricians who had been working in the dissecting room should wash their hands and change their clothes before

47

attending a confinement. Ignaz Semmelweis of Vienna went further. In 1847 he insisted that all students coming from the post-mortem or dissecting rooms must wash their hands in a solution of chloride of lime before entering his lying-in wards. The result was dramatic; deaths fell from 15 per cent, first to 3 per cent, and then to 1 per cent.

Measures for the prevention of hospital disease included the routine oral administration of sulphite of potash before operation, recommended by Professor Polli of Milan and used by Lister among others, although Lister himself had little faith in the treatment. Some hospitals not only passed a slow stream of chlorine gas through the wards during epidemics of infection, but 'disinfected' the surgical wards at regular intervals with chlorine. James Young Simpson thought the thread ligature to be the most potent cause of infection; he invented, to take its place, the method of securing bloodvessels which he named acupressure, tight fastening of the cut ends to the underside of the skin by means of metal needles.[7]

Simpson published a much more drastic suggestion for preventing hospital disease. He considered that large hospitals were specially dangerous because the mortality of amputation fell from an average 40·9 per cent in a hospital of 300 beds to 10·7 per cent in a private or single room and advocated the building of small temporary structures.[8] These might be of iron, which could be easily treated by flame when an outbreak of infection occurred, or even of wood which might be destroyed by fire and cheaply rebuilt. Miss Florence Nightingale produced from her fertile brain a plan that, although immediately useless, exerted a profound effect upon hospital architecture. She firmly believed that hospital disease could be ended by replacing the old block type of hospital with a series of small pavilions.[9] Such hospitals, a few of which were built in Germany, proved hopelessly impractical for ordinary purposes. The modified pavilion, consisting of a series of free ward blocks running from a connecting corridor, became the standard pattern of hospital design. But experience during the early years of the new St Thomas' Hospital, built largely according to the ideas of Miss Nightingale, showed that hospital design had little or no effect upon the incidence of hospital disease.

Theories to account for the prevalence of hospital disease

were many, some bizarre, some very close to the truth. During the latter years it was widely believed that miasma, a poisonous gas or exhalation, caused putrefaction. Miasma, generated from the foul contents of sewers and cesspits, entered the surgical ward to contaminate wound tissues. The foul smelling miasma of a gangrenous wound then spread to other wounds, contaminating them in turn. So the epidemic developed. This theory led to a most interesting and widely practised form of treatment based upon the tarnishing of silver spoons. A silver spoon tarnished quickly when left exposed to the sulphurous air of Victorian London. If such a spoon were frequently washed with cold water, tarnishing was delayed because the sulphide had no chance to form a thick discolouring film. Arguing that both tarnishing and infection were caused by miasma, the surgeon used quantities of the purest possible water, that is water which had been boiled and allowed to cool.

So came into being the 'cleanliness and cold water school', surgeons who used vast quantities of cold boiled water to cleanse the operation site, to soak their instruments, to irrigate and to dress the wound. Men such as Thomas Spencer Wells of the Samaritan Hospital in London and Robert Lawson Tait of Birmingham achieved remarkable results with this method, and Lister himself – we must remember that Lister was a 'pre-Listerian' surgeon for fifteen years – adopted the practice. But mere cleanliness is not sufficient to ensure an uninfected wound, even today; a hundred or so years ago strict cleanliness was impossible in a filthy city such as London.

Take one instance. On 26 June 1858 *Punch's Essence of Parliament* reported that the House of Commons had 'been taking some care of itself, having spray jets to kill the effluvium, emptying barges full of lime upon the mud before the terrace, and putting canvas wetted with chloride of zinc over the windows.'[10] This was the month of The Great Stink when, following an unusually hot and dry period, the Thames shrank to little better than a trickle between slimy banks of decaying garbage. Yet eighty-two million gallons of water continued to be pumped daily from the river into the cisterns of London houses – and hospitals – for all purposes of drinking and washing. This is but one instance: what chance had cleanliness in conditions such as these?

There was need for something far more powerful and drastic than the contemporary standard of cleanliness before the mortality of surgery could be reduced. There was another and a greater need. The surgeons had ideas on the cause of hospital disease but those ideas were very far from the truth. Until they knew the cause, any treatment which they employed must be empirical, a hit-or-miss shot in the dark, a blind attack upon an unknown and unseen enemy. Until they knew the cause they could not possibly know the correct method of prevention.

The cause was found as the result of some work done by the French chemist, Professor Louis Pasteur of Lille. The detail of Pasteur's experiments lies outside the field of this book; the fact that his findings are the fundamental basis upon which modern surgery rests must be emphasized; having emphasized that fact it is only necessary to tell the story in a very simplified form. Pasteur, having been called to investigate the accidental production of vinegar instead of alcohol from the fermentation of beet sugar, found by microscopical examination that the disaster appeared to be due to a foreign yeast of a living nature. This led him to enquire into the souring of wine and milk and, later, into the putrefaction of blood and urine. He found that the boiled fluids, sealed from the air, did not putrefy or sour. His most important finding, from the surgical point of view, was that 'pasteurized' fluids, contained in a glass tube with the ends drawn out into a capillary and bent at an angle, did not sour. Thus the contents of the tube were in contact with the air but whatever it was that caused souring could not pass the entirely stagnant column of air contained in the minute bore of the capillary. He understood that souring was due to a living particle of matter, a micro-organism too small to be seen by the naked eye, but at this time he did not know that there was any difference between yeasts, moulds, and bacteria. To these micro-organisms he gave the name of 'germs'. He described his experments at the Sorbonne University on 7 April 1864, and, telling of a flask of milk which he had kept sealed for some time, he first enunciated the Germ Theory:

'And I wait, I watch, I question it, begging it to recommence for me the beautiful spectacle of the first creation. But it is dumb, dumb since these experiments were begun several years ago; it is dumb because I have kept it from the only thing Man cannot produce, from the germs which float in the air, from Life, for Life is a germ and a germ is Life.'

Pasteur's theory was the starting point for Joseph Lister's great work. Lister applied Pasteur's findings to disease; having satisfied himself that infection must be caused by a microscopical living body carried in the air, he was quickly enabled to find a means of prevention.

Joseph Lister was born at Upton House in Plaistow, then in Essex but now part of the borough of Newham in Greater London, on 5 April 1827. He came from an old and undistinguished Yorkshire family who had joined the Society of Friends or Quakers in 1705. His father, Joseph Jackson Lister, was a wine merchant, but had a special interest in the microscope and was elected Fellow of the Royal Society in 1832 for his achievement of making the first achromatic instrument. Father and son were devoted to each other; there can be no doubt that the father's hobby strongly influenced the son's approach to scientific problems.

Joseph entered the Arts Faculty of University College, London, in 1844, graduated BA in 1847 and started his medical course at University College in October 1848. He is said to have been present at Liston's first operation under anaesthesia but the story must be regarded with some suspicion, because Lister was not even a medical student at the time. He qualified MB London in 1851 with honours and a gold medal; in the same year he became a Fellow of the Royal College of Surgeons of England. After serving as house physician and house surgeon at University College Hospital, he proposed to make a tour of various surgical centres, starting with Edinburgh. Lister intended to stay one month in Scotland, but in fact, remained there for twenty-four years.

He arrived at Edinburgh in September 1853, became Syme's assistant and house surgeon (Lister was the only man with whom Syme never quarrelled) and married Syme's daughter Agnes on 24 April 1856. Having 'married out of the persuasion' he was forced to leave the Quakers and became a member of the Church of England, a defection that had momentous consequences in 1877. After his marriage he abandoned all the peculiar Quaker mannerisms but continued to use the 'thee and thou' when writing to his father.

In the autumn of 1856 Lister was appointed assistant surgeon to the Edinburgh Royal Infirmary and remained on the staff for just over three years. During this first Edinburgh period he published two papers, one entitled *The Early Stages of Inflammation* and the other on the coagulation of blood, which show that his mind was already turning to the problem of wound-healing. It is also noteworthy that both papers depended upon microscopical work.

In January 1860 he received the appointment to the chair of surgery in the University of Glasgow and was elected surgeon to the Royal Infirmary eighteen months later. The nine years at Glasgow are the most important period in Lister's career, for it was in Glasgow that he put Pasteur's theories into practice. It is more convenient to outline the rest of his life here and then return to a detailed history of his discovery.

Lister does not seem to have been happy at Glasgow; he was overburdened with routine work and lecturing. Twice he applied for other appointments, but without success. One of these was the chair of systematic surgery at his old school, University College; it is said that he lost the appointment by only one vote. In April 1869 James Syme suffered a stroke and was forced to relinquish his chair of surgery at Edinburgh. He greatly desired that his son-in-law should succeed him, a proposal endorsed in a letter signed by one hundred and twenty-seven Edinburgh medical students. On 19 August 1869 Lister was informed that he had been elected professor of clinical surgery at Edinburgh in Syme's place, and he left Glasgow in the following October.

The next seven years proved to be the happiest period of his life, perhaps the only truly happy time. As the success and the fame of his methods grew, surgeons from all countries flocked to the Edinburgh Royal Infirmary; his lecture rooms were packed by an enthusiastic mob of students; he lived as busy a life as at Glasgow but he was not so burdened with routine work. He had time for research and for foreign travel.

In 1877 Lister was invited to accept the chair of surgery at the Anglican King's College Hospital, an appointment which could not have been offered to a non-conformist. It is too often said that London paid no attention to Lister's work and that he met nothing but apathy and unfriendliness at King's. For this reason it is important to emphasize that King's College Hospital in London was the only institution in the world which had the courage and the foresight to *invite* Lister to accept a professorship. It had always been his ambition to return to London and at last, after twenty-four years, King's gave him his chance. He laid down conditions before accepting the chair, conditions that were necessary but somewhat arrogant, and there is no doubt that he was not well-received when he came to King's in October 1877. But that unpopularity was of short duration.

Many well-deserved honours came to him during the next years; honorary degrees from Oxford and Cambridge in 1880, a baronetcy in 1883, the coveted German order 'Pour la Mérite' in 1885. In 1885 the Royal College of Surgeons invited him to accept the presidency but Lister, immersed in research and uninterested in medical politics, decided that the heavy duties of England's premier surgical office would interfere with his real work and declined the honour.

He was due to retire from King's under the age limit in 1892, but the hospital asked him to stay on for another year. In April 1893 his wife, Agnes, died after a very short illness while they were on holiday at Rapallo in Italy. Agnes had been Lister's mainstay for all their married life, acting as his confidential secretary (she had learned to imitate his handwriting), helping with his experimental work, preparing his intruments for private operations. Without her, he was lost. After he retired from King's at the beginning of October 1893, Lister performed no more surgery.

His friends, understanding that Lister must be given work to occupy his mind, persuaded him to accept the post of foreign secretary to the Royal Society. After much hesitation he unwillingly agreed to do so and, two years later in 1895, he was elected president. In 1896 he served as president of the British Association at its Liverpool meeting.

Lister was created a peer in 1897, the first surgeon to be so honoured. Shortly afterwards his health started to fail, but he partially recovered after a trip to South Africa. Lord Lister was one of the surgeons called into consultation when King Edward VII developed acute appendicitis just before the date fixed for his coronation. After the postponed ceremony Lister was sworn of the Privy Council and made one of the twelve original members of the newly instituted Order of Merit.

His eightieth birthday, 5 April 1907, was celebrated throughout the world but Lister felt too ill that day to meet his visitors for more than a quarter of an hour. In the following June he received his last honour and made his last public appearance when admitted to the Freedom of the City of London. A month later his sister-in-law, Miss Syme, who now kept house for him, took Lister to Walmer in Kent; there he remained for the last years of his life.

These years of seclusion were not happy. He always hoped to return to London; there is a story that his horses and carriage were kept ready at his house in Park Crescent for a summons from Walmer. He had been almost stone deaf for some years and in the summer of 1909 his sight began rapidly to fail. After nearly three years in a world of darkness and of silence, Lord Lister died from pneumonia on 10 February 1912.

Lister's true character has been concealed with a cloak of hero-worship thrown over him by his biographers. It is clear that even those who were most closely associated with him never got to know him well. The men who followed his teaching became his devoted disciples but they did not become his intimate friends. William Watson Cheyne, Lister's assistant for many years, remarked that he 'always stood in awe of Lister'. One of his students wrote that 'a strange atmosphere of inaccessibility always enveloped him'. Another said 'we were never quite at our ease and never quite at our best with him'.

Lister is presented to us as a saint: the only acknowledged blemish upon his character is his inveterate, and very discourteous, lack of punctuality. He was even twenty minutes late when due to deliver the Croonian Lecture of the Royal Society. There is no doubt that he was a fine man but he was also a strange man. He was a magnificent doctor, at his best with children; he inspired confidence in his patients and did everything in his power to ensure their comfort. For instance he made it a strict rule that an instrument tray must never be left uncovered in sight of the conscious patient; he had a very real sympathy with his patients and on many occasions he, himself, paid their fees in a private nursing home if they were unhappy in the crowded hospital ward. Lister was not an outstanding surgeon; indeed there are those who say that he fumbled his operations. He was certainly a slow and nervous operator; if difficulty arose he sweated so profusely that a nurse was always stationed beside him to wipe his forehead with a towel.

A truly religious man, he believed himself to be directly inspired by God in his work, and he turned to Him in all moments of perplexity. He stood for a minute in silence with his head bowed before starting any operation that promised to tax his skill. But there is another side to this picture; he was sanctimonious and practised the virtue of Christian resignation to a point which must have been infuriating. 'Lister sighed' is a constantly recurring theme in his biographies. Opposition to his views, an experiment ending in failure, disobedience to his orders, a request to see a patient at an inconvenient time, all evoked a gentle sigh of submission.

Lister was always polite in his manners and speech and seldom reproved his assistants for their errors – he sighed instead – but he possessed little tact and no sense of humour. It has been already mentioned that he made stringent conditions when he accepted the chair at King's College Hospital; these conditions were necessary but they antagonized the students, the nurses, and his colleagues. A more tactful, more subtle man would have imposed his will without arousing the hostility of nearly every section of the hospital community. His lack of humour is notable; he is said never to have laughed and in all the biographies there is recorded only one joke, so feeble that it will certainly not be repeated here.

Shyness gives us the keynote to his strange character. Lister made few friends; his shy, withdrawn nature would not allow him to make the first difficult approach. Because of this his life was not outwardly a happy one, but it is probable that he knew the true inward happiness which does not always reveal itself upon the surface. There is something attractive in this shy, gentle, good man, but there is none of the firework brilliance which makes Fergusson a 'character'. The difference between them is shown by two small, similar, incidents that occurred in the operating theatre of King's College Hospital. Fergusson did a certain operation in record time, and the audience loudly applauded him. He turned to them and bowed again and again, like an actor acknowledging his ovation. Lister performed the same operation with more than his usual speed and dexterity – and the large audience applauded him. He hushed the on-lookers into silence with the words 'Gentlemen, gentlemen – remember where you are.' To Fergusson the operating theatre was a theatre indeed and he was the star actor; to Lister it was a temple and he was there as the humble servant of mankind.

We now return to Glasgow in the year 1864. The new surgical block in which Lister's wards were housed had been opened only a few months before his appointment in 1861. A fine large building, well ventilated, it had been designed on the most modern lines; the managers were confident that outbreaks of hospital disease would be greatly diminished, if not entirely ended. As at St Thomas', the hope proved vain. Lister's two accident wards, the male accident ward on the ground floor and the female above, gained a reputation as bad as any in the United Kingdom. Lister attributed the high incidence of hospital disease to a disused burial ground supposed to lie beneath the block.

Lister, in common with many other surgeons, believed that hospital disease was caused by 'something in the air', but he was not satisfied with the theory of miasma. He doubted whether the cause could be simply ascribed to some unknown noxious gas but he held the spread of disease to be by means of air; it was not a contagion, passed by physical contact from patient to patient. At one time he thought that the causative agent must be solid matter, a fine impalpable dust resembling pollen. There is no evidence that he suspected this dust to be living, but his idea of invisible particles is of great interest for it shows that his outlook upon disease had already been affected by his early work with the microscope.

In an endeavour to prevent the entry of miasma, or of his impalpable dust, Lister tried the fairly common practice of covering wounds with an impermeable dressing, metal foil or gutta percha sheeting, a logical plan which entirely failed in its purpose for reasons hidden from him but patent to us. About 1860 he started dressing wounds according to the precepts of the cleanliness and cold water school. 'He used kettles of boiled water, often mixed with Condy's fluid, with which he tried to wash out the putrefying discharges and, in addition, Lister administered sulphite of soda, as recommended by Polli.'[11] Basins of cold boiled water and piles of towels appeared in his wards and he made strict rules to enforce cleanliness. But all these methods failed, and his results were poor. Lister states that until 1865 his amputations and his excisions of joints carried a mortality of over forty-five per cent.[12]

Some surgeon would undoubtedly have been led in due course to a realization of the importance of Pasteur's work. Lister heard of it quite by chance. At this time he read little and, although fluent in German and French, never read foreign medical or scientific journals. On a day between March and August 1865 he was walking with Dr Thomas Anderson, professor of chemistry at Glasgow University, when Anderson casually mentioned Pasteur's work and, seemingly, suggested that it might have some bearing upon medical and surgical problems. Lister was one of the few surgeons of that day who, because of his familiarity with the microscope, possessed the type of mind to accept Pasteur's findings without question.

These findings came as a revelation to Lister, for they exactly fitted his theories and his scanty knowledge of hospital disease. The existence of living 'germs', so closely resembling his postulated 'disease dust', explained everything by their essential fact of life and consequent power of generation. They teemed in the air and they multiplied in the wound. The wound inflicted by a street accident was already full of germs before ever the patient arrived at hospital. A means must therefore be found of killing the germs in such a wound, and of preventing the ingress of germs into the wound deliberately inflicted at operation.

Pasteur had killed his germs by heat but this was a means that could not be applied to the patient. Lister's mind turned to an incident of 1864, widely reported in the press. In 1863 Jules Lemaire of Paris introduced crude carbolic as a wound dressing, having already used it for other purposes. In the following year cattle, pastured on a sewage farm near Carlisle, became infected with entozoa; at the same time there was an increase in the number of cases of typhoid occurring in the city. When the sewage was treated with carbolic, both the cattle sickness and the number of typhoid cases rapidly diminished.

In the same year, 1864, the surgeons of St George's Hospital in London tried carbolic as a specific during a severe outbreak of hospital disease. This trial of carbolic, although a failure, had been reported in the *British Medical Journal*.

It is possible that Lister had already tried carbolic as a wound dressing without success. In March 1865 he dressed a compound fracture with the crude acid, but nothing is known of this experiment except that it failed on account, in Lister's phrase, 'of improper management'. We do not know the exact date of Lister's talk with Anderson, so we do not know whether this first use of carbolic took place before or after he had read Pasteur's work. The balance of probability inclines to the former.

Lister now evolved a plan for the use of carbolic in the light of his new-found knowledge of the existence of germs. His scheme of treatment required the formation of a scab, the natural method of wound healing. No doubt this was put into his mind by the work that he had already done upon the coagulation of blood. Until now the scab, being a coagulum of blood, had constituted both a protection and a danger. It was a protection so long as it remained uninfected but, once infected, the scab formed a certain pathway to the underlying tissues. So the scab itself must contain a means of destroying the invading germs at site; only thus could it form an effective natural barrier.

Lister first tried his new method on 12 August 1865, in the case of an eleven-year-old boy named James Greenlees, who had suffered a compound fracture of the tibia when knocked down by an empty cart in a Glasgow street. He seemed an ideal subject for this first experiment. The wound was a small one and did not lie directly over the site of fracture; thus there was a good chance that the extravasated blood around the bone ends had not already been infected. In such a case, although the danger of infection remained and amputation often became necessary, it was common practice to wait in the hope that the limb might be saved.

Here is Lister's own account of what was done. 'My house surgeon, Dr Macfee, acting under my instructions, laid a piece of lint dipped in liquid carbolic acid upon the wound, and applied lateral pasteboard splints padded with cotton wool, the limb resting on its outer side, with the knee bent. It was left undisturbed for four days, when, the boy complaining of some uneasiness, I removed the inner splint and examined the wound. It showed no sign of suppuration, but the skin in its immediate vicinity had a slight blush of redness. I now dressed the sore with water having a small proportion of carbolic acid diffused through it; and this was continued for five days, during which the uneasiness and the redness disappeared, the sore meanwhile furnishing no pus, although some superficial sloughs caused by the acid were separating. But the epidermis being excoriated by the dressing, I substituted for it a solution of one part of carbolic acid in from ten to twenty parts of olive oil, which was used for four days, during which a small amount of imperfect pus was produced from the surface of the sore, but not a drop appeared from beneath the skin. It was now clear that there was no longer any danger of deep-seated suppuration, and simple water-dressing was employed. Cicatrization proceeded just as in an ordinary granulating sore. At the expiration of six weeks I examined the condition of the bones, and, finding them firmly united, discarded the splints; and two days later the sore was entirely healed, so that the cure could not be said to have been at all retarded by the circumstances of the fracture being compound.'[13]

Success in a minor compound fracture such as this could hardly be regarded as conclusive evidence in favour of the new method; in fact Lister himself wrote that the injury might have healed without carbolic treatment. Ten months later, on 19 May 1866, a far more serious case was admitted into the Glasgow Royal Infirmary. 'It is one of compound fracture of the leg; with a wound of considerable size and accompanied by great bruising and great effusion of blood,' wrote Lister to his father. 'Though hardly expecting success, I tried the application of carbolic acid to the wound, to prevent decomposition of the blood, and so avoid the fearful mischief of suppuration throughout the limb. Well, it is now eight days since the accident, and the patient has been going on exactly as if there was no external wound, that is as if the fracture were a simple one. Thus a most dangerous accident seems to have been entirely deprived of its dangerous element.'[14]

Lister dressed this wound by a different method which

became, for a time, his standard technique. As much blood clot as possible was squeezed out and the wound thoroughly swabbed with crude carbolic. Lister then applied a piece of lint soaked in carbolic to the wound surface, with an overlap of half an inch on every side. Next he covered the lint with a thin sheet of malleable tin and strapped the whole dressing to the leg with adhesive tape. The wound was then packed round with absorbent wool and the limb splinted in the usual manner. Subsequent 'dressing' simply entailed lifting the metal protection and painting the lint surface with carbolic.

The wound never became infected and the fracture united without trouble. By means of the blood and carbolic soaked lint, Lister had attained his desired result, an antiseptic impregnated coagulum or scab through which Pasteur's 'germs' were unable to pass. He had not only by means of carbolic killed the bacteria which had already invaded the wound, but he had erected a barrier through which new bacteria were unable to pass. This is the essence of the Listerian Principle which he called Antisepsis.

Broadly speaking, antisepsis means destroying bacteria. Asepsis, the term used for the modern surgical technique, implies that bacteria are never allowed the chance to invade the wound. Lister's *method* depended upon the antiseptic drug carbolic and his *method* was therefore antisepsis. But his *principle* was to erect a barrier through which bacteria could not invade the wound; his *principle* is therefore asepsis by means of an antiseptic drug. It is most important to understand this. His fundamental aim remained constant throughout his many subsequent changes in detail. It was not enough simply to use an antiseptic; the constant aim must be to erect an antiseptic barrier in order to ensure an aseptic site. That is what so many of his contemporaries failed to understand, and this essential part of his teaching is still not fully appreciated today.

Progress was slow at the start. Eighteen months after his first use of antisepsis, when he published his historic monograph in the *Lancet* of 16 March 1867, his results depended upon only eleven cases of compound fracture. But the figures of even this small series spoke for themselves. Of his eleven patients, only one had died and that not from sepsis but from haemorrhage due to the fractured bone puncturing an artery. Two cases had been attacked by hospital disease. One of these recovered with conservative treatment and the second, which had developed while Lister was absent from Glasgow, recovered after amputation of the limb. The remaining eight patients all made uneventful recoveries.

Meanwhile, in October 1866, Lister had started to use carbolic in the treatment of abscesses. Here the barrier took the form, in his own term, of an antiseptic curtain. A piece of lint, soaked with one part of carbolic in four parts of boiled linseed oil, was laid over the area. The upper edge of the lint being held in place by an assistant, Lister raised the lower edge and inserted his scalpel, previously soaked in carbolized oil, beneath the protective covering. Pus was allowed to flow from below the antiseptic curtain which, in the case of large abscesses, might be momentarily raised to allow insertion of a pledget of carbolic soaked lint to act as a drain.

By now he had changed the method of dressing. Instead of painting lint with carbolic, he used a stiff paste of carbolic and linseed oil mixed with carbonate of lime. This was spread to a thickness of a quarter of an inch on suitably shaped pieces of sheet tin or tin-foil reinforced by adhesive plaster. The 'putty' slowly released carbolic acid to the wound surface while the metal covering prevented wasteful evaporation into the air.

In April, 1867, Lister commenced the use of antisepsis during operations. The first patient, a sick old man, suffered from a large tumour deeply embedded in the upper arm. Lister employed the same technique of his 'antiseptic curtain', but he also irrigated the wound with carbolic lotion. The patient made an uneventful recovery, and Lister was able to write to his father 'nothing could have been more satisfactory'. By August 1867 his results had proved so good that he could tell the British Medical Association 'since the antiseptic system has been brought into full operation, and wounds and abscesses no longer poison the atmosphere with putrid exhalations, my wards, although in other respects under precisely the same circumstances as before, have completely changed their character, so that during the last nine months not a single instance of pyaemia, hospital gangrene, or erysipelas has occurred in them.'[15]

CHAPTER 4

The Exciting Years

Lister had satisfied himself that antisepsis worked, but he had still to convince the world. Anaesthesia is an obvious advance; antisepsis not so obvious. We have seen that, within a year of the introduction, hardly a single major operation was performed in the civilized world without anaesthesia; antisepsis did not gain general acceptance until nearly fifteen years after Lister's first experiment in 1865. During these years he went on quietly working, improving his methods, teaching his visitors and his students, writing articles, preaching the gospel of antisepsis. By 1877 his methods bore little resemblance in detail to those of ten years before. Crude carbolic had given place to the pure crystallized acid, dissolved in olive oil or water. The messy putty of linseed oil and whitening was superseded by carbolic impregnated lac plaster and carbolized paraffin gauze; sutures were carefully prepared and steeped in carbolized oil. Wounds were no longer drained by hanging threads but by lengths of plaited horsehair, strips of carbolized lint, or the perforated rubber tubes introduced by the French surgeon Chassaignac. The dangerous thread ligature had been discarded in favour of absorbable catgut, carefully prepared and sterilized by carbolic. The antiseptic curtain of lint, under which Lister passed his scalpel to make a virtually blind incision, had been replaced firstly by massive syringing with carbolic lotion and then by the spray which surrounded wound, instruments, and surgeon in a fine cloud of antiseptic mist.

The carbolic spray, though not an essential of his method, is so intimately linked with Lister's name that a paragraph must be devoted to its story. A picture of the final model appeared upon stamps commemorating the 1965 centenary of his first use of antisepsis, although he did not invent it until after 1871. In fact Lister was not the first to use the carbolic spray; Thomas Nunn of the Middlesex Hospital introduced 'a modification of Richardson's spray' in 1868.[1] Lister also used a Richardson's spray, much like an ordinary scent bottle worked with a hand bulb, but he found that the jet was not sufficiently powerful. He therefore designed a much larger model, worked by a hand lever and standing on a tripod. So bulky and clumsy was the 'donkey engine', as it came to be called, that a Listerian surgeon could always be identified as such by some part or other of his spray sticking out of the carriage window when he travelled to an operation in a private house. Lister described this model at the Plymouth meeting of the British Medical Association in 1871.[2] In the next year he replaced the donkey engine by a much more compact spray consisting of a spirit lamp, a boiler, and a container for carbolic lotion; a steam jet crossed the open end of a tube leading into the carbolic and thus drew up and threw a fine spray of carbolized droplets into the air. There were two sizes, a small one for use when changing dressings, and a larger one capable of throwing a jet for a distance of twelve feet or of filling a room with a cloud of carbolized steam.

By a strange but fortunate chance a description of how a room was prepared for a Listerian operation has been preserved in the King's College Hospital case notes. It is believed to be the only description on record. The operation notes were written by a student named H. Dudley Ryder. They are very long-winded, enter into quite unnecessary detail, and end with the words 'Dr Playfair performed the operation and was assisted by Mr Rose, Dr Hayes being present. The nursing arrangements being in charge of and performed by Sister Jessie.' The kind of notes written by Mr Ryder on previous pages lead one to surmise that he had been reproved by his chief for scrappy note-taking and was using this ingenious method of getting his own back.

'No. 8 Ward in which the operation was performed was purified two days previously with sulphur fumes. Subsequently walls and floor washed with 1:20 carbolic lotion and two carbolic sprays were turned on for two hours immediately previous to the operation. The patient was also prepared for the operation by being dieted on milk for two days previous to operation. All instruments were soaked in 1 :20 carbolic lotion and warm 1 :40 was used throughout for sponges, etc. All other antiseptic precautions were in accordance with those adopted by Sir Joseph Lister.'

Such was the Listerian technique when he at last returned to London, as professor of clinical surgery at King's College and surgeon to King's College Hospital, in October 1877. London was still not convinced; the twelve years that had elapsed between his first use of antisepsis and his return to London had been a time of discussion and trial which grew into a warfare that divided surgeons into Listerians and non-Listerians. We catch a glimpse of the battle in Conan Doyle's story *His First Operation*. The new student, chaperoned by a senior, enters the operating theatre for the first time, takes his seat, and looks around him with frightened interest.

'Who are the two men at the table?' he asks.

'Nobody – dressers,' answers the senior man. 'One has charge of the instruments and the other of the puffing Billy. It's Lister's antiseptic spray, you know, and Archer's one of the carbolic acid men. Hayes is the leader of the cleanliness-and-cold-water school, and they all hate each other like poison.'

Conan Doyle set this little scene in Edinburgh where he had been a student. The general opinion appears to be that, while the rest of the world accepted Lister's teaching with eagerness, London alone held back and refused to have anything to do with antisepsis. Nothing can be further from the truth. There was opposition in Glasgow; hardly had Lister left for Edinburgh when Professor James Morton of Glasgow, who had used antisepsis in his wards, denied that the results were any better than with other methods and stated that the antiseptic principle was founded on false premises.[3] There was opposition in Edinburgh; as late as 1875 Professor Spence 'persistently rejected the antiseptic plan of treatment' and claimed that, by using only tepid water and plain lint as a dressing, he had achieved the low mortality of 4·76 per cent in amputations.[4] There was opposition in France, where the surgeon Després stated in 1879 that he would like to establish a 'cordon sanitaire' against Lister's method – that importation from England which, during the last few years, had made a tour of the world, invaded France, and there ravaged like an epidemic.[5] In America the majority of speakers at the June 1882 meeting of the American Surgical Association were still opposed to anti-sepsis.[6]

Of course there was opposition in London too. In 1879 William Savoury of St Bartholomew's Hospital delivered the address on surgery to the annual meeting of the British Medical Association at Cork; he took the opportunity to launch a violent attack upon Lister.[7] That colourful person William Fergusson is said to have 'snarled like a dog' whenever he met a Listerian surgeon in the corridors of King's College Hospital.

Lister had his disciples in London just as he had disciples in all other parts of the world. Howse of Guy's, Croft and Mac-Cormac of St Thomas', Marcus Beck of University College Hospital regularly used antisepsis almost from the earliest days. So did John Wood of King's; his case books clearly show that he followed Lister's advances in technique step by step, yet he is usually represented as one of Lister's most bitter opponents.

The trouble was that the antiseptic technique, although basically very simple, depended for success upon meticulous observation of a number of small details. Lister, isolated in a far corner of the United Kingdom, could only show these details to those who came to visit him; we cannot altogether blame the busy surgeons of London and other centres if they were unable to find time to visit Glasgow and Edinburgh. Then Lister continually changed his methods as his experience grew; there are complaints from surgeons that they could hardly keep pace with these changes.

Most of them tried their hand at the antiseptic technique. A very interesting survey made by the *Lancet* in 1868–9 shows that carbolic dressing was being used in nearly every large London hospital, and there are reports from many provincial hospitals too.[8] But the results, and the opinion based on those results, was very varied. This is hardly to be wondered at, for the majority of surgeons did not understand the underlying princi-ple; they can therefore hardly be blamed if they made a sorry hash of an unfamiliar technique and discarded it as useless. The surgeon, whether he succeeded with carbolic or not, was stimulated to take a much greater interest in the detail of

65

wound dressing; this is probably the first benefit that Lister's work brought to surgery; it is certainly the reason for the good results obtained by men like Spence who refused to accept antisepsis.

Opposition became fierce in 1869 when the medical profession – not surgeons only – began to understand that Lister's technique depended upon Pasteur's germ theory. A new theory will never be accepted without question, and Pasteur's theory was revolutionary for it upset all preconceived ideas of the causation of disease. The microscope was an unfamiliar instrument; Shephard Taylor in his *Diary of A Medical Student* records that the professor of physiology and morbid anatomy threatened to have *the* microscope locked up when his class became unruly.[9] The germ theory was a theory only; no one had yet been able to prove any association between disease and bacteria. A discussion held by the Pathological Society of London in 1875 gives some idea of the muddled thinking then prevalent.[10] One speaker believed that bacteria are produced by disease, not disease by bacteria. Another, who claimed to be a strong advocate of the germ theory, made the surprising remark that no such advocate regarded bacteria as being the cause of disease. At this time it was fashionable to make the parrot-joke, 'Shut the door quickly, or Professor Lister's germs will get in.'

The germ theory was the stumbling block. Many surgeons, and, it seems, particularly London surgeons, found themselves unable to accept the idea that wound infection can be caused by minute living particles which, at that time, had not been isolated. Some surgeons continued to practise antisepsis; they held it possible to accept Lister's method while denying the principle. Others abandoned antisepsis entirely and fiercely denied that any method depending upon the absurd germ theory could be useful. Many simply waited; they were apathetic in the sense that they did nothing; but they were waiting for proof that antisepsis was a much better way of treating wounds than any other.

That proof did not come for some years. Again and again the *Lancet*, which championed Lister, suggested that a special ward should be set aside in a London hospital and that strict antisepsis should be used in the ward.[11] Thus it would be easy to compare the results of antisepsis with other methods. But this sensible suggestion was disregarded. Again and again the *Lancet* pressed Lister to publish his figures and to confute his opponents, but Lister held that statistics could be made to prove anything, or nothing, and obstinately refused to publish his figures. He had some justification for, when he left Glasgow, he had written an account of the change in operative mortality wrought by antisepsis and the accuracy of his figures had been publicly challenged in a letter to the *Lancet* from the secretary of the Glasgow Royal Infirmary.[12]

Lister was not a magnificent operating surgeon of the type of Liston or Fergusson. He did little to widen the field of surgery. An analysis of his King's College Hospital case notes for the years 1877–93 shows that of 2,702 patients admitted into his wards, 647 received only very minor surgery or no surgery at all, 567 were operated on for accidents of various kinds, 323 for tuberculosis, and 276 for deformities of the bones. Thus 1,813, or 70 per cent of his patients, were treated by the type of surgery commonly practised by any surgeon of the pre-Listerian age. Among the remaining thirty per cent – a mixed bag – there is only one operation, the attempted removal of a brain tumour, which would certainly not have appeared in a pre-Listerian operating list. Two quite remarkable operations, one upon the heart and one to remove gallstones, have been found in other case books; the patients were admitted under a physician and Lister was called in to operate. Lister did not 'invent' any of these three operations; they had all been done at some time before.

Examination of his case notes reveals that his overall surgical mortality was 4·2 per cent (in comparison with the 9 per cent surgical mortality of a pre-Listerian surgeon quoted on page 44) and that his mortality from operations was only 1·5 per cent (compared with 9 per cent on page 44). Antisepsis had greatly decreased the mortality of surgery; but the figure of 1·5 per cent for Lister's operative death rate makes it clear that most of his operative surgery must have been of a minor nature.

We do, however, find a 'new' operation among the accident series and it was this operation, quite a simple one, which finally proved the usefulness of antisepsis. It was the wiring, by open operation, of the fractured patella or kneecap. Lister first wired a fractured patella on 26 October 1877, some three weeks after his arrival at King's College Hospital. Most broken bones will unite if the ends are steadily maintained in close apposition; it must be plain that, if they for some reason fail to unite properly, the most sensible thing to do is to cut down on the broken ends and rivet them together with wires, plates and screws, or grafts of bone, just as a broken piece of valuable china is sometimes riveted. But, to the pre-Listerian surgeon, this was most certainly not the obvious thing to do. He well knew that a simple fracture, in which the protective skin covering is not injured, carried no risk to life. He knew that a compound fracture, in which the protective skin covering has been wounded, was one of the most dangerous accidents which could happen.

Lister, faced with a simple broken kneecap which failed to unite when ordinary splinting methods were used, decided to cut down upon the site of fracture and to join the two pieces of broken bone together with silver wires. This manoeuvre broke the strictest rule of the pre-Listerian surgeon; Lister was proposing to change a simple fracture, involving no risk to life, into a compound fracture, carrying a grave risk of amputation or even of death. There were those who declared that, if he failed in this unwarranted experiment and the patient lost his life, Lister should be indicted on a charge of manslaughter. Lister did not fail; although the end result of operation was not good by modern standards, the patient Francis Smith retained not only his life but a useful limb.

The success of this unheard-of operation, repeated six times by Lister in the next six years, convinced London of the essential need for antisepsis. Lister's teaching and example drove the lesson home. Lister had won his battle by patience; he knew that he was right, that there was no necessity for drama, that his ideas must in the end be accepted. By 1880 the antiseptic method, if not the principle underlying that method, had received general approval.

But his success in London had come too late to save London's pre-eminence in the field of surgery. Initiative had already passed to another nation than Britain, and it was as the direct result of a paper written by Lister that this change came about.

On 15 July 1870 Germany, or more precisely the Kingdom

of Prussia, declared war on the French Empire of Napoleon III. On 2 September Napoleon surrendered at Sedan, but the war went on for another four months. On 3 September 1870 Lister published *A Method of Antiseptic Treatment Applicable to Wounded Soldiers in the Present War* in the *British Medical Journal*. The method which he described was a complicated one requiring large quantities of carbolic, lint, oiled silk, and gutta percha. He gave the warning 'the earlier the case comes under treatment, the greater will be the prospect of success, but even after the lapse of thirty-six hours it need not be altogether despaired of.'[13]

No doubt Lister's treatment would have proved excellent, but it was impossible to put the method fully into practice. Field surgeons, scanty in number, could not have carried the vast store of dressings and carbolic which the full treatment demanded. In this war of movement, the casualty, transported by his comrades or by slow horse ambulance, must have counted himself lucky if he arrived at a well-equipped base within thirty-six hours of receiving his wound. An additional difficulty lay in the quite extraordinary nature of the medical attention, the most heterogenous collection of men and women ever found in a battle area. Under the new flag of the Red Cross worked doctors from Holland, Belgium, Austria, America, and Great Britain, besides those of Germany and France; nursing duties were performed by sanitary corps orderlies from both armies, prisoners of war, dressers from the London hospitals, French and German Sisters of Mercy, the Anglican Sisterhoods of St John and of All Saints, gentlemen of the German Order of St John, Lutheran Diaconates and Orthodox Sisterhoods from Russia. Agreement on one standard – and complicated – method of dressing wounds would have been impossible among these varied sects and tongues.

The French hospitals paid no attention at all to Lister's suggestions. 'Antiseptics and ventilation alike are greatly neglected' wrote a *Lancet* correspondent. 'Pyaemia, dysentery, and diarrhoea abounded in all these places.'[14] The French surgeon Lucas-Championnière, who had studied under Lister at Glasgow in 1868, was ordered by superior authority to return unopened the bottles of carbolic which he had brought to a field hospital.

The Prussians made some attempt to put Lister's ideas into practice. The *Lancet* correspondent reported that, in the hospitals near Sedan, a modified form of antisepsis was being used with not very good results; 'as for dressing exactly according to Mr Lister's plan, I saw none of it anywhere'.[15] The same was true of hospitals at Aix-la-Chapelle, Saarbrucken, and Coblenz. Further back, in the tented hospitals of the Rhine, 'a most extensive use' was made of carbolic acid for dressings. Liberal applications of carbolic and chloride of lime to bedding and working surfaces helped to combat hospital disease and to ensure general cleanliness.[16]

As Lister had not published his recommendations until nearly two months after the outbreak of war, it was possible for the German surgeons to make comparisons. The results of antiseptic treatment were not good, but they were far better than when no antisepsis was used. Two facts emerged during these last months of the war. Firstly, the French wounded soldier eagerly surrendered, because he knew the Prussian medical treatment to be better than his own. Secondly, a wound healed more quickly when carbolic dressing was used; thus the military surgeon fulfilled his duty of returning cannon fodder to the battle field as swiftly as possible.

Before 1870 the German surgeon worked in an institution, often enormous in size, that fell far below the standards of hygiene of even a nineteenth-century English hospital. We know from the accounts of English travellers that the general state of cleanliness and sanitation in Europe was quite revolting when compared with the amenities of a London that we should regard as indescribably filthy. The war of 1870 taught the German surgeon that wounds healed more quickly under clean conditions; cleanliness, carbolic, and Lister became interwoven in his mind. There followed a spate of expensive hospital reconstruction, and there also followed an enthusiasm for Lister's technique. Germany, alone among nations, accepted Lister's teaching whole-heartedly, and a rapid advance in surgery developed as the result. In the twenty years after the introduction of antisepsis, London ceased to be the centre of surgery; initiative passed into the hands of the German-speaking peoples.

We shall meet many of these German surgeons, and consider the advances they made, in the chapters dealing with surgical specialities. But in June 1875 Lister made a tour of the larger surgical centres in Germany and received everywhere a great ovation. Let us go with him on this trip and introduce ourselves to some of the men whom he met. There was Richard von Volkmann, professor of surgery at Halle and Leipzig, a brilliant operator, mainly interested in the surgery of bones and joints, but also the first man to excise the rectum for cancer in 1878. Friedrich von Esmarch of Kiel, primarily a military surgeon, wrote treatises on first aid and, in 1861, organized a scheme for the proper siting of field hospitals and bandaging stations in relation to the battle line. Esmarch's bandage, a long rubber strip used to render a limb bloodless by compression, is still a necessary piece of surgical equipment, although first introduced as long ago as 1873. Not many surgeons can claim kinship with an emperor, so it may be of interest to mention that Esmarch was uncle, if only by marriage, to Kaiser Wilhelm II.

Karl Thiersch of Erlanger and Leipzig is a name remembered today by the Thiersch graft, a very thin graft of skin in common use. He invented this method in 1874. Thiersch arranged to perform a demonstration operation for Lister (and the King of Saxony) at Leipzig. It was to be the removal of a loose body from the knee joint and he therefore proposed to render the leg bloodless by applying an Esmarch's bandage. As this was an important occasion, a brand new one had been provided. Needless to say, it snapped at the crucial moment, which should be a salutary reminder that demonstration operations never go smoothly.

From Leipzig Lister moved on to Berlin, where he met Professor Bernhard von Langenbeck, whom we mentioned in the second chapter. Langenbeck, now in his sixty-fifth year, made Lister's visit the occasion of his first use of antisepsis, an example of delicate tact. The case was one in which excision of the knee joint might have been found necessary. Seven years later, in 1882, the elderly Langenbeck was succeeded in the chair of surgery by Ernst von Bergmann, a Baltic Russian born at Riga, who was to be largely responsible for converting anti-sepsis into a technique approaching our present day asepsis.

Among other German-speaking surgeons of this time was Vincenz Czerny of Freiburg and Heidelberg, the first man to remove the uterine new growths known as fibroids or myomata

71

through an incision in the abdominal wall. This was in 1881. Then there was the German Pole J. von Mikulicz-Radecki, whose name is usually simplified to Mikulicz. He held the chair of surgery at Königsburg from 1887 and at Breslau from 1890 until his death in 1905. Mikulicz devised many new operations, particularly upon the oesophagus, and one that has become known as Paul's or Mikulicz's operation which consists of bringing a cancer of the large bowel to the surface of the abdomen and removing it at a later date.

Johann von Nussbaum was a particular friend and devotee of Lister's. An able surgeon, he worked in the immense *Allgemeines Krankenhaus* at Munich and described his experiences with antisepsis there in a book published in 1879. The hospital had previously, he wrote, been a 'pest house' for hospital diseases. In the five years before 1879 hardly a single case had developed although, but for antisepsis, no alteration of any kind had been made. He claimed that one of the most remarkable advantages of the method was in the lesser time that a patient needed to stay in hospital. Those rare cases of amputation which recovered in the days before antisepsis remained in the wards for at least a hundred and forty and perhaps for as long as a hundred and eighty days. By the use of antisepsis the patient could be discharged after thirty or forty days; some had left hospital completely cured after fourteen days, having been dressed only four times.[17]

Anton Wölfler of Graz, who moved to Prague in 1895, has the distinction of being the first man to perform, or to report having performed, the famous operation of gastro-enterostomy, which consists of joining the stomach to the upper end of the small intestine so as to bypass an obstruction or an ulcer. He did the operation in a case of advanced cancer of the pylorus, the valved opening through which the stomach contents pass into the duodenum or first part of the small intestine. He reported this at the German Surgical Congress of 1881; in the same paper he mentioned three similar operations performed by Theodor Billroth. Two of the four patients had survived.

Although Wölfler was the first to report this particular operation, it should be associated with the name of the last and the greatest of our German surgeons, Theodor Billroth, who may justly be called the father of abdominal surgery. Born on the Island of Rügen in 1829, Billroth graduated from Berlin University in 1852. It is said that he wanted to devote his life to music but was persuaded to take up medicine against his will; he retained his interest in music and took a leading part in the fierce disputes between the partisans of Brahms and of Wagner. A great, genial, bear of a man, singularly like Tennyson in appearance and in his manner of dress, he also resembled William Fergusson in his enormous zest for life, his lavish hospitality, his colourful personality.

After graduating, Billroth became Langenbeck's assistant at Berlin, was appointed professor of surgery at Zurich in 1860, and moved to Vienna seven years later. It is not too much to say that he founded the famous Viennese school of surgery entirely through his own example and effort. A brilliant operating surgeon and a man of rare intelligence, he at once understood the importance of Lister's work. All his life he taught and practised the detail of Lister's technique but, by some strange quirk of thinking, he became an agnostic in regard to the germ theory. Like some of his London contemporaries, he believed it possible to follow Lister's practice accurately while preserving an open mind as to the principle. There is no doubt that he succeeded, but Billroth was an exceptional man.

The list of his advances in surgery makes impressive reading but only one or two need be mentioned here. In 1872 he resected the oesophagus; in the following year he performed the first total excision of the larynx for cancer; in 1881, as has already been mentioned, he performed the operation of gastro-enterostomy, at the same time resecting the pylorus. Early on he turned his attention to cancer of the rectum and, between 1868 and 1876, removed no less than thirty-three of these new growths. The years between 1878 and 1892 were filled with cases of intestinal resection and with the group of operations then known as 'enterorraphies', the short-circuiting of one part of the bowel to another. The special method of stitching bowel, the sero-muscular suture, which had been invented by the French surgeon Antoine Lembert, did not come into more than limited use before Billroth started his series of operations. It is of some interest that, at a meeting of the Clinical Society of London in 1879, Howard Marsh of St Bartholomew's Hospital reported two cases in which Billroth had divided the bowel and united the cut ends by Lembert sutures. 'Such suture of the divided bowel,' said Marsh, 'promises good results.' Here is a clear indication of Billroth's influence during his lifetime. A well-known medical historian, Arturo Castiglione, writes of him 'by his work and through his pupils, he was the most important single influence in the development of surgical knowledge'. Lister made surgery safe; Billroth, by the time of his death in 1894, had shown how, through Lister's work, the field of surgery could be enlarged.

It is true that the surgeons of victorious Germany led the field in these years following the Franco-Prussian war, but we must not be led into the mistaken belief that the surgeons of other countries were standing still. In France, humiliating defeat had brough in its train a hatred of all things foreign and, particularly, of all things German. There was a tendency to look upon antisepsis as a theft of French ideas; Pasteur had developed the germ theory, Lemaire had introduced carbolic, Chassaignac the india-rubber drainage tube; Lister's sole contribution had been the carbolic spray which was useless – and his results were 2 per cent worse than under any other form of treatment. The French surgeon, Perrin, who cited this figure at a meeting of the Paris Societé de Chirurgie in 1879, did not say where he had obtained his facts or support them with any evidence.[18]

But Lister had his friends in France. Lucas-Championnière has already been mentioned; a fine surgeon, he published the first textbook of antiseptic surgery (first in any land) in 1876. He had been the pupil of another great French surgeon, Paul Broca, who is sometimes regarded as the founder of modern neurosurgery, and was particularly interested in trephining of the skull. Plastic and orthopaedic surgery owe much to Louis Ollier who followed Lister's teaching, albeit somewhat half-heartedly. Another French Listerian, Jules Péan, was one of the first surgeons to remove the uterus through the vagina (vaginal hysterectomy) and he also introduced a most useful little instrument for securing blood vessels during operations. A few years later two urologists, J. C. F. Guyon and J. Albarran, made the Necker Hospital in Paris a world centre for surgery of the urinary tract.

Across the Atlantic the United States of America engaged

themselves in mending the havoc of civil war. American medicine depended largely upon post-graduate study in European centres – the time had not yet come when American teaching and research facilities would be the envy of the world. National bankruptcy and preoccupation with internal troubles led to a withdrawal from Europe during the eighteen sixties. Antisepsis did not make any decided impact upon American practice until 1876, when Lister attended the International Congress of Medicine at Philadelphia as president of the surgical section. After the Congress, Lister toured the surgical centres, but he met with a mixed reception; only in Boston and, to a lesser degree in New York, was he received with enthusiasm.

The first American treatise on antisepsis did not appear until 1888. It was written by Arpad Gerster, who had been born at Kassen in Hungary and had emigrated to America. But America could boast some very good surgeons at this time. Another European emigrant, the Swiss-born Nicholas Senn, achieved fame as a follower of Billroth in abdominal surgery; in 1886 he suggested that it might be possible to remove a diseased pancreas, but he never attempted the operation. One of Senn's introductions was a method of suturing bowel so as to prevent leakage of the contents, a disaster that can cause fatal peritonitis. We shall meet Senn again in another chapter.

H. O. Marcy of Massachusetts is credited with the introduction of antiseptic ligatures used in the repair of hernia (1878) and another surgeon, Christian Fenger, was a pioneer in the operative treatment of brain abscess; at a later date he made advances in surgery of the bile duct and of the ureters. H. J. Bigelow of Boston, who had been present at Morton's first public demonstration of anaesthesia, is remembered for his method of extracting stone fragments from the bladder, a most important advance in technique which is almost unchanged today although he published a description of his operation in 1878. Samuel David Gross performed laparotomy, an exploratory opening of the abdomen, in the case of a ruptured urinary bladder as early as 1867, but there is no evidence that he used any antiseptic precautions. We met Gross in the second chapter, where we also met James Marion Sims. Sims, who died in

1883, headed an Anglo-American ambulance unit to the Franco-Prussian war and did very good work.

Sir John Erichsen, Lister's chief at University College Hospital, is supposed to have said in 1874: 'The brain, the thorax, and the abdomen will forever remain closed to the hands of the wise and humane surgeon.' In fact the only evidence that Erichsen made this remark seems to depend upon a memory by the throat surgeon Sir St Clair Thomson – and Thomson was only fifteen years old in 1874! But there is no doubt that many British surgeons thought the largely experimental operations performed by the Germans and others to be quite unjustifiable. Opinion was mixed. C. F. Maunder of Charing Cross Hospital declared himself opposed to interfering with the abdomen on the grounds that rough handling of the viscera must of itself always result in disaster. But at the same meeting, in 1879, at which Maunder expressed his opinion so strongly, Howard Marsh of St Bartholomew's took the opposite view. He insisted that early operation must be performed in all cases of intestinal obstruction. Only thus could the patient's life be saved; this, he implied, was the surgery of the future.[19]

Six months later Robert Lawson Tait of Birmingham, one of the more controversial figures in surgery, boldly declared that he 'made it a rule to open the abdomen in all doubtful cases – as to the nature of the tumour – where there seemed a possibility of benefit from operative proceedings and, in between fifty and sixty cases . . . had had no reason to regret the proceeding.'[20] This was in the year 1879, just about the time that Billroth, the father of abdominal surgery, was starting his series of operations.

From the above it will be seen that the forward movement of surgery was by no means confined to Germany alone; it was a world-wide advance which gathered momentum as the years passed until, by the end of the nineteenth century, progress had become more rapid than in any field of medicine, before or since, and perhaps more rapid than in any sphere of human endeavour. The abdomen, the brain, the lungs, and the heart; operations upon all these organs were recorded before 1900; the surgery of today has its roots in the work done by the surgeons of the last quarter of the nineteenth century.

This world-wide forward thrust would not have been possible

without contacts between the nations. Increased ease of communication is as important a part of the history of surgery as is anaesthesia or antisepsis. The Age of Steam made travel more rapid and more comfortable; travel demanded a knowledge of foreign languages; knowledge of a foreign language stimulated interest in the scientific journals of another country. The London surgeon read of the work done in a Berlin clinic and found himself anxious to see that work with his own eyes. At the beginning of the nineteenth century a journey to Berlin would have entailed an absence of weeks or even months from his London practice. Now it was easy; he did not so much as need a passport; there were no currency restrictions or difficulties. With a few golden English sovereigns in his pocket, he could be in Berlin two days after making up his mind to go – and he could be back in his London consulting room within the week.

Consider this little incident, compiled from the diaries of Miss Emma Durham, a nurse whom we met in the first chapter. On a day in 1901 she was on leave in Essex, drinking a cup of tea with a friend after lunch, when a telegram came from her nursing institute 'Be at Burwood Place at four to start for Russia. Urgent.' It was then two o'clock; she hastily packed her bag, caught the two-forty train to Fenchurch Street, drove in a hansom cab to the Bank, boarded a horse-bus for Burwood Place, and was on the doorstep of her nursing institute at five minutes to four. There she received her instructions and was told to go to Regent's Park to meet the patient's mother. That evening she and the mother took the boat train from Charing Cross, arrived at Ostend at midnight, and immediately boarded the trans-European express. Next evening they stayed the night in Vienna. Twenty-four hours later they came to Volochynsk, the frontier town of Imperial Russia, and reached their destination, Kiev, early on the following morning. Today the actual journey by air would be much quicker; but could anyone except a Very Important Person – which Miss Durham was not – suddenly decide to leave Essex at two o'clock on a Tuesday afternoon and be in Russia early on the Friday morning?

It was this speed of travel which made interchange of surgical ideas and experience possible. Just as international fairs, expositions, and exhibitions became increasingly frequent during the years between 1840 and the First World War, so the international medical and surgical congress became commonplace. These congresses provided great opportunities for advance; here surgeons met their foreign colleagues in person, discussed their hopes and their difficulties, and came away with a broadened knowledge of their subject. Nor did contact end with the last session of the congress, for a better postal service enabled exchange of thought to be maintained. The number of medical journals steadily increased; foreign correspondents regularly made reports of new advances in the various centres.

We rightly attribute this widened scope of surgery to Lister's introduction of antisepsis although as we shall see in the next chapter, progress did not depend upon Lister's work alone. During the last decade of the nineteenth century and the first decade of the twentieth, a gradual change took place in the method of applying Lister's principle to surgery. Antisepsis, killing of bacteria by an antiseptic drug at the site of the operation wound, gave place to a mixed technique in which large quantities of antiseptic drugs were still used, but some attempt was also made to render the materials prepared for operation 'sterile'; that is, certain instruments, towels, sponges, and other things were pre-treated so that they came to the operation free of bacteria. In the end this mixed technique gave place to our modern asepsis, in which everything is rendered sterile, free from bacteria, before operation and is maintained in a sterile state during the operation. In order to understand how this change came about, we must return for a moment to Lister's introduction of antisepsis.

From the beginning Lister believed infection to be primarily air-borne. He accepted Pasteur's dictum that 'every speck of dust carries at least one germ'. His belief was strengthened by the work of Professor John Tyndall, begun in 1869 and published in 1881, which showed that the amount of dust carried in apparently clean air is very large. Lister knew of Tyndall's findings and repeated Tyndall's experiments with a beam of light at least as early as 1871.[21]

Lister introduced the carbolic spray on the assumption that the cloud of antiseptic mist would kill the infecting organisms carried on the dust in the air and so give a bacteria-free operating field. Bacteria is a more modern term; at this time Lister did not clearly understand that there are different types of micro-organism; he probably regarded the 'germ of hospital disease' as a single entity, little if any different from a yeast or mould. Advances in the science of bacteriology made it apparent that the vast majority of air-borne organisms are not harmful; they are non-pathogenic, that is they cannot cause disease, in contradistinction to the pathogenic organisms which are the cause of infections.

In 1883 Elie Ilya Ilyich Metchnikoff, born near Kharkoff in Russia and afterwards Pasteur's assistant, propounded his theory of phagocytosis, based on his observation that the white corpuscles of the small water shrimp, Daphnia, form giant cells in order to deal with invading spores of a vegetable organism. The human large white corpuscles, to which the name phago-cytes or eating cells was given, can engulf and digest foreign organisms which find their way into the bloodstream. It became clear that a healthy individual could cope with the few pathogenic organisms normally found in clean air; wound infection was not air-borne but occurred as the result of massive invasion from dirty hands, unsterilized instruments, or con-taminated dressings. On the face of it Lister's spray, which he had introduced to 'clean' the air, was useless. We must, how-ever, question whether the spray did not form a necessary – or advisable – part of Lister's practice. His reasoning was faulty but he, and at that time all surgeons, operated without caps, masks, or gloves. Thus the spray may have been essential to prevent massive invasion from the hair, from the hands, or by droplet infection from the nose and throat.

Lister himself discarded the spray in 1887 when its usefulness had already been challenged for several years, notably by the German surgeon Viktor von Bruns in 1880. In England the tendency was to adopt, or to partially adopt, Lister's method while questioning the principle. The case was the reverse in Germany; the German surgeon, trained in a more academic and coldly scientific fashion than his British colleague, accepted the principle but soon started to question the method. In 1875 Carl Eberth of Halle showed that many bacteria are harboured on the skin, in the sweat glands, and in the hair follicles. This seemed to be an argument in favour of the spray, but Eberth found that the deeper skin layers, and so the glands and follicles, could not be sterilized by means of antiseptics. A few years later Hermann Kümmell of Hamburg showed that equally satisfactory results, and fairly adequate protection, could be attained by simple scrubbing of the hands and fore-arms with soap and water.

A further advance or change came in 1880, when another German, Merke, resurrected Pasteur's original finding that micro-organisms can be easily destroyed by boiling. This led, in 1881-2, to the introduction of methods of steam sterilization by the bacteriologist Robert Koch and his assistant Wolfhügel. Steam sterilization did not, at first, give very good results and could not be used, as it is now, for the sterilization of almost everything required for an operation; the modified Listerian method, as it returned from Germany to England in the mid eighteen eighties, took the form of a mixed 'antiseptic-aseptic' technique. The surgeon scrubbed up; towels were treated by steam heat; some instruments were boiled; sharp instruments, such as scissors and scalpels were still soaked for twenty minutes in carbolic; hands, face, and hair went uncovered; antiseptics such as carbolic and mercuric chloride were freely used. Dressings consisted of one or other of the various impregnated gauzes which are commemorated in a King's College Hospital song of about 1887:

'There is a worthy baronet who once took up the cause
Of Antiseptic Surgery and Antiseptic Gauze.
First there was a yellow one, then there was a blue;
Then there was a red one and a white one, too.
Next there was a violet one, so we thought he'd go
Right through all the colours of the bright rainbow.'

Lister had coloured his experimental gauzes with various dyes; the most satisfactory and most widely used were the blue, impregnated with the double salt of mercury bichloride and ammonium chloride (sal alembroth) and the violet, coloured with rosanilin and containing the double cyanide of mercury and zinc.

In 1886 the chief advocates of this mixed or near-aseptic technique were C. B. Lockwood of St Bartholomew's, Gustav Neuber of Kiel, and Ernst von Bergmann of Berlin. About 1890

Ludwig Lautenschlager, a pharmacologist of Freiburg, introduced an improved apparatus for steam sterilization by means of which Bergmann was enabled to practise an almost purely aseptic technique in 1891, first described by one of his assistants, Kurt Schimmelbusch, in a book published 1892. Attempts at a purely aseptic technique must, however, have been appallingly dangerous while the surgeon worked with naked hands, hair, and face. This was soon understood and various protective coverings were introduced.

A covering for the hands had been suggested by Thomas Watson, a physician, in 1843, first implemented by J. von Mikulicz-Radecki, who used cotton gloves about 1885. The modern rubber glove was introduced, but not invented, by William Stewart Halsted of the Johns Hopkins Hospital, Baltimore, in 1894. There is a nice little story that these rubber gloves were not first used by Halsted for the protection of the patient but of his theatre nurse, who had developed a nasty rash of the hands from contact with antiseptics. Whether the story be true or not, there is no doubt that Halsted later married the girl. Many surgeons opposed the wearing of rubber gloves on the ground that they constricted the hands and made delicate work impossible.

Halsted seems also to have introduced, or at least popularized, the wearing of caps to cover the hair. Gauze face-masks were first worn by either Mikulicz or the French surgeon Paul Berger in 1896–7, but did not come into general use for many years; some surgeons preferred absolute silence in the theatre, which they incorrectly thought would be enough to prevent droplet infection. The operating gown in its present form seems to have originated in Italy although Berkeley Moynihan of Leeds claimed to have been the first surgeon to wear a gown; he also claimed that he was the first British surgeon to wear gloves. But many surgeons wore protective clothing of various kinds long before the days of asepsis; Thomas Beddoes of Bristol wrote of 'the surgeons in their dresses' in 1803. Rubber boots were first used in the operating theatre by Richard von Volkmann and his assistants in the eighteen eighties; they had been found essential because of Volkmann's custom of having carbolic poured from watering cans all over the floor during an operation.

The first British surgeon to use an aseptic, as opposed to a clean or an antiseptic, technique was Cuthbert Wallace. Immediately on his appointment to an assistant surgeoncy at at St Thomas' Hospital in 1897, Wallace introduced rigid asepsis and induced the hospital governors to make the necessary alterations in theatre equipment and methods of sterilization. His excellent results drew surgeons and representatives of hospital management committees from all parts of the world to seek his advice on the problems of asepsis. Another who did much to popularize the aseptic method in these early years was William Arbuthnot Lane of Guy's, who is also credited with the logical advance commonly known as the 'no touch' technique. Here nothing in contact with the wound is ever touched by the hand, even when gloved; needles are held in specially designed holders and towels are draped around the operation site with forceps, for example.

But it would be an error to suggest that there was a swift change-over from antisepsis to asepsis; the two methods persisted side by side and in modified forms for years; many surgeons still practised a mixed 'antiseptic-aseptic' technique after the First World War. Nor did modern full asepsis, in which no person may enter a theatre for any purpose unless properly gowned, capped, masked, and booted, become general until the risk of cross-infection (which means the spread of infection from, say, the throat of a nurse to the throat of a surgeon and from the throat of a surgeon to the wound of his patient) was clearly understood from experience gained during the years 1939–45. The author remembers that, when he was a surgical dresser in 1931, students on his 'firm' did not wear masks in the theatre unless they were assisting the surgeon at the operation.

So surgery advanced and so the detailed technique which made that advance possible gradually changed until it bore no resemblance to the methods used by Lister. His contemporaries (and many of his successors) used carbolic because it is a powerful antiseptic. Lister used the dangerous carbolic because it was the most efficient means he knew to produce an aseptic operating field. This is the difference. Lister's 'treatment' has gone for ever, as all treatments are at some time replaced by others. But his principle of a barrier erected between the wound and the invading bacteria of disease remains unchallenged. Presumably it will remain unchallenged so long as operations are performed and wounds are dressed. Therein lies his unique contribution to surgery.

CHAPTER 5

Science Comes to the Aid of Surgery

Many surgeons of the author's acquaintance would dislike the title of this chapter, for they prefer to call the various medical specialities upon which they depend by the name of 'ancillary departments'. But the title is correct; during the latter half of the nineteenth century a number of scientific discoveries, not directly connected with surgery, helped the surgeon in his work. Indeed, we have already seen that Lister's antisepsis depended upon Pasteur's findings which were, at first, solely concerned with the problem of why vinegar was produced during the fermentation of beet sugar.

Until almost the end of the nineteenth century the diagnostician, whether surgeon or physician, depended largely upon his senses; sense of touch, of hearing, of sight, even of smell and of taste. He had a few aids; the stethoscope described by the French physician René Laennec in 1818 (a nineteenth-century doctor could often be identified by the bulge which the wooden stethoscope made in his top hat); the clinical thermo-meter, largely introduced into medicine by James Currie of Liverpool at the end of the eighteenth century; one or two other pieces of apparatus to test the capacity of the lungs and to make a tracing of the pulse-beat. Beyond these, he had little more than his 'clinical acumen', which was simply experience based upon minute observation.

Some of these practitioners became wonderful diagnosticians. Of such was Joseph Bell, professor of surgery at Edinburgh, who taught Conan Doyle and whom Conan Doyle acknowledged to be the original of Sherlock Holmes. Bell trained himself so well in the observation of detail, and thereby became so able in 'spot diagnosis', that he could tell a patient's work from the state of his hands and the district in which he lived by the colour of the mud on his boots. It is related of a famous physician, Lionel Smith Beale, that he was once called in to advise on a case of some mysterious fever which had puzzled the family doctor. 'Typhus,' said Beale when he came to the sick-room door. 'You haven't even seen my patient yet,' protested the doctor. 'No, but I've smelt him,' answered Beale. 'Typhus fever always smells of mice.'

From very early times the clinician has tried to check his diagnosis and to trace the course of disease by the examination called in the old days 'anatomies', now known as autopsies or post-mortems. Attendance in the hospital post-mortem room formed as important a part of the nineteenth-century student's curriculum as did his work in the dissecting room. In the latter he learned the anatomy of the normal human being; in the post-mortem room he learned morbid anatomy, the changes in normal anatomy wrought by disease.

The nature of a fatal illness can often be demonstrated by the gross, easily seen changes in certain organs. For instance, Giovanni Battista Morgagni of Padua, sometimes looked upon as the founder of the science of morbid anatomy, showed that the presence of the disease pneumonia, diagnosed during life, can be confirmed after death. The lung is consolidated instead of aerated; if placed in a vessel of water it will sink and not float. But the body was a single entity made up of various easily demonstrable structures such as the muscles, the nerves, bones, blood-vessels, and viscera. In 1800 Marie Francois Bichat of Paris published a new idea; he believed that disease affected, not organs, but tissues or 'membranes' as he called them, and he classified twenty-one different membranes in which the ravages of disease could be shown.

This concept of tissues was an advance and increased the interest in morbid anatomy. Great strides were made; Carl Rokitansky of Vienna himself performed at least thirty thousand autopsies, and he examined specimens from an equal number done by others. He published the results of this great survey in a series of beautifully illustrated books. A brilliant pathologist, he described the post-mortem appearances of many diseases. But Rokitansky's descriptions depended entirely upon what he could see with the naked eye; he could only describe the grosser manifestations of disease.

In the middle of the nineteenth century two German scientists, the botanist Matthias Schleiden and the anatomist Theodor Schwann, propounded the theory that living organisms are made up of cells; Schwann drew attention to the similarity between animal and vegetable tissues, in that both show a cell-structure under the microscope. Their idea was investigated by a number of German physiologists and anatomists, outstanding among whom is Rudolf Virchow of Würzburg and Berlin, the founder of the science of cellular pathology. He was a versatile man, who designed the sewerage system of Berlin, organized the Prussian ambulance corps in 1870, and served as a member of the German Reichstag. Born at Schievelbein, Pomerania, in 1821, he graduated from Berlin in 1843, founded one of the most influential of all medical journals, *Virchow's Archives*, in 1847 when aged only twenty-six, and three years later was appointed professor of pathology at Würzburg, removing to the Berlin chair in 1856. He died in 1902.

In his *Cellular-Pathologie*, published 1858, Virchow defined the body as 'a cell-state in which every cell is a citizen'. He wrote that there is no such thing as a disease-cell, but that diseased cells are only modifications of normal cells. A new growth of cells, he said, presupposes already existing cells. This dictum radically altered the age-old concept of the human mechanism. No longer was the body a single entity or a collection of tissues, the different parts of which were clearly visible to the naked eye and easily demonstrable by gross dissection. Now the body was a collection of cells, each endowed with individual life and capable of undergoing change. The disease process could be shown by the changes in these cells. Thus the surgeon, who had depended solely upon his knowledge of naked-eye anatomy, entered into a new world revealed by the microscope; thus was born the science of surgical pathology. As the knowledge of cell changes increased, so the surgeon leaned more heavily upon the pathologist. The surgeon cuts a small piece from the tissue which he suspects and sends it to the pathological laboratory; the pathologist cuts sections from the specimen, stains them, examines them under the microscope,

86

and gives the answer to the surgeon. When Julius Cohnheim, Virchow's pupil, introduced his method of quick frozen section in 1870, the surgeon was thereby enabled to have his answer while still in process of operating upon the patient. In fact this method did not come into more than limited use until 1905, when L. D. Wilson improved Cohnheim's technique. Now the specimen can be hardened by freezing with solid carbon dioxide, and the result can be telephoned to the surgeon in the operating theatre within a very few minutes.

No man did more for the advancement of surgical pathology than James Paget of Bart's, whom we briefly encountered in the second chapter. 'His greatest achievement, perhaps, was that he raised the surgeon in public estimation and caused surgery to hold its present high position in the social scale. A few surgeons before him had been gentlemen,' wrote the great historian and surgeon Sir D'Arcy Power of Paget.[1] It is an undeniably great achievement to raise a surgeon to the status of gentleman, but Paget should be given credit for more than this. Paget showed that cancerous tissue can be recognized by microscopical examination.

This remarkable – and charming – man was born at Great Yarmouth on 11 January 1814, the eighth of the seventeen children of a brewer. He had a hard struggle against poverty for many years. In 1830 he was apprenticed to a surgeon in Yarmouth and entered St Bartholomew's Hospital as a student in 1834, qualifying MRCS in 1836. For the next five years he supported himself by coaching and by medical journalism. He never applied for the post of house surgeon, being too poor to afford the 'dressing fee' demanded by St Bartholomew's – at that time house surgeons received no salary and were often expected to pay for the privilage of working in the hospitals – but acted as a clinical clerk to a member of the staff, Dr Latham. The fact that he had not served as a house surgeon nearly lost him his election to an assistant surgeoncy at the hospital eleven years later. This is a good example of the difficulties which beset the man without private means who wished to specialize in the mid nineteenth century and for many years to come.

Meanwhile he had been appointed curator of the museum and demonstrator in morbid anatomy at St Bartholomew's. In 1848 Paget prepared a scholarly catalogue of the anatomical and pathological specimens in the museum and, from 1846–9, he made a similar catalogue of the specimens in the Hunterian Museum of the Royal College of Surgeons. He was elected assistant surgeon to St Bartholomew's Hospital in 1847, became full surgeon in 1861, and resigned from the active staff to be elected consulting surgeon ten years later. He rapidly gained a large practice and acquired many honours. On the death of Fergusson in 1877, Queen Victoria appointed Paget to be her Sergeant Surgeon.

Paget took as his pattern the teaching of Johannes Müller, a great physiologist who is regarded as the founder of scientific medicine in Germany and who was one of the first to apply the microscope to distinguish between various types of tumour. Müller died in 1853; so far as is known the two never met, but Müller's influence is clearly to be seen in the nature of Paget's work. As early as 1835, when still a student, Paget discovered the nematode or round worm, *Trichina Spiralis*, while examining specimens of muscle fibre under the microscope. In 1842 he published an important paper *On the Chief Results Obtained by the Use of the Microscope in the Study of Human Anatomy and Physiology*. From 1851 until 1887 he wrote a number of equally important papers on cancerous and other malignant tumours. His name is attached to two different diseases; Paget's disease of the nipple, which is an early stage in cancer of the breast, and osteitis deformans, a general overgrowth of bone most noticeable in the skull, which is commonly called Paget's Disease.

Paget was a man of wide interests and wrote on many subjects. Like Tennyson, he loved simple words and made effective use of them. A typical example, seventy-eight consecutive words of one syllable, is to be found at the end of his Presidential Address to the Pathological Society of London: 'One sees that, as men grow old and wish for rest, they are prone to ask, 'Where are we to stop?' I do not know more than this: that we must not stop where we are; we must go on and on, and we may be sure that those who work to find the truth will not work in vain – sure that, with true work, true good will come. So I will hope that it may be here during my presidency.' It would be a good thing if some medical authors of today were to follow Paget's example, instead of trying to bury their ignorance of the English tongue under a heap of polysyllables.

James Paget was not only a fine surgical pathologist and a great diagnostician, but a delightful character. He lived very simply, despite the large income that he earned, and he worked hard until the end of his long life on 30 December 1899; always punctual, never appearing hurried, he managed to pack an immense amount into his busy day by careful organization. He possessed the scrupulously honest mind of the true research worker and, with all his success, he remained a modest, retiring man. Happily married, he believed in the family holiday and rarely travelled without his wife or children. Paget's sons inherited some of his intellect; one, Stephen, became a surgeon of merit and two others ended as bishops.

The science of bacteriology had its beginning at a later date than the science of morbid anatomy or pathology, but is of equal importance in the development of surgery. We have seen the start in an earlier chapter, when Pasteur understood the existence of living micro-organisms. Bacteriology became a science when it was possible to differentiate one organism from another and to show that the isolated organism always caused a distinct disease.

Two organisms were discovered by Louis Pasteur who, in 1878–9, described a 'microbe en amas de graines' which is now known as a staphylococcus, and a 'microbe en chapelet de graines' which we now call streptococcus pyogenes. But the association of these and other bacteria with disease was not definitely proved until Robert Koch grew pure cultures outside the body and transmitted disease by inoculating animals with his cultures.

Robert Koch was born at Klausthal in Hanover, then an independent kingdom, in 1843. He graduated from Göttingen and, after serving in the Franco-Prussian war, settled as a kind of state-supported general practitioner in the country district of Wollstein. He had no proper laboratory and no special training but he was interested in the microscope and spent much of his spare time examining specimens. In April 1876 Koch reported to the botanist Ferdinand Cohn of Breslau that he had made a special study of the large anthrax bacillus which is particularly common in horses and cattle and can be transmitted to man. Koch did not discover this bacillus; it had been seen many times before and had been accurately described by Pollender in 1849.

But Koch managed to isolate it by making a culture. At Cohn's invitation, he demonstrated that the bacillus is always present in the recognized disease, that a culture can be grown through several generations outside the body, and that the descended generation is capable of producing the recognizable disease in animals. This new concept of 'an *in vitro* descent', that is, existence and generation outside living body tissue, was violently opposed by those who did not believe the germ theory and, particularly, by the great French physiologist Paul Bert; but Koch's findings were confirmed in the laboratory by Louis Pasteur who succeeded in growing the anthrax bacillus through some twenty generations *in vitro*.

Karl Weigert coloured preparations of bacteria in 1871, so that they could more easily be observed under the microscope; in 1875 he introduced aniline dyes as stains for this purpose. Making use of Weigert's method, Koch described the staining of different types of bacteria and was able to photograph his specimens. In 1878 he identified six different forms of surgical infection by stained preparations and proved that each of the six organisms bred true through several generations *in vitro* or by inoculation into animals. Three years later, in 1881, he succeeded in producing pure cultures (they had previously been more or less contaminated with other organisms) by transplanting selected generations grown on glass plates covered with a nutrient medium of gelatine and meat infusion.

Koch's most widely remembered discovery is that of the tubercle bacillus which bears his name. He described the organism as the cause of tuberculosis in 1882 and, in the same paper, he laid down those rules of the relationship between bacteria and disease which, although originally outlined by Jakob Henle, have become known as Koch's Postulates:

1. The organism must be found in all cases of the disease under discussion and its distribution in the body should be in accordance with the lesions observed. (For instance, in the case of a quinsy, the organism must be seen if pus from the tonsillar abscess is examined under the microscope.)

2. The organisms should be cultivated outside the body of the host in pure culture for several generations.

3. The organism isolated in this way should reproduce the disease in other susceptible animals.

Application of these postulates proved the relationship between bacteria and disease. They are valid today.

His discovery of the tubercle bacillus led Koch to the error which cast a cloud over his life until he died in 1910. The idea, that once the cause of disease is known a cure will quickly be found, had been growing in men's minds for some time. Tuberculosis being the most prevalent and devastating of all diseases, Koch naturally strove to find the cure. His reasoning seems to have been that over-population will produce a poison capable of killing the individual; he tried to manufacture an autotoxin lethal to the tubercle bacillus. In 1890 he prepared tuberculin, a filtered and concentrated glycerine broth in which tubercle bacilli had been grown for six to eight weeks. After a prolonged trial and many over-optimistic reports, there came bitter disappointment; tuberculin was found to be not only useless but actively dangerous. Had tuberculin proved successful in 1890, the story of surgery during the next fifty years would have been very different. In time tuberculin came to be used as a 'patch test', a local reaction showing whether or no the subject is susceptible to tuberculous infection.

Among other bacteriologists who advanced the knowledge of surgical infections may be mentioned Friedrich Fehleisen, who discovered the causative organism of the 'hospital disease' erysipelas in 1883, Arthur Nicolaier who discovered that of tetanus or lock-jaw in 1884, Theodor Escherich who described infection by bacillus coli, the troublesome and often dangerous infection caused by contamination with faeces, and W. H. Welch who, with G. H. F. Nuttall, discovered the commonest organism of the mixed infection gas gangrene in 1892. It will be remembered that gas gangrene, one of the worst of wound infections, may have been the 'hospital gangrene' so feared in pre-Listerian times.

The next great boon to surgery, X-rays, was discovered in 1895. The present day surgeon must surely find it difficult to understand how his forefathers came to any diagnosis at all without this modern essential. The story is a quite simple one.

Wilhelm Konrad Röntgen, born at Lennep, Rhineland, in 1845, held the chair of physics successively at Strasbourg, Giessen, and Würzburg. In November 1895, ten years after his appointment to the Würzburg chair, he was investigating cathode rays by means of a Crookes' tube when he noticed that strange shadows were being cast by various objects in the room. He surrounded the Crookes' tube with a close fitting shield of black paper, thereby cutting out a possible source of light, and found that the shadows were thrown by objects in front of a platino-barium screen, standing about nine feet away, which shone with a greenish fluorescent glow. This was a kind of radiation that Röntgen had never before observed. The shadows varied in intensity; some objects were quite opaque and so threw dark shadows; others, although not normally translucent, appeared only faintly outlined against the phosphorescent glow of the screen. There is a story that Frau Röntgen, coming to see what delayed her husband from his supper, laid her hand on a photographic plate and thus produced the first X-ray picture of her bones and of her ring.[2]

Röntgen communicated his discovery to a meeting of the Würzburg Physico-Medical Society in a paper which was published in their *Proceedings* on 28 December 1895. A translation of this paper, by Arthur Stanton, appeared in the British scientific journal *Nature* on 23 January 1896.[3] The earliest known photograph is that of Professor Albert von Kölliker's hand, taken at Röntgen's first public demonstration on 23 January. Another very early and very interesting positive is that of Lister's hand, also dating from 1896, in the possession of King's College Hospital Medical School. The first X-ray photographs in the *Lancet* appeared on 25 January 1896, only two days after the translation of Röntgen's original paper in *Nature*. The photographs were experimental, one of the human hand and one of a frog skeleton, made by A. Campbell Swinton in his laboratory at 66 Victoria Street.[4] Less than a month later, on 22 February, there appeared in the *Lancet* an account of the first diagnostic use, the localization, followed by removal, of a bullet or airgun pellet in a boy's wrist.[5] The surgeon concerned was Robert Jones, whom we shall meet again, and the photographs were taken by Oliver Lodge, professor of physics at Liverpool. Here is a dramatic example of interchange of ideas between nations and of the speed of advance made possible by easier communication.

At the Würzburg meeting, Röntgen suggested that, as the nature of his new rays was unknown, they should be given the name of X-rays 'for the sake of brevity'. Professor von Kölliker, a distinguished anatomist and physiologist, at once appreciated and forecast the importance of Röntgen's discovery in medicine. He moved the only fitting name to be 'Röntgen Rays', a proposal carried unanimously by the meeting. The term X-rays, commonly used in Britain, is therefore incorrect. But, after so many years, it would be pedantic to insist upon the correct terminology – and the English 'X-ray Department' is surely better than the clumsy 'Department of Roentgenology.'

Kölliker's forecast proved right; the use of X-rays for diagnosing fractures and foreign bodies in the tissues entered medicine very quickly. Improvements and new techniques followed in rapid succession. Walter Cannon, afterwards professor of physics at Harvard University, introduced the heavy metal bismuth, which is radio-opaque and can be given in the form of a 'meal' to outline the stomach, in 1897 while he was still a student. He published his first study of stomach movements, revealed by the bismuth meal, in 1898 and followed this by a study of the movements of the intestinal tract in 1902. Cannon's experiments were made on animals; in 1906 E. J. Beck of Chicago applied Cannon's idea to the human patient. Bismuth proved to be rather toxic and, at a later date, was replaced by barium, which is used today.

Then X-rays began to be tried in the cure of various diseases. It is interesting that the first therapeutic use of X-rays was suggested, or at least wondered aloud, by Sir Joseph Lister. In his presidential address to the British Association of 1897, he cited cases of the use of X-rays in the diagnosis of fractures and the detection of foreign bodies, and then remarked: 'There is another way in which the Röntgen rays connect themselves with physiology and may possibly influence medicine. It is found that if the skin is long exposed to their actions it becomes very much irritated, affected with a sort of aggravated sunburning. This suggests the idea that the transmission of the rays through the human body may not altogether be a matter of indifference to internal organs but may by long continued action produce, according to the condition of the part concerned, injurious irritation or salutary stimulation.'[6]

Leopold Freund of Vienna was probably the first man to employ X-rays in this way (1896) for the simple removal of unwanted hair. Next year X-rays were applied to the treatment of the skin disease lupus, which Virchow had shown to be a form of tuberculosis; the treatment was popularized by the American dermatologist W. A. Pusey in 1900. Indiscriminate use of X-rays is very dangerous, as had been suggested by Lister's remarks; they could not be applied with any safety until Guido Holzknecht and Robert Kienböck of Vienna worked out a dosage system between the years 1900–2. Deep X-ray therapy followed in 1902 through the researches of G. C. Perthes of Leipzig and was used in the treatment of tuberculosis, uterine haemorrhage, and uterine tumours by Holzknecht and others during the years 1906–10.

Meanwhile the modest professor of physics, Wilhelm Röntgen, had found himself enveloped in a blaze of world-wide fame. In 1899 he was appointed to the influential chair of Munich and he received many honours, including a Nobel prize (1901). Shortly after this award a rumour started that it was Röntgen's assistant, and not Röntgen himself, who had made the discovery. In the wrangle that followed Röntgen developed a morbid hatred of publicity. He shrank into himself, becoming almost a hermit, refusing to see anyone but his students and a few friends who had never questioned his claim. The First World War added to his deep distress for, from the beginning, he had no doubt of Germany's inevitable defeat. He died, a dispirited and lonely man, on 10 February 1922, ten years to the day after that other great benefactor of surgery, Joseph Lister.

In 1895, just before Röntgen's discovery, Niels Finsen of Copenhagen had used concentrated ultra-violet light in the treatment of lupus. Interest began to be focused on the properties, and medical value, of light rays in general. In France, Henri Poincaré, attracted by the fluorescence of Röntgen's platino-barium screen when submitted to the rays of a Crookes' lamp, started to investigate the phenomenon. The work was taken up by Antoine Henri Becquerel who in 1896 discovered that salts of the rare metal uranium spontaneously emitted a hitherto unknown type of ray. A salt of uranium, having been kept in darkness for some months, proved capable of creating an image upon a photographic plate, even though entirely surrounded by black paper.

Marya Sklodovski, born in 1867 at Warsaw in Russian Poland, had grown up with a hatred of Imperial despotism and had migrated to the freer air of France in 1891. For four heroic years this brilliant girl managed to exist as a student of the Sorbonne University in Paris on about five pounds a month. In 1895 she married a remarkable physicist, Pierre Curie, laboratory chief of the School of Physics and Chemistry of the city of Paris. During the summer of 1897 Marie Curie studied Henri Poincaré's work and, in February 1898, she started an investigation into the source of energy which Becquerel's discovery had proved to exist in uranium. She had chosen this subject, almost at random, as her thesis for the degree of doctor of science.

In the course of her examination of many mineral specimens in the School of Physics collection, Marie Curie discovered a most surprising fact. Certain ores – only a few – produced emanation of rays, 'radioactivity', far greater than could be accounted for by their content of uranium. She realized that radioactive emanations could only come from a hitherto unknown element. With the help of Pierre (who left his own important work on crystallography) she set about the task of isolating this element.

The most strongly radioactive ore which they had so far found was one of uranium, called pitchblende, used commercially in the manufacture of glassware. By fractional analysis they prepared two extractions of pitchblende, both abnormally radioactive, but differing in chemical behaviour. The difference indicated that there were two new elements and not just one. By July 1898 they were so reasonably certain of the nature of one of these elements that they decided to give it a name. Marie chose 'polonium' in honour of her fatherland.

There remained the second element, which seemed to be even more strongly radioactive than polonium. In December 1898 Marie Curie decided to give this new element the name of 'radium'.

The discovery was received with scepticism because the

Curies had not as yet been able to isolate their two new elements. It was obvious that an enormous quantity of pitch-blende would have to be treated in order to extract a minute amount of radium. The couple now decided to divide their efforts. Pierre studied the chemical and physical properties of radium. Marie renewed her efforts to isolate the element.

She started with a ton of pitchblende residues from the St Joachimsthal mine in Austria; this was soon exhausted and further ton loads were delivered at frequent intervals. All this mass of material she treated, kilogramme by kilogramme. In 1902 she succeeded in preparing one decigramme (approximately one ten millionth part of a ton) of radium chloride. After four years of incessant work the Curies' postulated element had at last become a tangible chemical salt. On 25 June 1903 Marie Curie presented her long-delayed thesis *Researches on Radio-active Substances* to the examining board and was awarded the degree of Doctor of Physical Science of the University of Paris.

Meanwhile, radioactive substances had been shown to have certain effects upon human and animal tissue. The work was begun by two Germans, Walkhoff and Giesch, in 1900. Pierre Curie tried the experiment of exposing his arm to the emanation of a highly radioactive concentrate. The skin reddened over an area of six square centimetres and, within a few days, broke down to form an open wound. Healing started on the forty-second day but was not complete until five weeks later. Marie Curie had accidentally sustained a radium 'burn' and Henri Becquerel was also burned by carrying a small tube of radioactive material in his waistcoat pocket. Pierre Curie noted that the fingers of both his and Marie's hands became hardened and painful after working with radioactive concentrates.

These findings were published by Henri Becquerel and Pierre Curie in June 1901. In the same year Pierre collaborated with Professor Charles Bouchard and Professor Balthazard in a study of the action of radium emanation on animals; they came to the conclusion that there might be a therapeutic use, possibly in the treatment of malignant growths. In 1903 Holzknecht and Gottwald Schwartz of Vienna described their experiments with animal tissues. Exposure to radium caused degenerative changes in skin cells, in the cells of the walls of small blood vessels, and in the hair-like capillary blood vessels.

At the same meeting Exner showed a patient who suffered from the cancerous skin tumour known as a malignant melanoma. The tumour had been excised some three years previously, but a number of small secondary tumours had appeared in the skin of one shoulder. These, which had been present for eight months, were exposed to three milligrammes of radium bromide for from three to twenty-five minutes each. All those exposed for more than fifteen minutes became smaller after ten days and disappeared by the end of a month.[7]

Exner reported success in other cases and W. J. Morton of New York also tried radium in malignant disease. The first use of radium in Britain seems to have been at the Cancer Hospital, Fulham Road, in 1903–4, the radium having been bought through the generosity of Lord Iveagh. It was quite an extensive trial, seventeen patients being treated. All suffered from advanced cancers; treatment ended in most disappointing failure. In every case the effect was negative, either no change or an increase in the size of the tumour.[8]

There is little doubt that Marie Curie and her co-workers believed that they had, in radium, discovered the 'cure for cancer'. This belief was shared by many in the first quarter of the twentieth century. The hope proved vain. Prolonged trials have shown that radium and radioactive substances, though extremely useful in selected cases, do not provide a complete answer.

A short recapitulation is here in order. We have traced in broad outline the story of surgery from the time when it was little better than barbarity, through the years when it became a relatively painless but highly dangerous art, through the opening of the Listerian epoch, into the days when the art was joined to science, when pathology, bacteriology, radiology and radiotherapy each added something to treatment, to diagnosis, and to the detail of operative technique. All these made for rapid advance; we saw the beginnings of that advance in the last chapter; now, with these new aids, the pace quickened until, by 1914, the work of a general surgeon had become very similar to that of a general surgeon today, and entirely different from that of the surgeon of 1890.

The nature and extent of this change can best be seen by taking the work of one man. William Watson Cheyne, although

97

he became president of the Royal College of Surgeons, can be counted an example of a first-class, everyday surgeon. For this reason the scope of his practice provides a more revealing picture than would that of a genius.

We can first trace in his case-books the new skills which have already been outlined. Surgical pathology opened the way to more exact description, dependent upon microscopic examination. The old, confused 'necrosis and caries', although still used at the beginning of the Cheyne series of notes in 1889, soon gives place to the more modern terminology of 'osteo-myelitis' and 'tuberculosis'. The first reference to the quick method of frozen section occurs in 1908, three years after Wilson reintroduced the method in 1905.

Advances in bacteriology are reflected in the examination of sputum for tubercle bacilli (1890) and the inoculation of a guinea pig with suspected tuberculous fluid in the same year. In 1891 there is the first mention of the treatment of skin tuberculosis, lupus, by 'Koch's Fluid' which was the un-successful tuberculin. An interesting advance of 1896 is the treatment of an infection with antistreptococcal serum. Koch's tuberculin had stimulated a search for antisera or antitoxins which might have the effect of destroying various types of bacteria.

The first mention of X-rays comes in 1896, less than a year after Röntgen made his discovery. A bullet was found with their aid and, a month or two later, Cheyne is reported to have removed two toes 'relying on Röntgen photographs'. A quite remarkable case is recorded in 1903. The patient, nicely described as a master-mariner, tried to commit suicide by shooting himself with a revolver in the public lavatory of the Temple underground station. Admitted unconscious into Cheyne's ward, his skull was duly X-rayed. The plate revealed not one but two bullets lying between the substance of the brain and the skull. The old sea-captain recovered consciousness, was questioned, and explained that he had been shot in the head during a battle with Malay pirates some twenty years before. He was discharged from hospital with both bullets still in his head.

The first reference to a bismuth meal for an examination of the stomach comes in 1909, and the photographs are inserted in the notes. The first X-ray picture to be found is six years earlier, in 1903 – unfortunately not that of the master-mariner. Mention of photographs is a reminder that ordinary photography has proved a boon to surgical and medical records. In Cheyne's notes a number are pasted in, the first being in 1890. But the earliest photograph in the whole series of hospital case notes is to be found in one of the physician's books. Dated 1857, it is still remarkably clear.

In 1901 there is mention of the X-ray treatment of a rodent ulcer, but there is no record of the use of radium until 1911, when two cases of cancer, one of the mouth and one of the lip, were treated by submission to the emanation from radium bromide. Two years later, in 1913, comes the first mention of a radium burn.

The above shows us how the new extension of scientific knowledge was turned into practice by the surgeon. We can also find in the case-notes clear, almost dramatic, evidence of the change which this advancing knowledge wrought in the techniques of surgery. That change can best be shown by summarizing the figures and presenting them in the form of a table. All the cross headings, Accident, Tubercle and so on, refer to operations performed. The column headings refer to the total operative surgery performed by Lister during the years 1877–93 and to the total operative surgery performed by Cheyne between the years 1889–1912. The latter has been divided into four columns as follows: his two first years as a surgeon with charge of beds 1889–90, the six years 1892–98, the central year in the series 1901, and the ten years 1902–12. The records for the years 1891, 1899, 1900 are not complete (Cheyne was absent at the Boer War in 1900) and so have not been included.

The cases referred to as 'other' need a little explanation. These case-notes were kept by medical students and medical students vary in both aptitude and diligence – even today. Sometimes it is impossible to decide on the exact nature of a disease or treatment from the very scrappy notes. There are also a large number of very minor 'operations', the type of treatment that we should not call an 'operation' nowadays. Most of this minor work would fall under a heading 'sepsis', opening of boils, treatment of carbuncles and of cuts which have become infected. This type of surgery was, of course,

	Lister 1877–93	Cheyne 1889–90	Cheyne 1892–8	Cheyne 1901	Cheyne 1902–12
	%	%	%	%	%
Accident	29	9	9·2	11	9·4
Tubercle	16	26	20·5	20·5	10·9
Orthopaedic	14	13	7·2	8·5	6·1
Malignant Disease	9·5	4	8·5	15·5	9·5
Surgery of Repair	3·5	3·5	8·4	2·5	3·9
Haemorrhoids	1·5	4	4	1	2·5
Osteomyelitis	5	1·5	1·6	1·5	1·5
Varicose Veins	2·5	6·5	3·8	3	3·1
Benign Tumours	2·5	—	2	1	2·2
Repair of Hernia	2	5·5	9·4	7	11·9
Surgery of Syphilis	1·5	3	1	·5	·5
Strangulated Hernia	1	1	·4	1·5	·5
Surgery of Thyroid	·5	—	1·6	1·5	1·2
Urological	1	—	1·7	—	2·3
Plastic Surgery					·3
Abdominal Surgery	—	·5	4·3	10	16·5
Other	21·5	22·5	16·4	14	15·2

important but it remained unchanged throughout the period that we are now considering.

There emerges a picture of swift advance. We see that, in his first two years on the full staff, Cheyne performed a type of surgery little different from that of Lister, which itself was little different, but for the lower mortality, from that of the pre-Listerian surgeon. The three major divisions, Accident, Tuberculosis, and Orthopaedics, account for 59 per cent of Lister's practice during the years 1877–93, and for 48 per cent of Cheyne's practice during the years 1889 and 1890. Thereafter the numbers decline until we reach the figure of 26·4 per cent in 1902–12. It is noteworthy that Lister, particularly interested in the treatment of fractures, had no less than 29 per cent of accidents admitted to his wards. During the twenty-two years under consideration, Cheyne's figure is remarkably constant; approximately 10 per cent of his patients were victims of accident.

In the first two years Cheyne did rather more operations on haemorrhoids (piles) and varicose veins than during the remainder of his career. Here is an interesting point; even today this type of surgery is commonly performed by a junior surgeon. Already, in 1889–90, his percentage of hernia operations is over double that of Lister, and this percentage rises until it reaches 11·9 per cent in 1902–12. In the first two years there is only one 'new' operation that was not performed by Lister; 'Abdominal Surgery ·5 per cent' represents a single abdominal operation performed by Cheyne in 1890. It was an open operation for the relief of intussusception, a condition in which part of the bowel becomes invaginated causing acute obstruction, and it was an unusual enough case to be reported in the *Lancet*.[9]

There is an increase in urological surgery and in surgery of the thyroid gland. But it is the two lines, abdominal surgery and the surgery of hernia, which provide the most striking evidence of over-all change. Hernia rises from 2 per cent to 11·9 per cent; we shall see the reason for this in a later chapter but we should note here that this is not the surgery of strangulated hernia, that essential operation performed even before the days of anaesthesia; it is the repair of hernia, which is an operation for the convenience and comfort of the patient.

Not a single abdominal operation is mentioned in Lister's case notes. He did perform one such operation but it does not occur in the Lister series. Abdominal surgery accounts for a mere half of one per cent in Cheyne's record for the years 1889–90; it rises to 4·3 per cent for the years 1892–8; to 10 per cent in the central year 1901; and at last to no less than 16·5 per cent for the period 1902–12. Here is a dramatic change if ever there was one. By 1912 abdominal surgery has become the highest percentage figure in the whole of Cheyne's surgery and the revealed picture of 1902–12, entirely different from that of 1889–90, is not unlike the general surgery of today.

We find echoes of world events and changes in these notes. There is a casualty from the Boer war in 1900, and the first mention of a motor-car accident comes in 1906 – quite late in the devastating career of the automobile. Then there is an aeroplane crash in 1912; the victim Marcel Desoutter, well known as an early aviator, survived amputation of both legs and afterwards joined the family firm of surgical instrument and appliance makers. He died in 1952.

We have not carried the analysis of Cheyne's notes into 1913 because in that year King's College Hospital, at which Cheyne worked, moved from Portugal Street to its present site on Denmark Hill in South London. The notes for this year are scrappy, partly because the students were temporarily attached to Charing Cross Hospital and partly because no operations, except emergencies, were done for over three months. But there is one very interesting note for 1913. It is a case of an operation for the relief of duodenal ulcer, called Finney's operation because it was first performed and described by John Finney, a surgeon of Baltimore in the United States. At the end of the operation note, the student adds that Dr Mayo of Rochester, USA, was among those present in the theatre.

In 1845 William Worrall Mayo, a native of Eccles who had read chemistry at Owens College, Manchester, emigrated to America where he became a doctor. William Worral had two sons, William James who was born at Le Sueur on 29 June 1861, and Charles Horace, born on 9 July 1865, at Rochester where William Worrall had settled in practice. Both sons studied medicine; William qualified in 1883 from the University of Michigan, Charles from the North Western University in 1888.

From early boyhood they assisted their father in his practice. Will wrote 'My brother and I grew up to be physicians just as boys on a farm grow up to be farmers. We began by taking care of father's horses, keeping his office clean, and riding about the country with him on his calls. From the age of sixteen I was his first surgical assistant and Charlie began giving anaesthetics when he was a lad of twelve. Father performed as many post-mortems as he could and Charlie and I always attended.'[10] Charlie's obituary notice mentions that he became his father's 'house surgeon' at so early an age that he had to stand on an upturned biscuit box in order to see over the table when assisting at operations.

In 1883 a devastating storm swept Rochester, causing much damage and loss of life. W. W. Mayo, with his two sons and the Sisters of the Order of Saint Francis, did valiant work among the injured. The Mother Superior of the Order decided to commemorate their work by building and endowing a small hospital of fifty beds in Rochester. The hospital of St Mary opened in 1889 with fifteen patients, attended by five nursing Sisters, Sister Mary Joseph as surgical assistant, and Mother Alfred as Sister-in-Charge. The Mayo family formed the entire medical staff.

This hospital was not a charitable institution. From the start, every patient had to pay according to his means. But patients from charitable organizations were accepted without charge, and the patient's own word was regarded as sufficient guarantee of the scale upon which he would be required to pay. Rochester, even today, is only a small town; in 1889 it was a village, served by no important road and not on a main railway line. For ten years the Mayos worked quietly in something that was no more than a cottage hospital. Then, about the year 1900, William sent a paper to the American *Annals of Surgery*. His paper contained particulars of so many cases of successful treatment of gallstones that the incredulous editor came to see for himself. He was the first of many thousands of visitors to Rochester.

The brothers had kept well abreast of all the advances that had so recently been made; they were perhaps the first to understand that these advances were not only of great importance but had added to the complexity of medicine. They realized that if these 'ancillary departments' were to be fully used, they must be housed under one roof. They found that exact diagnosis demanded complete investigation; it was not enough to pass a hand over the abdomen if a patient complained of indigestion; all the systems, the alimentary system, the heart, the lungs, the kidneys, must be carefully examined, and expert advice upon each system must be readily available. This became their basic principle; a painstaking, complete investigation of the patient by highly trained experts in a single clinic. At first the Mayos had to make themselves the experts; as their fame increased they trained others in their method until they had their team. Neither brother was any kind of a specialist at the start. It was not until after 1900 that they devoted their whole time to surgery; as the years passed 'Will' became the more expert in surgery of the abdomen, 'Charlie' in surgery of the head and neck.

They made a perfect combination, bound together by a most unusual brotherly love and confidence, which manifested itself in the use of a joint wallet on which each urged the other to draw more heavily. Will was the better administrator, somewhat withdrawn, with a tendency to descend from on high to put all things in order; Charlie was the more original in thought, with a witty, friendly temperament that made for a happy and cooperative staff. Both brothers showed themselves remarkably shrewd in choosing their colleagues. It says much for the Mayos that they were so successful in building up and in keeping together their large staff, for Rochester was no cultural nor social centre; the clinic and the work of the clinic had to be all-sufficing.

This work rapidly increased as their fame spread. By 1906 Will had performed one hundred and fifty resections of the stomach for cancer with a 10 per cent mortality and a three year survival in nearly thirty per cent of cases; in the one year 1906 he did thirty-six of these operations with only one death (Cheyne did his first in 1905). As the clinic grew in size the medical staff rose in numbers until there were more than one hundred and fifty full-time members and twice that number of young graduates under instruction. The original small hospital expanded until the beds numbered between fifteen hundred and two thousand; in 1938 just over one thousand patients registered in a single day.

The Mayos firmly believed in international exchange of knowledge and ideas. They and their staff travelled widely and they encouraged visitors to make use of their experience at Rochester. The brothers introduced a standard case-taking form, at a time when medical recording was still haphazard, on which all details of each patient were entered. The records were open for consultation and discussion to every member of the staff; from these discussions resulted the *Proceedings of the Staff Meetings of the Mayo Clinic*, in which many new advances and discoveries have been described.

As patients paid fees, often large fees, to the Clinic, a surplus of cash rapidly accumulated. In 1913 the brothers offered a sum of a million and a half dollars to the University of Minnesota for the purposes of medical education and research. Incredible though it may seem, the State Legislature made difficulties and it needed an impassioned address by Will before the scheme got under way. The Mayo Foundation, which does so much for research and post-graduate instruction, opened in 1915.

The two brothers, who had worked closely and successfully together, were not long separated by death. Charlie died on 26 May, 1939, and Will two months later on 28 July. Their

Clinic and their methods became the model for similar ventures in America. As we have seen, that great country could boast some excellent surgeons during the nineteenth century; it is largely through the efforts of the Mayo brothers that the United States of America has made such great strides in surgery during the past sixty years.

CHAPTER 6

Wars and Wounds

It is a distressing but easily explained fact that the disaster of war has added much to the knowledge of surgery. The surgeon's primary duty in warfare is to heal wounds. He therefore requires to know how a wound heals and how he may most quickly cause it to heal; he requires to know how infection of the wound occurs and how he may prevent that infection; he requires to know why the victim of a wound is put in peril of death through pain and loss of blood, and how that 'shock' may best be treated. War has brought progress in many other techniques of surgery, but these are the three great advances most directly attributable to the specialized conditions of war, and these are the wartime advances which will most lastingly benefit the civilian patient.

The knowledge of and the answer to these three problems, wound healing, infection, and shock, is still by no means complete; research continues today. But the results of wound treatment, which embodies rapid healing without infection and the successful combating of shock, are much better than they were at the beginning of the twentieth century, and these improved results depend largely upon knowledge gained in the World Wars. So in this chapter we shall consider the type of wound inflicted and the treatment accorded to the wound in the two wars. In order to understand what happened it is necessary to go back again to the nineteenth century.

Lister's method of antisepsis was always successful when applied to the deliberate wound of a planned operation. Antisepsis could also be successful when the wound was accidental, always provided that treatment was applied before bacteria

106

had a chance of invading the deeper layers of tissue, for anti-septic drugs are only able to deal with micro-organisms by direct contact. The method of asepsis is always successful when applied to the wound of a planned operation – in both contexts 'always' must be qualified with the words 'provided there is no error of technique'. But asepsis alone is useless against even a lightly infected accidental wound; obviously, for asepsis does not depend upon bacteria-killing drugs and the term itself implies that no bacteria are ever allowed to be present. The problem is twofold; to prevent a wound becoming infected and to deal successfully with a wound that is already infected. War, by providing wounds in huge numbers, brings these problems to the urgent notice of the surgeon.

As we have already seen, antiseptics were first used in the treatment of war wounds by the Prussians during the campaign of 1870. William MacCormac, a surgeon on the staff of St Thomas' Hospital and one of Lister's first disciples in London, volunteered his help at the outbreak of the Franco-Prussian War. Suspected by the French of being a Prussian spy, he was arrested at Metz and sent back to Paris. This unfortunate experience did not deter him, for he joined the Anglo-American ambulance unit as second in command to the American surgeon Marion Sims, and organized a hastily prepared hospital of 384 beds at the battle of Sedan. Here he practised as good a Listerian technique as shortage of supplies allowed, and his results, though by no means good, satisfied him that antisepsis was an advance on any other method. In the Russo-Turkish War of 1876–7, MacCormac served as commandant of a National Aid Detachment formed by the Stafford House Committee. The Committee provided quite adequate medical supplies and the antiseptic treatment of wounds, better understood and simpli-fied, became possible as a routine. MacCormac, using anti-sepsis, achieved remarkably good results at the battle of Alexinatz in September 1876.[1]

On the outbreak of the Boer War in 1899 MacCormac, although over sixty years of age, was appointed consulting surgeon to the South African Field Force. Experience in South Africa confirmed him, and the majority of his fellow Listerians, in the belief that antisepsis had solved the problem of wound infection. They had made a terrible mistake which, although of no importance at the time, was to have devastating consequences fifteen years later. In the Boer War, the large majority of battle injuries were simple penetrating wounds caused by the high-velocity Mauser bullet, a long thin missile which passed straight through the body tissues and, provided that it missed any vital organ or large blood vessel, did remarkably little damage. The terrain over which the two armies fought consisted in the main of sunbaked rock and sandy waste, a sterile uncultivated land in which the risk of soil-borne infection was abnormally low. If a man were hit in the brain or the heart, he was usually killed outright, but penetrating wounds of the lungs and of the abdomen often healed with very little trouble. MacCormac concluded that operation upon such wounds did more harm than good; antiseptic dressings and conservative treatment seemed to give the best results.[2]

Not everyone agreed with MacCormac. His advice was followed by most surgeons, because he was counted a great authority on wounds and had more practical experience of war than the majority. But Colonel W. F. Stevenson, professor of surgery at the Army Medical School, Netley, challenged MacCormac's view. In 1897 Stevenson had published a book, *Wounds in War*, and had advocated that a wound of the abdomen should always be explored by open operation,[3] because of the risk that the bowel may have been punctured and the bowel contents have escaped into the abdominal cavity, when the very dangerous infection of peritonitis would almost inevitably follow. A few surgeons put Stevenson's teaching into practice, but their results were neither so good nor so bad as to suggest that either method of treatment was the better.

Such was the position when MacCormac died in 1901, before the Boer War had ended. Three years later (9 February 1904) the Japanese launched an unheralded but provoked attack upon the Russian Empire of Nicholas II. Whatever may be the alleged faults of Tsarist Russia, her medical services in time of war were second to none in devotion – if not in efficiency – and her ambulance trains were better organized than those of any other country. Many Russian surgeons were women; in 1876 MacCormac somewhat ungallantly wrote 'there was also a Russian lady doctor whose scientific pretensions were, I hope, greater than her personal ones'.

Princess Vera Ignatievna Gedroitz was a Russian surgeon who had studied medicine in Germany. At the end of 1904 she managed to bring a well-equipped ambulance train close to the front line and was thereby enabled to operate upon battle casualties in good conditions and within a short time of wounding.[4] She adopted a policy of operating for early penetrating wounds of the abdomen and her results were better than any that had yet been attained. Further back at the base hospitals results were still poor; the point to be noted is that Princess Gedroitz, by means of her ambulance train, was able to operate upon her patients within a very short time of wounding.

Surgeons therefore entered the 1914 war with mixed views on the best way of treating the wounded. The official policy favoured non-intervention (or 'conservative' treatment) in wounds of the head, abdomen, and chest; in fact, war surgery would still be limited to the classical dressing of wounds, amputation or excision, and the setting of fractures. On one point everyone was agreed. Antiseptics had proved their worth in the Boer War and antisepsis must once again be the method of choice in 1914. It was now that the fatal mistake made by MacCormac and his followers became apparent.

The war of 1914 was fought under quite different conditions from those of the Boer War. The first difference lay in the nature of the terrain. Flanders and the eastern border of France is an intensely cultivated area of long standing, highly manured, and so rich in pathogenic organisms. The two armies dug themselves deep into something that was little better than a nutrient medium for bacteria, and lived for four years in conditions of squalor unknown since the Middle Ages. Secondly, the type of wound proved to be quite different from that of the Boer War. After the opening and very short battle of movement, plastering of trenches with shrapnel and high-explosive shells caused many more wounds than did bullets, from which dugouts and sand-bag parapets provided more or less adequate protection, except when troops attacked across the intervening ground.

In these changed conditions antiseptics were soon found to be worse than useless. The army surgeon, who had pinned his faith on the proved value of antiseptics in the Boer War, had lost sight of the fact that even the most powerful antiseptic drug cannot destroy organisms deep in the tissues or invading the blood stream. He may never have read Lister's clear statement that, to be effective, antiseptic treatment must be applied as soon as possible and, at the most, within thirty-six hours, but it is quite extraordinary that the basic principle of Lister's teaching had been forgotten in so short a time. The sole object of the spray, the irrigation, the carbolic dressing, was to kill bacteria before they had a chance of entering the wound; the whole object of swift antiseptic cleansing was to destroy bacteria while they yet remained upon the body surface.

Antisepsis had apparently succeeded in the Boer War because of the type of missile and the relatively sterile terrain. But the essentials of antisepsis could not possibly be attained in the conditions of the First World War. The shrapnel shell, exploding in mid-air and throwing down a conical shower of bullets, had the effect of rending the body rather than of causing a simple punctured wound. High explosive, besides causing gross destruction of tissues, riddled the casualty with earth, fragments of clothing, and foreign bodies derived from any obstruction between the victim and the blast. All clothing was saturated with the mud of trench warfare, and those trenches were dug through soil heavily contaminated by centuries of cultivation. Thus all wounds were massively and deeply invaded by pathogenic organisms from the moment of infliction. The easily solved problem of preventing a clean wound from becoming infected in a clean countryside gave place to the urgent necessity of finding some means to combat massive and deep invasion of the tissues by pathogenic organisms.

The initial failure resulted in the reappearance of diseases which had hardly been seen for a generation. All wounds suppurated; compound fractures of the femur carried a mortality in the region of eighty per cent[5]– as bad as in the American Civil War. Septicaemia, pyaemia, gas gangrene, and erysipelas became as rife and as fatal as in the eighteen fifties. The method which had so signally failed was the mixed antiseptic-aseptic technique in common use. The cry now arose 'Back to Lister'; the demand was for more rigid antisepsis, treatment by stronger antiseptic drugs at an earlier stage.

An antiseptic drug, a bactericide, kills the organism by direct contact. It is a protoplasmic poison and, as such, can cause destruction of human body cells within its reach. Wounding, particularly the gross type of wound inflicted by high explosive, damages the blood supply to the part wounded by tearing the blood vessels. The tissues become devitalized because the blood supply has been interrupted. Tissues that are devitalized will not heal easily, and healing is further delayed by the additional damage sustained when an antiseptic drug is used.

The attempt to use stronger antiseptics failed utterly. A bitter controversy now developed between the exponents of antisepsis and the antagonists, the latter faction being led by Almroth Wright of St Mary's Hospital.[6] Wright, assisted by a younger man named Alexander Fleming, established that even the strongest antiseptics lose bactericidal power in the presence of blood and serum and that, being protoplasmic poisons, they actively damage tissues already partially devitalized by inter-rupted blood supply. Research proceeded along three lines; firstly, to encourage the human body itself to deal with infec-tion; secondly, to find an antiseptic capable of exerting bactericidal action in the presence of serum and which would not delay healing by damaging the tissues; thirdly, to explore the advantages of excising damaged and devitalized tissue.

Considerable progress was made in all three lines of research. Wright advised dressing with 'lymphagogues', solutions such as strong hypertonic saline, which would produce a copious flow of serum by simple osmosis and so concentrate the body's natural defence, the antibodies, at the site of infection. A hypertonic solution of magnesium sulphate was found more effective. Blander antiseptics such as iodoform, the famous bismuth–iodoform–paraffin–paste or BIPP, and the flavine compounds, acriflavine and proflavine, did not harm the tissues to the same extent as did carbolic acid and mercuric chloride. Richard Charles, among others, showed that the excision of all hopelessly damaged tissue, leaving a widely opened wound, lessened the incidence of infection by removing a breeding ground for bacteria. This form of treatment came to be known as 'debridement', a rather interesting word first used by the French surgeon Pierre Joseph Desault in 1799. Although many people think it is derived from 'debris', the derivation is in fact from the French 'brides', English 'bridles', and therefore implies unbridling, the removal of a barrier to free drainage.

The French army had encountered similar troubles with their wounded. At Compeigne, Alexis Carrel, an authority on the healing of surgical wounds, obtained promising results by irrigating war wounds with a solution of sodium hypochlorite, but the strongly alkaline chemical proved too irritating for routine use. In 1915 Henry Drysdale Dakin, an English chemist who settled in New York, buffered or neutralized the alkaline sodium hypochlorite with boric acid. Single treatments were too short-lived to be effective; Carrel introduced a method of continuous irrigation. So came into being the famous Carrel-Dakin method of dealing with wounds. As finally evolved, it consisted of thorough debridement and the insertion of thin perforated rubber tubes into all parts of the wound, the tubes being kept in place by loosely packed gauze and the skin protected from the still somewhat irritating solution by layers of paraffin gauze. The tubes, connected to a container of Dakin's solution, were flushed through every two hours. Dressings were changed daily and a close watch kept on infection by taking swabs for culture. The wound was not sutured in the first instance; it was left open until little or no infection remained (secondary suture).

Another problem arose when the United States entered the war in 1917. The Carrel-Dakin treatment was a lengthy business, and morale demanded that the wounded soldier, faced with prolonged illness, should be returned to his native land as soon as possible. In the case of the American, a journey to his native land could only be made by crowded hospital ship with a limited number of medical attendants to carry out a time-consuming treatment. The United States surgeons were therefore forced to evolve a simpler method. They made little attempt to deal with infection; the wound was packed with vaseline gauze and the whole skin area smeared with vaseline or covered by a quite thin layer of vaseline gauze. The limb was then encased in plaster of Paris without further padding or any material to absorb discharges. The results were surprising. The leading advocate of this method, Hiram Winnett Orr of Lincoln, Nebraska, found himself quite amazed by the fact that so little sepsis developed under this simple form of treatment. Thus began the treatment of wounds by 'immobilization' with plaster or firm splinting.

By the end of the war it had become apparent that the excision of devitalized tissue, the breeding ground of bacteria, is the most important single part of wound treatment. Provided that the casualty arrived in the clearing station within a few hours of receiving his wound, the surgeon could stitch that wound up (primary suture) after excision of damaged tissue, without undue risk of severe infection. The problem remained of wounds already grossly infected or which became grossly infected after early treatment. Once bacteria had established themselves, it was impossible to remove them; only the human mechanism itself could win the battle, and the surgeon's sole duty was to give such aid as he could. Any attempt at direct attack by antiseptics resulted in disaster. The answer to that problem did not come until the Second World War.

The lessons of the First World War taught the surgeon that damaged tissue is dangerous. Gentle surgery, already advocated by Halsted and Lane among others, reached its peak with the 'caressing of the tissues' preached by Berkeley Moynihan. Antisepsis had fallen into disrepute, although a few of the old guard Listerians refused to abandon it entirely. The surgeon adopted strict measures to exclude bacteria, relying upon the bactericidal power of the healthy patient to kill such stray pathogenic organisms as might fall upon the operation wound. He was particular to guard against pockets of damaged tissue, and he therefore insisted upon the importance of clean cutting and the obliteration of all dead space. Understanding that blood clot and foreign bodies are a potent cause of sepsis, he took great care to secure blood vessels and he used the finest suture material possible. For these reasons the post-war surgeon tended to operate more slowly and deliberately than had his predecessors.

The risk of infection, though lessened, still remained. Any wound which became infected, either through accidental infliction in dirty conditions or by error of surgical technique, endangered the patient's life; until after 1935 there was no known drug capable of destroying the organism once it had entered the patient's blood stream. From time to time chemists searched for 'the perfect antiseptic', one which could be safely swallowed or injected without harm to the patient yet would be capable of killing pathogenic bacteria. Most medical men thought that such a drug must be an impossibility.

In 1906 Elie Metchnikoff published his theory that soured milk is an intestinal disinfectant, a belief still shared by many laymen. Metchnikoff's idea stimulated search for an antiseptic that could be absorbed through the gut or safely injected into the blood vessels. In 1909 Paul Ehrlich, a German scientist, and his Japanese assistant, S. Hata, introduced a new form of drug originally known under its laboratory number '606' and afterwards named salvarsan.[7] This was the first 'systemic antiseptic', one which could be injected into the human system without undue harm (it had some quite nasty side-effects) and which was effective against pathogenic micro-organisms in the human tissues.

Salvarsan deserves the vogue phrase 'a major break-through'. Ehrlich himself called it his 'magic bullet'; salvarsan was hailed as a miracle-working drug, lethal to every kind of pathogenic organism. It soon became clear that this arsenical preparation is only effective against the spirochaete, which causes syphilis and some tropical diseases. Despite this limitation, salvarsan is of major importance in the history of medicine, for here was the first realization of the concept that it might be possible to attack infection from within the body. Salvarsan was widely used in 1914–18; after the failure of antisepsis, a number of commercial firms intensified their efforts, in a somewhat haphazard manner, to find a similar 'perfect antiseptic' effective against other types of organism. Certain dyestuffs, notably the aniline group, were already in use as external antiseptics and these seemed to provide one promising line of research.

Early in 1935 Gerhard Domagk, a chemist working for the large German organization, Bayer's or I. G. Farbenindustrie, discovered that a derivative of the dye chrysoidine, prontosil rubrum, cured mice which had been artificially infected with streptococci. Prontosil R was placed on the market as a systemic antiseptic; Bayer's started to experiment with other dyestuffs, patenting such products as seemed hopeful. In the same year three French workers at the Pasteur Institute, Tréfouel, Boret, and Nitti, submitted this complex dye derivative, Prontosil R, to test and found that it contained an active, simpler constitutent called sulphanilamide, the existence of which was already known. Leonard Colebrook of the Medical Research

Council in London and Meave Kelly of Queen Charlotte's Hospital carried out comparative trials of sulphanilamide and prontosil in cases of puerperal fever, caused by a streptococcus, and found them to be equally effective.[8]

Sulphanilamide, the first of the sulphonamide or 'sulfa' drugs, is therefore the second worth-while systemic antiseptic, given orally or into the blood stream and exercising an effect at the site of infection. It is not a true antiseptic or bactericide, but rather a 'bacteristatic' which keeps the organism in a state of enfeebled existence and so assists the normal body mechanism to deal with the organism more efficiently. Sulphanilamide is by no means the perfect drug for it has a toxic action – sometimes a very uncomfortable action – but the damage which it inflicts upon the micro-organism is out of all proportion to its toxicity. Sulphanilamide proved of value in the treatment of gonorrhea, peritonitis, and cellulitis; a modified sulphonamide effective against the pneumococcus, the famous May and Baker 693 or sulphapyridine, was discovered by A. J. Ewins in 1938 and successfully used in the treatment of pneumonia.[9] Other drugs of the same class followed, sulphadiazine, sulphadimidine in 1941.

Meanwhile armies of the right had rebelled against communist rule in Spain, and a new form of wound treatment evolved during those years of misery. This treatment was a combination and modification of two techniques which depended upon the findings of the First World War and had come into limited use during the inter-war years. The method of prolonged immobilization of infected wounds in plaster, although not generally popular in the United States, had been successfully used in the treatment of osteomyelitis by Winnett Orr among others. Lorenz Böhler of Vienna discarded the old-time padded splints and applied plaster of Paris directly to the skin when treating fractures. During the Spanish Civil War of 1936–9 Joseph Trueta of Barcelona (who afterwards became professor of orthopaedic surgery at Oxford) modified and combined the techniques of Orr and Böhler to meet the needs of casualties, especially of air-raid casualties. After a thorough debridement, he united the upper and lower parts of the wound by primary suture and packed the intervening wound space with moist gauze. Any fracture was accurately set. Trueta then covered the wound with close-mesh gauze, padded such bony prominences as might become chafed, and applied plaster of Paris directly to the skin and to the wound surface, including in his plaster the joints above and below the wound, so as to maintain immobilization of the wounded area.

The wound was left untouched for from four to six weeks; plasters were changed every second month until the wound healed. In his own hands, Trueta's method gave magnificent results; of his first 1,073 cases only six patients died; by the end of the war he and his assistants had treated nearly twenty thousand casualties with only four amputations and under a hundred deaths. Not everyone was so successful; when Trueta's method was used in the Second World War, it was soon found that it could lead to disaster in less experienced hands.

The Second World War posed problems very different from those of the First. From 1914 to 1918 the battle front was to all intents and purposes static; a down-the-line evacuation of wounded could be organized and practised with little fear of interruption save from the ordinary hazards of a countryside under bombardment. By 1939 speed of evacuation had been considerably accelerated but so had the speed of advance and retreat; the war of fast movement made it necessary to push properly equipped centres further and further back from a wavering front line. Thus the main duty of the forward surgeon became that of ensuring a surgically safe journey of the casualty to a distant base.

The war can be divided into three phases from the point of view of wound treatment. The first, the short and disastrous campaign of 1940, may be regarded as a continuation of the 1914–18 war, fought over a similar terrain, aided by knowledge gained in the inter-war years, and hampered by the unexpected speed of movement. Wound excision and, if necessary or possible, immobilization in plaster gave good results; but, in this opening phase, the surgeon learned anew that primary suture carries a grave risk unless preliminary debridement is thorough and unless it is possible to keep the patient under constant supervision. In the emergency of rapid retreat neither prolonged operation nor after-supervision were possible. The new magic sulphonamides proved disappointing in the prevention of wound sepsis, not sufficiently effective when applied to the wound site and too fraught with unpleasant side effects when administered by mouth.

The second phase opened in North Africa, a terrain even more sterile than that of the Boer War. Here the sulphonamides were more successful than in Europe, possibly because of a different type of infection or perhaps because of greater experience in their use. The big problem was the fluid battle line and consequent need to push well-equipped centres very far back. Immobilization in unpadded plasters was found to be dangerous owing to the long, rough journey and lack of supervision.

In 1943 the theatre of war shifted again to Europe and the third phase began. Once more the terrain was a moist, well-cultivated soil instead of dry sterile sands, and the battle line became increasingly static. Wounds were more heavily contaminated with pathogenic organisms, better surgical facilities could be provided, and evacuation of casualties was easier. Surgeons now closed wounds by a two-stage operation. The forward surgeon removed blood clot and foreign bodies, excised grossly contaminated and devitalized tissue, and made free drainage of the wound possible by incisions through the skin and underlying fascia. The casualty was then evacuated to a base hospital where the second operation, closure of the wound, took place between the third and fifth day.

This dull and somewhat technical account masks a picture of intense effort. That cannot be described, for it is made up of a long series of individual trials, successes, and disappointments. The reader is asked to appreciate that this was a battle as great as any fought in the two world wars. The battle was seemingly for a quite small thing; the clean healing of a wound. Victory brought with it a benefit to the human race greater than any that has been conferred by all the wars that have troubled the world.

Part of the victory was won by an entirely new form of drug, first used experimentally in 1941. Penicillin belongs to the group of products known as antibiotics, a word often loosely used and misunderstood. Antibiosis, the antonym of symbiosis, was originally applied to the destruction for food of one living creature by another; the lion eats the deer which eats the grass which smothers the more weakly growing plant and feeds on the humus so formed. It is quite an old idea in the science of bacteriology and here originated with Pasteur's suggestion that it might be possible to set micro-organism to make war upon micro-organism. He and Jules Joubert observed the phenomenon when they saw that the large bacilli of anthrax are destroyed by what they described as 'common' bacteria. This was in 1887.

Ten years before Pasteur's observation, in 1876, Professor John Tyndall reported that the mould *Penicillium glaucum* caused the death of bacteria in 'sour' mutton broth infusions. The mould covered the broth in a thick, tough layer – anyone who has left a bowl of Irish stew too long in a warm larder will have seen it – and he thought that the bacteria died, or perhaps only became dormant, because the impervious coat deprived them of oxygen from the air. The same observation was made by other workers, among whom Lister is said to have been one. Lister certainly stated 'bacteria occasion putrefaction in the fluid, and when this has advanced to a certain degree, the growth of the penicillium is arrested.'[10] But whether he ever saw the converse example of antibiosis, as Tyndall did, is open to some doubt.

Nothing more happened until 1928 when a quiet, almost unknown little Scotsman, Alexander Fleming of St Mary's Hospital, noticed that a culture dish (petri dish) impregnated with staphylococci had become contaminated by a mould. In his original paper he described this mould as *Penicillium rubrum* but it was, in fact, *Penicillium notatum*. He found that where the spreading patches of penicillium mould touched the colonies of staphylococci, the colonies of staphylococci were shrinking. Struck by this unusual happening, Fleming isolated the mould and grew it in broth, when the broth became bright yellow in colour with a dark green felted mass on top. He filtered off some of this yellow broth and found that it would kill staphylococci. He tried growing thirteen different moulds, including eight strains of penicillium, but only one penicillium produced a lethal filtrate. 'In the rest of this article,' wrote Fleming in the *British Journal of Experimental Pathology*, 'allusion will constantly be made to experiments with filtrates of a broth culture of this mould, so for convenience and to avoid the repetition of the rather cumbersome phrase "Mould broth filtrate", the name "penicillin" will be used.'[11] Fleming not only discovered penicillin in 1928 but gave it the name by which it is known today. He tried his crude penicillin solution on various pathogenic organisms, finding that some were killed and some unaffected. The most important of those killed were staphylococci, streptococcus pyogenes, gonococci and pneumococci. Here is a good range of pathogenic organisms: gonococci cause gonorrhea; pneumococci cause pneumonia; staphylococci cause boils, carbuncles, pyaemia, and osteomyelitis; streptococcus pyogenes causes septicaemia and erysipelas. One of the unaffected organisms was bacillus influenzae, sometimes known as Pfeiffer's bacillus.

Fleming discovered that his filtrate was not toxic. 'The toxicity to animals of powerfully antibacterial mould broth filtrate appears to be very low,' he wrote. 'Twenty c.c. injected intravenously into a rabbit were not more toxic than the same quantity of broth.' In the summary of his findings he described penicillin as 'an efficient antiseptic for application to, or injection into, areas infected with penicillin-sensitive microbes'.

The work had been done. Crude penicillin had been prepared and found lethal to some of the most dangerous wound organisms; Fleming had found that animals could tolerate injection of the crude drug; he had made the direct suggestion that it might be injected or applied to the infected site. But no one took any notice. It is sometimes argued that Fleming buried his discovery in the pages of a specialist journal, an example of the folly of divorcing the laboratory worker from the clinician. Others hold that the emergence of sulphonamide drugs, only a few years later, blinded the medical profession to the importance of his discovery. Neither of these explanations seems to supply the correct answer for, after all, laboratory workers are ready enough to provide weapons for the clinicians and the clinicians are ready enough to receive those weapons, while the very existence of the sulphonamides should have awakened, and did awaken, renewed interest in the battle against infection. Possibly the neglect was just an unlucky chance. Equally possibly, Fleming's unfortunate use of the words 'efficient antiseptic' in the extract quoted above suggested that penicillin was just another and somewhat bizarre addition to 'antisepsis', a method well on its way to death and burial.

Fleming himself seems to have been quite unmoved by his

discovery. It goes against the grain to say that so great a bene-factor was lacking in intelligence, but he must have had some queer gap in his mental processes. Shy, taciturn, reserved as he was, it is yet astonishing that he made no mention of his re-markable findings in ordinary conversation to his colleagues across the luncheon table. Had he done so, someone must surely have grasped the importance of his work. He and a few others made some use of his penicillin broth. For ten years it remained a 'laboratory antiseptic', used to differentiate various strains of bacteria. At that time there was much discussion on the subject of Pfeiffer's bacillus, whether or not it was the cause of influenza. As this particular organism is penicillin-resistant, penicillin was used to produce a culture uncontaminated by other bacteria. One or two people did a few investigations; the yellow colouring matter, chrysogenin, was isolated in 1932 but found to have no bactericidal action;[12] R. D. Reid failed to prepare pure penicil-lin from the crude broth but was able to describe some of its properties in 1935.[13]

Howard Florey, Ernst Chain, and others commenced a study of penicillin at the Sir William Dunn School of Pathology, Oxford, in 1939. During the course of the next year they managed to obtain from the crude broth a brown powder which was soluble in water and stable in solution. They understood that this was not pure penicillin but a contaminated con-centrate. They found that this concentrate had great anti-bacterial effect. It was tested *in vitro* and on rats, mice, and cats. In 1940 Florey and his colleagues were able to publish their conclusion 'The results are clear cut, and show that penicillin is active *in vivo* against at least three of the organisms inhibited *in vitro*.'[14]

Next year, in August 1941, they published a lengthy survey of progress which included administration of crude penicillin to human patients, under the supervision of C. M. Fletcher. Between 12 February and 26 July, six patients were treated orally or by intravenous injection and four by local application. The first patient, a forty-three-year-old policeman, had been admitted to the Radcliffe Infirmary with a quite small cut near his mouth, which had become infected with both a staphy-lococcus and streptococcus pyogenes. This resulted in a par-ticularly lethal form of septicaemia, for which the sulphonamide drugs proved useless. On 12 February 1941, as the patient's condition was clearly hopeless, Florey decided to make trial of penicillin. After administration of eight hundred milligrammes of the crude drug in twenty-four hours, there came a dramatic improvement, but the small supply ran out and treatment had to be interrupted while penicillin was recovered from the patient's urine for reinjection. Steady improvement continued until 17 February, when the supply of penicillin was entirely exhausted. The patient's condition remained stationary for ten days, but thereafter deteriorated rapidly until death on 15 March. Treatment of the second patient, a child, commenced with penicillin recovered from the policeman's urine. Florey and his colleagues summed up their findings in the words 'Penicillin was given intravenously to five patients with staphylococcal and streptococcal infections and by mouth to one baby with a persistent staphylococcal urinary infection. It was also applied locally to four cases of eye infection. In all these cases a favourable therapeutic response was obtained.'[15]

The production of penicillin is a slow process. It still had to be prepared in sufficient quantity for a large-scale trial and, in 1941, British industry was stretched to the limit in a frantic endeavour to re-equip the armed forces after the disaster of 1940. Florey turned to the United States. He persuaded American industry that penicillin was not only a weapon of war but is also a drug of lasting benefit to the human race. The Department of Agricultural Research Laboratory, Illinois, discovered a far more productive form of penicillium mould, *Penicillium chrysogenum* (said to have been isolated from a rotting canteloupe melon picked up by one of their female assistants in a food shop) and also found that the production process could be speeded by the addition of corn-steep liquor, a waste material from the manufacture of corn starch, to the nutrient broth. Improved methods rapidly increased production and, with an increased supply at command, it became possible to produce a pure form. In 1942 hardly enough of the crude drug was available for clinical trial on one hundred patients; in 1958 more than four hundred and forty tons of pure crystallized penicillin was produced by America alone; in 1943 a sufficient supply had been built up to allow a limited use, under strict control, by the medical personnel of the allied forces. An unpleasant side of this story is the immense black market in penicillin which grew up just after the war.

From the treatment of wounds we turn to the treatment of shock caused by wounds. Surgical shock, one of the greater dangers of large wounds, is a term first used to denote collapse from injury or operation by James Latta in 1795. It has puzzled and exercised the brains of the medical profession for centuries, and the exact cause of certain types of shock is still open to some doubt. Shock may develop for a number of reasons. There is the patient who, in the newspaper report, is always admitted to hospital 'suffering from shock' and who has been through a frightening experience but is quite uninjured; there is shock due to pain alone; there is shock which develops as the result of damage, particularly crushing damage, to the tissues; and there is shock due to loss of blood. In all types of shock the clinical picture, essentially that of a lowered blood pressure, is the same.

There is no need to go in to the various theories of shock which have been put forward from time to time, for here we will consider the treatment of only the simplest form, shock due to a wound which causes pain and loss of blood. It must be obvious that, when a patient is shocked due to blood loss, the most effective treatment is to restore the blood. But, although it sounds simple, there are a number of difficulties to be overcome before blood transfusion can be a safe procedure.

Transfusion of blood is a very old idea. Much of the earlier part of the story belongs to legend rather than to history, but it may be mentioned that Christopher Wren and his colleagues of the Royal Society watched Richard Lower transfuse blood from one animal to another; at about the same time (1664) Major of Leipzig managed to introduce blood into the vein of a man and, three years later, Jean Baptiste Denys of Montpellier transfused lamb's blood into a youth of fifteen. This type of experiment aroused much hostility; transfusion of human blood has been forbidden by Act of the French Parlement and laid under Papal Interdict.

The more recent part of the story starts with James Blundell, lecturer in midwifery to Guy's Hospital, who, after animal experiment, transfused a man dying of cancer of the stomach with human blood on 26 September 1818. There was some improvement in the patient's condition but he died fifty-six hours later.[16] In 1824 Blundell bled a dog to the point of death and immediately transfused it with blood taken from another dog. The first dog recovered. A rumour started that Blundell proposed to transfuse women, endangered by haemorrhage following childbirth, with animal blood, a treatment that had already been often suggested and sometimes practised. His assistant, R. J. Linton, quieted these suspicions by stating that Blundell did not propose to introduce dog's blood into women, but human blood transfused directly from donor to recipient.[17]

Later in 1824 Blundell published his *Researches Physiological and Pathological* in which he stated that arterial blood is preferable to venous blood because of the ease of direction transfusion. (The arterial pressure being much higher than the venous pressure, arterial blood from a donor will enter the vein of the recipient if artery and vein are connected together.) But he said that venous blood might be safely transfused by means of a syringe, and he invented a kind of pump for the purpose. Experiment had shown him that it was not necessary to replace the whole volume of blood lost; an animal's life could be saved by transfusing a much smaller quantity than had been bled off. Blundell made a most important observation 'If the operation be performed on the human body, human blood only should be employed until some other blood be found which is equally congenial to the vessels.'[18]

Blundell's transfusion pump was of somewhat complicated design; in 1857 Higginson introduced a much simpler syringe, a rubber bulb with a tube at either end and non-return valves. One tube could be tied into the vein of the donor and the other into the vein of the recipient; by pumping the bulb, blood would be drawn from the donor and transfused into the recipient. Probably not one in a hundred nurses, who often use Higginson's syringe to pump fluid into the rectum or vagina, know that he invented it for quite another purpose. In 1872 J. H. Aveling invented a vein-to-vein cannula; one of the better known little anecdotes in the history of blood transfusion is that Aveling saved the life of a female patient by transfusing her with six and a half ounces of blood, the donor being the lady's coachman.

Clotting of the blood was the great problem in these early

transfusions. In 1869 J. Braxton Hicks of Guy's Hospital endeavoured to overcome this by adding sodium phosphate to the blood when it was passing through the pump (he used a Blundell's apparatus). He transfused four patients, but all four died. Death could have been due to the sodium phosphate, but we do not know how close to death the patients were when transfused and, of course, the wrong type of blood might well have been given. In 1901 Jules Bordet and Octave Gengou partially solved the difficulty by coating the interior of all syringes, tubes, and cannulae with paraffin wax. This made transfusion difficult because the wax often peeled off and blocked the lumen of the tube or cannula. In 1914 Albert Hustin of Brussels drew blood off into a vessel, added sodium citrate, and transfused the citrated blood into the recipient's vein. This method, which effectively prevents clotting, is used today.

We said above that the death of Hicks' patients might have been due to the wrong type of blood. Blundell had written that only human blood should be used to transfuse the human as early as 1824, but animal blood was often preferred during the next fifty years. Higginson noted a 'reaction' which he described as a rather severe rigor; he attributed this to the presence of air bubbles, but it must have been caused by the wrong type of blood. In 1874 Leonard Landois, a German physiologist, showed that the blood of one animal species can haemolyse, or break down, the cells of another and so cause death. Despite this important finding, a doctor named Hasse strongly advised that lamb's blood should be used in preference to human blood at the 1874 surgical congress in Berlin.

The next and greater advance came in 1901, when Karl Landsteiner of Vienna discovered the existence of 'agglutinins' in the blood and divided human blood into four groups. He found that the blood serum of one group might cause the red blood corpuscles of another group to clump together (agglutinate); that is, the blood of one group might not be 'compatible' with that of another. It is not generally known that the London pathologist M. Shattock independently discovered this fact in the same year as Landsteiner.[19] The present ABO blood grouping system is essentially the same as Landsteiner's; in 1907 J. Jansky of Norway introduced a 1, 2, 3, 4 grouping system and in 1910 W. L. Moss of Baltimore also introduced a numerical system which exactly reversed Jansky's. It needed the League of Nations to sort that problem out.

At the beginning of the First World War it was therefore possible to give blood without danger of agglutination or of clotting. Grouped, citrated blood was, in fact, first used therapeutically by Richard Lewisohn of New York and Louis Agote of Buenos Aires in 1915. But the shocked and wounded soldier of the First World War was more often treated with the intravenous infusion of saline than with blood. Intravenous saline had been used as long ago as 1832, when Dr Latta of Leith advised injection of large quantities to combat the stage of acute collapse in cholera.[20] Many surgeons relied upon saline for the treatment of surgical shock during operations. The accustomed use of saline and the difficulty of securing blood, when no organized donor service existed, resulted in the neglect of blood transfusion. In 1916–7 O. H. Robertson, a Canadian medical officer, started the use of citrated blood in the battle area, designing a special container for the purpose. Robertson also showed that blood can be refrigerated and kept in cold storage for up to a month with safety. Blood transfusion was first used on a fairly large scale at the first battle of Cambrai in 1917, but only as a desperate life-saving measure. Throughout the 1914–8 war the standard treatment of shock depended upon first aid control of haemorrhage and setting of fractures, morphia to relieve pain and apprehension, warmth to combat the chilly symptoms of lowered blood pressure. A cup of hot, sweet tea and a cigarette formed an essential part of this treatment, probably more appreciated by the casualty than anything else.

Saline continued to be used far more frequently than blood during the nineteen twenties. George Washington Crile of Cleveland, USA, and William Arbuthnot Lane in London did a great deal of work upon shock and were firm believers in the virtue of saline. J. B. Murphy of Chicago invented a 'drip' method of slow and continuous infusion in place of rapid pumping-in of a 'dose' of saline with a syringe. Murphy's drip was much improved by Rudolph Matas of New Orleans in 1902, who also advised the addition of glucose to the saline, a mixture often used today. His drip included a glass chamber, making it possible to count the number of drops given per minute and so to control and to measure the flow of saline accurately. This drip apparatus was first used for giving blood by H. J. Marriott and Alan Kekwick of the Middlesex Hospital in 1935. Their patient had a gastric ulcer which was causing a severe haemorrhage. They gave a continuous infusion of fresh citrated blood for some days, with very favourable results.[21] This was the first time that blood had been given continuously over a long period and not as a single 'dose'.

The difficulty was to find blood donors. Usually the blood was taken from a close relative of the patient; he was bled in an adjoining room and the blood immediately given to the patient in the ward or operating theatre. Early in the nineteen thirties Professor Shanov of Kharkov suggested the possibility of using blood drained from fresh corpses; the blood might then be refrigerated and stored. In 1933 Sergei Yudin of Moscow adopted Shanov's idea and formed a blood bank; four years later he reported success with this stored cadaveric blood, and the method is still used in Russia.[22]

Such treatment of the dead body, although logical, did not commend itself to western peoples who preferred to depend upon the generosity of voluntary, living donors. About the year 1920 a surgeon in Camberwell was faced with the problem of urgently finding blood for a patient who seemed to possess no living relatives at all. The hospital pathologist had the idea of appealing to the Red Cross. He rang up the Camberwell and Peckham branch and put the problem to their secretary, Percy Lane Oliver. Oliver hastily made a house-to-house search for volunteers and arrived at the hospital with a number of people prepared to give their blood. They were all 'cross-matched' to find one whose blood was of the same group as the patient's and a suitable donor was selected. The patient recovered.

Oliver decided that there was need for a better, more organized, method of providing blood donors. He collected a number of volunteers from whom a sample of blood was taken and whose group was noted. Oliver kept a list of his volunteers and of their groups. When the call for blood came, he set off on his bicycle, collected a suitable volunteer, and brought him to the hospital. His effort developed, after 1921, into the London Blood Transfusion Service, still so small and so primitive that the whole service could be run from Oliver's private house. Similar services were formed in other large cities.[23]

Blood was still taken from the donor and immediately transfused to the recipient; it was not until 1937 that Bernard Fantus of Chicago published an account of the scheme adopted at Cook County Hospital for storing a reserve of donated blood. At the beginning of the Second World War there existed a register of blood donors, organized by the Red Cross, and the blood could be stored with safety for from ten to fifteen days – Robertson's suggestion of a month had proved over-optimistic. Few surgeons had used blood to any large extent, and very few had any practical knowledge of blood transfusion, which was generally regarded as the province of the pathologist. A supply of blood for the armed forces was brilliantly organized by Lionel Whitby from a centre near Bristol, and two more collection and storage depots were set up near London. Some idea of the 'official attitude' in 1939 may be gained from the estimate that a daily supply of one hundred pints of blood would be ample for all purposes; by 1944 British donors were providing over twelve hundred pints a day.

In the first phase of the Second World War blood was still little used and most surgeons regarded a maximum of one pint in four hours as the safe limit, but experience with air-raid casualties in the 1940 blitz clearly showed that 'resuscitation', the recovery of shocked patients to a state fit for operation, was virtually useless unless a volume of blood almost equal to that which had been lost was replaced. The civilian doctor, dealing with air-raid casualties, taught this lesson to the army surgeon. In the army, large scale blood transfusion was first used at the battle of El Alamein on 26 May 1942 and proved its worth. Thereafter, largely through the work of C. H. Buttle, rapid and complete replenishment of blood loss became the essential of resuscitation. Twenty pints of blood and ten of plasma (the serum of the blood without red corpuscles) came to be regarded as the bare minimum requirement for every hundred casualties. Base units for collection and dispatch of blood were set up in the theatres of war. A surgeon writes of one in Bari, Italy, that it was improvised out of a disused brewery and that many difficulties, including an invasion of flies, had to be overcome. All donors were members of the British armed forces and all gave their blood freely, the only remuneration being 'resuscitation' with one pint of beer. A Dakota plane, affectionately known as the Blood Wagon, regularly transported up to three hundred bottles of blood daily to the Eighth Army front. No patient, friend or enemy, was ever refused a necessary blood transfusion.[24]

During the war another important fact about blood transfusion came to light. In 1940 Landsteiner, who had emigrated from Austria to the United States, discovered the Rhesus or Rh factor, while working at the Rockefeller Institute with Alexander Wiener. The Rhesus factor is of particular importance when transfusing blood to women. The mysterious name 'Rhesus' derives from the rhesus monkeys upon which the experiments were carried out. This is a graceful and unusual compliment to that forgotten member of the partnership, the laboratory animal.

The new types of wound commonly inflicted in both World Wars had a profound and lasting effect upon operative techniques. The major developments in plastic surgery and orthopaedics, in surgery of the brain and of the thorax, will be dealt with in their due place. But we have already mentioned that there was considerable difference of opinion on the subject of abdominal wounds at the beginning of the First World War. Treatment of abdominal wounds demands a somewhat different approach from the abdominal 'catastrophe' caused by disease, and may conveniently be briefly considered at this point.

The official policy in 1914 still remained one of non-intervention. The dreadful injuries caused by high explosive made it inevitable that this attitude soon changed; surgeons could not stand idly by when death must be certain if nothing was done. More than any other man on the allied side, Cuthbert Wallace of St Thomas' Hospital supported and encouraged junior RAMC surgeons in their efforts to deal with a type of abdominal injury which they had never before encountered. Many of these operations were marvels of improvisation, performed in conditions that would normally be regarded as impossible. John Campbell, who first operated successfully on a gunshot wound of the stomach; Owen Richards, who first successfully resected part of the small intestine; Claude Frankau, who performed the first successful resection of the colon; these and many others showed what the surgeon can do when faced with an entirely new type of emergency. Knowledge gained from this inevitably experimental surgery resulted in the planned operation for abdominal injury of the Second World War, typified by the method of Heneage Ogilvie. Ogilvie, when faced with a wound of the large intestine, opened the abdomen with a surgical incision, brought the wounded intestine to the surface through a second incision, and allowed the wound in the bowel to act as a colostomy or false anus. At a later date the opening in the bowel could be closed and the bowel returned to the abdominal cavity by a very minor operation. This procedure incorporated the important principle of 'resting the bowel', first advocated by John Ryle in 1920, in which a tube is passed by mouth into the stomach or small intestine; the bowel contents can then be aspirated at regular intervals, while intravenous infusion of saline or glucose-saline make it possible to give no nourishment by mouth. This method had come into use by 1939 and contributed largely to the successful treatment of abdominal wounds in the Second World War; it is now a standard treatment for the 'acute abdomen' caused by obstructed bowel.

Thus, between the years 1914 and 1945, the treatment of wounds and of the wounded underwent a radical change. It may seem to some readers that we have spent far too much time upon this point and have entered into too great detail. We have, indeed, only touched the fringe of the many problems, some of which are still unsolved. The wound is the essential of surgery; it matters not whether the wound is in the skin, in the liver, the bowel, the heart, the lungs or the brain. What matters is that this wound heals, wherever it is placed. The purposeful wound of an operation must be so inflicted that it does not cause un-treatable shock, that it heals cleanly and without infection. This is the aim of every surgeon.

By 1945 surgery had become a complex subject, so complex that no one man could possibly practise its many variations. Although the interwar years saw the heyday of the 'general' surgeon, he already regarded certain regions of the body as outside his field. For instance, he rarely operated upon the nose, the throat, the ear, or the eye. He often developed a special interest in certain diseases or in operations upon a particular body-system; the brain, the urinary tract, the skeleton are examples. As time progressed, he tended more and more to confine himself to his speciality. Thus developed the fragmentation which is so marked a feature of practise today, when specialization – perhaps overspecialization – has virtually divided surgery into watertight compartments. There are still many who call themselves 'general' surgeons, but they would acknowledge that 'general surgery' is merely a convenient name; it does not include a number of important specialities. For this reason we shall now cease to trace the story of surgery as a whole, and proceed to describe the individual histories of these various specialities.

CHAPTER 7

Lithotomists and Bone Setters

Urology and Orthopaedics

Urology, the oldest surgical speciality, derives from a single operation, removal of a stone from the urinary bladder, which our forefathers regarded as the highest test of surgical skill. Orthopaedics, in its modern sense of surgery of bones and joints, has developed largely from the practice of unqualified bone setters. There is no particular link between the two specialities except for the fact that they were the first to emerge from the 'general' surgery of the early twentieth century.

Cutting for the stone or lithotomy can boast a long history, being mentioned in the Hippocratic Oath 'I will not use the knife either on sufferers from stone, but I will give place to such as are craftsmen therein.', an early example of the intellectual physician passing on the actual treatment of a diagnosed disorder to the practical surgeon. Many of these 'lithotomists' were skilful operators and travelled widely; certain towns or cities became renowned for the operation; in England, Norwich was one of the better-known centres. A good lithotomist attracted apprentices and handed on his skill to them; the apprentice settled in the town and the 'centre' developed. So often does the operation seem to have been performed that it is sometimes said that bladder stones were much more common in the ages of horse-back riding, dietary indiscretion, and hard drinking. There may be something in the theory but against it must be set the fact that lithotomy has acquired its important place in ancient surgery for the simple reason that it was one of the few 'cutting' operations to be regularly attempted. Perhaps the best known example of an early lithotomy is the one performed by Thomas Hollyer of St Thomas' Hospital on 26 March 1658.[12]

His patient, Samuel Pepys, kept the day upon which he was successfully cut as an annual and solemn feast of thanksgiving.

A few details of this important technique may be of interest. In Europe, the original operation was a modification of one used by the Roman doctor Celsus, who lived 25 BC – AD 50, and has at various times been called 'cutting on the gripe', 'the perineal operation', or 'the lesser apparatus'. The last name gives us a clue to the simplicity of this method, only a knife to make the incision and a hook to remove the stone being needed. The surgeon operated at the perineum between the genital organs and the rectum, pushed the stone forward to the floor of the bladder by means of two fingers in the rectum, made a semilunar incision over the stone, and brought it out through the floor of the bladder. The wound often failed to heal and resulted in a fistula through which urine constantly dribbled away.

The next operation, known as the 'greater apparatus' because more instruments were required, was devised by John de Romanis of Cremona and popularized by his pupil Marianus, or Mariano Santo de Barletta, in the years 1520–37. At first called the 'Marian operation', it was later referred to as the 'old way' or the 'median incision', because the surgeon cut in the middle line of the perineum, through the prostate gland into the urethra, and pulled the stone out of the bladder with forceps. The word 'old' was applied when surgeons started to practise the 'lateral incision' or 'new way'.[2]

'Lateral lithotomy', also known as the 'approved operation', has an interesting little history. It is probably just as old an operation as the last, but it is unknown who invented the method. At the end of the seventeenth century, a Franciscan lay brother named Jacques Baulot, or Frère Jacques, travelled over most of Western Europe cutting for the stone. He was a Frenchman, probably born at Beaulieu in 1651, and had received little if any medical training. Frère Jacques at first used an operation which had been popular among Hindu surgeons and was introduced into Europe by Pierre Franco of Berne and Lausanne in 1556. In 1697 Jacques went to Paris; according to one story he was so successful that he aroused the jealousy of the Parisian surgeons and was forced to resume his travels in Europe. According to another version, his results were so bad that the king himself ordered Jacques to learn the elements of anatomy. There seems to be some truth in the latter account, for Jacques undoubtedly did study under the French surgeon G. C. Fagou, who attended the royal household. As a result of his anatomical studies, Jacques took up the 'lateral incision', in which the cut is not made in the midline of the perineum but to one side; healing is more certain when the cut is made in this manner and so the chance of a fistula is lessened. Jacques now modified and improved the operation by introducing a 'staff' or guide into the urethra and cutting down upon the staff with his knife. He only made his incision through the anterior wall of the bladder, and did not touch the posterior wall.

Frère Jacques next went to Holland, where he continued his studies under Professor Rau of Leyden. He showed his method to Rau, who probably replaced the round, probe-like, guide used by Jacques with a grooved staff, a much better instrument because the knife could be fitted into the groove and slid along it so as not to cause damage to adjoining tissue. Whether Rau invented the grooved staff or not, he certainly used it and he became the most successful lithotomist in Europe. Skilful lithotomists earned very large fees; Professor Rau naturally became a popular teacher and pupils flocked to learn the secrets of 'his' method.

Cutting for the stone lent itself to charlatanry. It was easy for an unprincipled surgeon to 'palm' a stone, to perform a bungling operation, and to show the palmed stone to the patient at the end. In France, where surgical practice was better regulated than in other countries, strict laws were enforced against such deceits; at least two 'surgeons' were executed for this type of fraud. Rau did not cheat his patients, but he did cheat his pupils by teaching them a dangerous technique. Frère Jacques had been careful to incise only the anterior wall of the bladder, but Rau taught that both the anterior and posterior walls should be opened. The posterior bladder wall lies close to the rectum and it was very easy, in the rapid kind of operation then necessary, to injure the rectal wall or to cut through the sphincter muscle of the anus. The former will result in a fistula between the bladder and the rectum, the latter in incontinence of faeces. Rau, although careful to practise the correct method himself, was so selfish and jealous of his own success that he purposely kept secret the most essential part of the Jacques operation.[3]

William Cheselden of St Thomas' Hospital learned of 'lateral' lithotomy or the 'new way' from one of Rau's pupils. He soon came to the conclusion that this cannot have been the method practised by Frère Jacques and, being a man of great brilliance, understood why Rau's operation, so successful in his own hands, often resulted in disaster when practised by others. The correct technique of lateral lithotomy was reintroduced by Cheselden about the year 1725, and is often called by his name.[4] His results were excellent for those days; his operative mortality did not exceed 17 per cent, whereas the mortality of most surgeons was in the region of 40 per cent; a swift but gentle operator, his record time is said to have been forty-five seconds, and it was the aim of every surgeon to beat this. S. F. Morand, a well known Paris lithotomist, said that he saw a stone removed by the lateral operation in twenty-four seconds; Morand watched Cheselden cut for the stone on twenty-seven occasions without the loss of a patient. Cheselden wrote an interesting little note on the subject of his success 'If I have my reputation in this way I have earned it dearly, for no one ever endured more anxiety and sickness before an operation, yet from the time I began to operate all uneasiness ceased and if I have had better success than some others I do not impute it to my knowledge but to the happiness of a mind that was never ruffled or disconcerted and a hand that never trembled during any operation.'

The danger of the open lithotomy operation caused surgeons to investigate the possibility of crushing a stone by means of instruments passed through the natural passage into the bladder. This operation, known as lithotrity, was attempted in 1626 by Sanctorius of Padua, but no real progress was made until the nineteenth century. Gruithuisen of Bavaria (1813) and Elderton in Scotland (1819) suggested that stones might be reduced to powder and washed out of the bladder; Gruithuisen made a strong metal rod ending in a pair of blunt scissors, by which the stone could be cut and partly crushed. Elderton advised preliminary drilling of the stone; in 1833 Baron Heurteloup of Paris invented a claw-like lithotrite which grasped the stone while a metal rod could be rotated to drill out the central part. A surgeon named Rigal proposed the opposite manoeuvre; the grasped stone was rotated and rubbed against a roughened surface so that the circumference became gradually worn away.

Jean Civiale of Paris had been experimenting with lithotrites since 1817. On 13 January 1824 he gave his first public demonstration at the Necker Hospital with an instrument consisting of two metal tubes, one inside the other; the inner tube ended in three metal prongs by which the stone could be seized. The inner tube being retracted and the stone thus held firmly between the prongs, a sharp-pointed metal rod was passed down the lumen and rotated by means of a bow. Civiale restricted the length of operation to five minutes, after which such fragments as had been bored away were washed out of the bladder. Thus several sittings (the approved term) were necessary for even a small stone. Civiale's demonstrations involved him in a clash with Heurteloup and another French lithotritist, J. Leroy d'Etoilles, both of whom claimed priority for the invention of his instrument. It seems fairly certain that, although a number of models had been designed for a proposed operation by Heurteloup and others, Civiale was the first to apply the theoretical idea of lithotrity to the living patient.

By 1835 Civiale had considerably improved both his method and his instrument. In 1820 John Weiss, a London instrument maker, produced a stone extractor (not a lithotrite or crusher) to the design of Astley Cooper; with this Cooper extracted no less than eighty small stones from the bladder of one patient. The Weiss extractor was modified into a curved, beaked instrument of two parts, one sliding in the groove of the other; a small saw could be inserted between the beaks if it was thought advisable to cut the stone. Civiale made this extractor into a serviceable lithotrite by strengthening the two beaked parts and by using a hammer or a hand-screw to crush the grasped stone. The hammer principle, orginally devised by Heurteloup, was very cumbersome in use, demanding a vice in which the instrument could be held while percussion was applied. Weiss invented the screw, by means of which pressure was gradually exerted upon the stone held between the beaks, but it was not sufficiently effective until modified by J. F. Charrière of Paris.[5]

Sir Henry Thompson of University College Hospital became the best known exponent of lithotrity in England. About 1860 he converted the Civiale instrument by replacing the hand-screw with a wheel-screw and grooving the beaked blades so that debris could be more easily removed. Although later improved by Guyon of Paris, Thompson's modified lithotrite is that in use today. Thompson gained a European reputation and may be looked on as the first English urologist worthy of the name. In 1863 he was called to operate upon Leopold I, King of the Belgians, eighteen months after Civiale had failed to crush the stone. In 1873 he started to crush a large stone in the bladder of ex-Emperor Napoleon III of France, but the emperor died at 10.45 in the morning of 9 January, one hour and a quarter before the third sitting had been planned to take place. Thompson quite well understood his own importance in the world. 'Sir,' he told a patient. 'I find that you have a stone in your bladder.' 'Oh, no, Sir Henry, that is impossible. I have just been examined by a very rising surgeon and he assured me that I have nothing of the kind.' 'Sir, *I* have risen!'

Thompson never prolonged operation beyond two minutes, and would submit his patients to as many as twenty-five sittings. These multitudinous sittings were thought necessary partly because of the belief that prolonged instrumentation of the bladder caused shock and partly because the surgeon found it difficult to wash out the small fragments of stone. The latter problem suggested a number of ingenious solutions. A continuous stream of water, by means of a double catheter inserted at the end of operation was advocated by Gruithuisen. According to William Fergusson, Gruithuisen attached the entry tube of his catheter to a reservoir on top of a two-storey house in order to get sufficient pressure. 'Perhaps with more mechanical ingenuity than surgical discretion,' remarked Fergusson.[6] In 1846 Sir Philip Crampton of Dublin invented a suction apparatus consisting of a glass bottle exhausted of air and connected to the catheter by a rubber tube and stopcock. The disadvantages were that the vacuum soon failed and the bladder had often to be refilled with water.

In 1878 H. J. Bigelow, professor of surgery in Harvard University, came to the conclusion that prolonged instrumentation is less dangerous than repeated operations which always left fragments of stone behind. Bigelow introduced the method known as litholapaxy. Lithotomy means cutting for stone; lithotrity means crushing the stone; litholapaxy means evacuation of the stone. It is interesting that the last word was coined by Oliver Wendell Holmes who also introduced the term anaesthesia. The only new part of Bigelow's operation was the evacuation of all stone fragments after crushing at one sitting.

The more important part of Bigelow's apparatus therefore consisted of a better type of evacuator. Evacuators had already been invented by J. T. Clover, a London anaesthetist, C. F. Maunder of Charing Cross and others, but none of these models were effective. Bigelow's evacuator, or syphon as he called it, consisted of a straight metal tube, as wide as possible, connected by a bayonet joint to a rubber ball communicating with a glass trap. The ball held ten ounces of water, of which five could be forced into the bladder by manual compression. Release of compression resulted in the backflow of water bearing fragments of stone which fell to the bottom of the trap.[7] Bigelow's evacuator has since been modified but the principle remains exactly the same. With the introduction of anaesthesia and antisepsis, the suprapubic operation, opening the bladder through the lower abdomen, came into common use for removal of large stones, while smaller stones were treated with Thompson's lithotrite and Bigelow's evacuator. Though the instruments have been slightly changed, the method remains the same today.

Until the eighteen sixties presence of a stone could only be determined by the patient's symptoms and by sounding the bladder with a metal probe. In 1805 P. Bozzini of Frankfurt tried to see into the bladder with a straight metal tube, open at both ends, illuminated by reflected light. This was quite ineffective; F. August Haken added a glass eye-piece in 1862 and F. R. Cruise of Dublin improved the method of illumination. With these aids A. J. Desormeaux of Paris, who had been experimenting since 1853, produced an instrument with which some kind of a view could be obtained. Desormeaux's instrument is the parent not only of the modern cystoscope for examining the bladder, but of all similar 'scopes' used to see into the trachea, lungs, oesophagus and stomach. Illumination was still by reflected light; in 1867 Julius Bruck, a dentist of

Breslau, tried to overcome this most inconvenient method by the seemingly extraordinary expedient of inserting an incandescent platinum loop into the rectum. This required a very complicated cooling system and the transmitted light was not really powerful enough to give a good view of the bladder. Max Nitze of Dresden and Joseph Leiter, a Viennese instrument maker, produced a much better instrument, incorporating a system of lenses, in 1879. This is generally regarded as the first 'modern' cystoscope but, like the Desormeaux instrument, it was designed for use in the rectum, the back of the throat, the nose, and even the stomach, as well as in the bladder. The Nitze cystoscope still depended upon incandescent platinum for illumination and required a cooling system which made it cumbersome in use. Seven years later von Dittel and Leiter adopted Edison's invention of the carbon filament lamp as a source of electric light; the difficulty of producing a 'mini-bulb' had delayed this advance for some years. An irrigating cystoscope, by which the bladder could be continuously flushed through with water, was introduced in 1888 and, by 1889, cystoscopy had become a sufficiently common procedure for E. Hurry Fenwick of the London Hospital to publish a monograph on *Electrical Illumination of the Bladder and Urethra*. Today cystoscopy is a routine examination.

When removing stones from the male, surgeons often found that the lobed prostate gland, which lies at the neck of the bladder, interfered with the operation. It was not so much that enlargement of the gland made lithotomy difficult, but that the forceps closed upon a lobe instead of upon the stone, or that both lobe and stone were grasped at the same time. Further, enlargement of the prostate was one of the commoner causes of retention of urine which could only be relieved by forcible dilatation with 'bougies' or by passing a catheter, methods which had certainly been known to the Arabian physician Avicenna, born in the tenth century. The man who suffered from an enlarged prostate, causing urinary obstruction, was condemned to a catheter life for the rest of his days.

Tearing of the prostate during operation could cause severe haemorrhage, and catheter life was dangerous because the bladder soon became infected and infection travelled up the ureters to the kidneys. Surgeons therefore made attempts to deal with the enlarged prostate, but the problem was a difficult one because of the risk involved by opening the bladder. In 1834 G. J. Guthrie tried to overcome the problem by means of a special knife, called a urethrotome, which could be passed up the urethra in order to 'scratch' some kind of a passage at the bladder neck. Three years later L. A. Mercier of Paris invented instruments with which some of the obstructing gland could be excised. In 1874 Enrico Bottini tried a cautery knife heated by a galvanic battery.

These methods involved operation by the natural passage of the urethra; we will finish with this route before considering the open operation. No further progress was made along these lines for over thirty years, when the famous American urologist H. H. Young of Baltimore introduced his 'punch' method, sections of prostate being pared out by a tubular, sharp-edged, instrument. Young first used the 'cold punch' in 1909, but he did not describe his technique until 1913. Recently a well-known London urologist has told the author that the cold punch is still popular in the 'wilds of Scotland, America, and St Thomas' Hospital'.

Meanwhile the high-frequency current had entered medicine through the work of Professor K. F. Nagelschmidt, a German physicist, and Professor Paul Oudin of France in 1893–4. Nagelschmidt first suggested the use of cutting 'diathermy' in place of the knife in 1909; he demonstrated a diathermy excision of a small tumour of the tongue at St Bartholomew's Hospital in 1910. Gosta Forsell of Stockholm excised cancers of the breast with the 'diathermy knife' in 1923; by 1939 some American surgeons were prophesying that the scalpel would be a forgotten surgical instrument within five years.

As early as 1910 Edwin Beer applied the high-frequency current to surgery of the bladder. Georges Luys of Paris introduced the operation which he called 'forage de la prostate' in 1918; this would now be termed 'fulguration' implying destruction of the gland by the electric current. In 1920 J. R. Caulk of St Louis substituted an electrocautery blade for the circular blade of Young's cold punch and thus made the 'hot punch' which burned its way through prostatic tissue. This had the advantage of cutting the gland and of coagulating blood vessels by heat at the same time. About 1921 Kenneth Walker of Bart's introduced a very similar method and, in 1923, another American urologist, C. W. Collings, adapted Caulk's simple electrocautery punch for the diathermy current.

All these methods suffered from the grave disadvantage of being blind operations, because the various instruments could not be passed through the necessarily narrow bore of a cystoscope. In 1924 Stern of New York invented an instrument resembling a cystoscope through which a looped wire could be passed; the loop carried the diathermy current and a cut could thereby be made under direct vision. Six years later J. F. McCarthy of New York, who had been experimenting with these cutting loops for twenty years, devised his resectotome, a loop which could be advanced and drawn back under direct vision, and described his technique of transurethral electroresection, excision of portions of the prostate gland by diathermy through the urethra, first used in Great Britain by Terence Millin in the same year, 1930. Some urologists thought that transurethral resection would replace all forms of surgical treatment of the prostate; others were not so sure. By 1937, when electroresection had been on trial for seven years (Caulk alone collected details of 15,448 cases) it had become generally understood that the method, while holding a very important place, did not give a complete answer.

Attempts had already been made to remove part of the obstructing gland by other routes. In 1848 William Fergusson 'partly tore and partly cut away' portions of the prostate during the course of a lateral lithotomy; the patient, aged 75, made a good recovery. When he exhibited this and other specimens at a surgical meeting in London, Fergusson overheard whispers 'about rough and improper proceedings in lithotomy'. Some similar kind of operation had been performed by the French surgeon J. Z. Amussat in 1836, but Fergusson seems to have been the first to suggest that prostatectomy might enter practice as a routine method. In 1870, having easily removed one or more lobes of the gland from an eighty-year-old patient, he wrote 'When stone is combined with enlarged prostate, who can say from which cause the distress is greatest? So if it happens that the surgeon is called upon to relieve his patient from stone, and finds an enlarged prostate at the same time, why should he not, in extracting the stone, when it seems in his power, as in the cases above referred to, take away a superfluous portion of the prostate at the same time?'[8]

The two greatest figures in urological circles, Jean Guyon of Paris and Sir Henry Thompson of London, were strongly opposed to any interference with the prostate; probably for this reason, Fergusson's suggestion was not adopted. Sixteen years later W. T. Belfield of Chicago removed, by open operation through the lower part of the abdomen (suprapubic incision), an outgrowth or lobe of the prostate from a man of seventy-three. It is of some importance in the history to notice that the piece removed was 'as large as a hazel nut'. Belfield performed a similar operation in the following year.

In November 1887 A. F. McGill of Leeds, a nephew and godson of William Fergusson, described three cases. His operation consisted of opening the bladder by suprapubic incision and removing such portion of the prostate as 'prevents the passage of the urine from the bladder into the urethral canal'.[9] The gland was removed partly by tearing with forceps and partly by cutting with scissors. At that time Berkeley Moynihan, afterwards Lord Moynihan of Leeds, was McGill's dresser and acting house surgeon. Typically, Moynihan wrote that McGill did not know what structure he was removing until told by his acting house surgeon! Moynihan also states that, at the 1889 meeting of the British Medical Association in Leeds, McGill showed a number of old men, seated in a row, each holding his prostate in a jar on his knees. But, despite this weighty evidence, there is little to suggest that McGill ever removed the whole prostate gland of set purpose. In nine of the twelve cases which he published, the amount of material removed is likened to a walnut, a bean, or a pea, and only one of his specimens, preserved in the museum of Leeds University, is a complete gland.[10]

McGill died from diabetes in November 1890, at the early age of forty-three. In the same month Belfield, of all people, attacked the suprapubic operation. Some eighty cases were known to him; 'in nearly one-third of the cases on record the radical operation failed to restore voluntary urination'. Surgeons now started to turn to the route suggested by Fergusson, the perineal approach commonly used in lithotomy. In 1873 J. W. S. Gouley of New York devised, but apparently never practised, a formal operation of this type, and in 1889 O. Zuckerkandl of Vienna actually removed the whole gland through a perineal incision. This is probably the first total prostatectomy. The perineal operation was perfected by H. H. Young of Baltimore and is still popular in America.

In 1893 treatment of the enlarged prostate underwent a dramatic change. That year the American Professor J. William White strongly advocated castration as a means of 'shrinking' the gland, on the analogy that removal of the ovaries will cause regression of uterine fibroids in the female. Peter Freyer, writing in 1901, remarks 'one of the most remarkable effects of castration is the decided improvement in the symptoms that sets in in many cases a few hours after operation.' This is interesting, because castration does not relieve the symptoms of an enlarged prostate. Apparent success was due to the fact that some of these were not simple, benign, glandular enlargements but were undiagnosed cancers of the prostate. The modern and very successful treatment of prostatic cancer depends upon the same principle; the patient is given the feminizing hormone, oestrogen.

For seven years attempts at prostatectomy were virtually abandoned. Then, on 1 December 1900, Peter Johnson Freyer of St Peter's Hospital for Stone in London performed his first 'total extirpation of the prostate', using the suprapubic route. The patient, a man of sixty-nine, made an excellent recovery and was shown by Freyer to be in perfect health at a meeting held in London on 26 June 1901.[11] By 1904 Freyer had performed 107 operations with ten deaths, only four of his patients being under sixty years of age.

After some opposition, Freyer's prostatectomy came into general use and reversed the revolution effected by White's suggestion of castration. But his operation was not a very good one, being to all intents a blind removal. He used a small incision and, with one finger in the rectum to steady the gland, enucleated the prostate with the fingers of his other hand, keeping one nail specially sharpened for the purpose. 'It is astonishing through what a comparatively small suprapubic wound a very large prostate can be delivered,' he wrote.[12] The blind operation resulted in a good deal of sepsis and, in a large number of cases, dangerous bleeding after the patient had been returned to bed. Many surgeons remarked on the strange fact that this bleeding did not occur immediately after the prostate had been removed, but came on an hour or two later. We now understand that the blood pressure had been lowered by shock and that bleeding did not start until it rose again.

Sir John Thomson-Walker of St Peter's and King's College Hospitals reported that 1,276 Freyer operations had been performed at St Peter's between the years 1901 and 1918. Of these, 104 or just over 8 per cent had died. 'It is not my object to decry a procedure so patently successful,' he wrote. 'My idea is that improvement may be made even in this successful operation.' Thomson-Walker turned the blind Freyer method into a much better operation by means of a larger incision, a specially designed instrument to retract the wound edges, and stitches or slings inserted at the brim of the cavity from which the prostate had been removed. This is an example of the kind of obvious and simple improvement which, in all branches of surgery, helps to change a dangerous operation into a safe one. The much wider exposure enabled Thomson-Walker to control bleeding points at the time and to remove shreds of damaged tissue which, as we saw in the last chapter, are breeding places of infection. In the eleven years 1919–29 Thomson-Walker performed 472 prostatectomies for simple enlargement of the gland with a mortality of 5·2 per cent.[13] A very similar and equally good operation was devised by E. S. Judd of the Mayo Clinic in 1917.

In 1927 S. Harry Harris of Sydney, Australia, started to perform a somewhat different operation, more difficult but more successful than the Freyer or Thomson-Walker. The essentials were, or are, complete control of bleeding by suture and obliteration of the cavity left after removal of the gland. In a series of 371 cases between 1927 and 1932 Harris experienced ten deaths, a mortality of only 2·7 per cent.

Wilson H. Hey of Manchester advocated an operation which he called 'aseptic suprapubic total prostatectomy' in 1945, and claimed that it was the simplest, easiest and safest method yet devised. Also in 1945 Terence Millin, then of All Saints' Hospital, London, introduced a quite new approach in which the prostate was not removed through the bladder but by an incision made into the space which lies between the bladder and the pubic bone.[14] Known as the retropubic operation, it is perhaps the method of choice in suitable cases today.

The one operation of lithotomy has therefore developed into a quite complex series of techniques. And this is not all, for the removal of stones from the bladder led to operations on the ureters and on the kidneys. There is a legend that the Italian surgeon Domenico Marchetti successfully extracted a stone from the kidney of an English consul named Hobson in 1633. The first man to remove a kidney itself (nephrectomy) was an American, E. B. Wolcott, in 1861. He had set out with the idea of performing an entirely different operation, and his patient died fifteen days later. The first to remove a kidney successfully and of set purpose was Gustav Simon of Heidelberg on 2 August 1869. Simon used no antiseptic precautions at all and it is not surprising to learn that his next nephrectomy, in 1871, died of pyaemia.[15]

There is no space to describe the histories of the many other operations and examinations which make up the operative work of the urological specialist, but it will be convenient to end this section with a few notes on the development of radiotherapy, which is particularly well demonstrated by changes in the technique of treating bladder cancer. The first attempts to remove new growths of the bladder were by an Englishman, Warren, in 1761, and by P. J. Desault of Paris who twisted off a cancer with forceps when performing lithotomy. In 1875 Billroth removed a bladder tumour by the suprapubic route, and in 1877 Professor G. M. Humphry of Addenbrooke's Hospital, Cambridge, excised a new growth from the bladder of a twenty-one-year-old man by a lateral lithotomy incision.[16] The lad recovered after two months of intense agony, barely controlled by three grains of morphia a day (half a grain of morphia is a large dose). Removal of that part of the bladder invaded by growth (partial cystectomy) began to come into use during the early years of the twentieth century through the work of Bastianelli in Italy, Hurry Fenwick in England, and Gardner, Watson, and W. J. Mayo in America.

In 1910 Edwin Beer introduced the important method of transurethral fulguration, which has been mentioned in connection with the prostate; this is still commonly used for the simple type of bladder growths known as papillomata. Also in

1910 the French pioneer of radium therapy, Henri Dominici, advocated the burying of radium into the substance of a bladder cancer through a suprapubic incision. The American W. F. Braasch advised 'dropping' radium into the bladder, rather than implanting it into the tumour, in 1918, while H. H. Young and W. A. Frontze of Baltimore devised a special instrument for passing radium per urethram under direct vision in 1919.

Radium is scarce and costly. In 1900, before Marie Curie had isolated radium salts, Lord Rutherford demonstrated that radioactive emanation can be collected from strongly radioactive solids. G. Failla of America 'bottled' radium emanation in glass capillaries, and these unprotected tubes were used to a certain extent in surgery after 1921. The International Committee on Chemical Elements advised substitution of the name 'radon' for 'radium emanation' in 1923. Three years later Joseph Muir of New York started to use capillary glass tubes of radon encased in platinum to prevent too powerful an action; these are 'radon seeds'. In 1934 B. S. Barringer of New York, who had been a staunch supporter of radium therapy in the treatment of bladder cancer since 1917, advocated that as much as possible of the tumour should be removed and radon seeds be inserted into the invaded bladder wall. Cystoscopic implantation of radon seeds followed, largely through the work of H. H. Young.

Radioactive fall-out engendered by nuclear fission suggested the use of cheaper radioactive isotopes in place of the costly emanation and salts of radium. During the years 1946–50 J. S. Mitchell and W. V. Mayneord worked with the metals tantalum and cobalt. In 1951–2 Professor D. W. Smithers and his colleagues at the Royal Cancer (Royal Marsden) Hospital investigated tantalum and gold. The result of these investigations was the introduction of radioactive tantalum wire, in the form of 'hairpins', as a substitute for radium, and of radioactive gold, in the form of 'grains', as a substitute for radon seeds. A repeater 'gun' for the introduction of these grains into the tissues was designed by H. J. Hodt in 1951.

Gold grains do not appear to have been used in the human patient until 1955 when R. C. Ledlie of the Royal Marsden Hospital implanted them in a case of cancer of the stomach. In the same year they were used for treatment of cancer of the lung and of the bladder. Radioactive cobalt or caesium 'bombs' are another means of treating cancer on the same principle.

The treatment of bladder cancer now consists of excision in suitable cases combined with implantation of small seeds of a metal that has been rendered radioactive by exposure to the emanation of an atomic pile. It is of interest that we here see the first influence of the atomic age upon surgery. And so we must end this section on urology, for we have left history behind and are fumbling into the future.

Urology has been described with special reference to the evolution of operative techniques; just as many and as important operations have added to the usefulness of orthopaedic surgery. Although a few of these advances will be mentioned, the history of the speciality will here be told with the emphasis upon the development of a service, which started with the bone setter and has grown into the centre for treatment and rehabilitation of persons who would otherwise be crippled.

The English bone setter acquired his special skill because England is a seafaring nation. No doctors were carried in the Merchant Service; sprains, dislocations, fractures had to be dealt with by an ordinary member of the crew who had attained, or who pretended to have attained, some ability in their treatment. The loblolly boy and the surgeon's mate of the Royal Navy learned the tricks of the trade from the ship's surgeon who, be it remembered, was himself not infrequently recognized rather than trained. Such men found that they could supplement their incomes in retirement by manipulating the limbs of their neighbours. Few of them depended upon bone setting for their livelihood; the village blacksmith, a farmer, his shepherd, any of these and many others might engage in the craft as a profitable sideline.

There were, too, many bone setters who passed their art down through properly indentured apprentices, and there was a distinct tendency for the trade to be familial; among known families to have practised bone setting for several generations are those of Hutton, Thomas, Taylor, Crowther, and Mason. Women often became as proficient as their brothers; Sally Mapp, sometimes known as Mrs Mabbs, proved so much in demand that the town of Epsom paid her a retaining fee to live there in the eighteenth century. When she visited London to attend the quality at a well-known coffee house, she drove in a magnificent coach and four with liveried footmen and postillions. Nearly a century later Ann Thomas, one of the four daughters and three sons of Richard Evan Thomas who all practised bone setting, carried her art across the Atlantic and became renowned for her skill when she settled in Wisconsin.

Some of them, living in country districts, usefully undertook duties which the qualified practitioner, bound by the ethics of his profession, could not contemplate. The successful horse-doctor often applied his knowledge of animal disabilities to man; equally the bone setter, having learned upon the relatively valueless human being, found himself called in by the squire to advise upon the treatment of an expensive beast. His training – such as it was – stood him in good stead when it came to the treatment of animals, for he relied almost solely upon sense of touch. The patient's history or the symptoms of disease meant little or nothing to him; his hands showed him that the bones were or were not in the right places, that a joint was either too freely mobile or too firmly fixed, that the covering skin was hot or cold.

He tried to correct deformities by manipulations, irons, splints, and bandages stiffened with various gums and starch. Until about the middle of the nineteenth century he commonly set fractures and reduced dislocations but, as the surgeon took over more of this part of his practice, he contented himself with treating the after-effects caused by injury, disease – or surgery – with exercises and rubbings. The wise man never touched a 'hot joint', for he had learned from experience that inflammation is best left at rest. There existed a solid core of skilful practitioners who did much good work in their limited field. But there were also a number of true 'quacks' who brought bone setting into disrepute by advocating their rubbings and manipulations as a cure for every kind of disease.

The bone setters flourished alongside and often worked in conjunction with the medical profession. Just as the modern orthopaedic surgeon sends his patient to a masseur and – occasionally – advises him to consult an osteopath (all three of these are descended from the bone setter) so the nineteenth century surgeon frequently referred patients to his unqualified rival. It is well to remember that, although rivalry existed, there was also co-operation. William Cheselden wrote that he recommended a patient 'not knowing how to cure him myself' to a bone setter, Mr Presgrove of Westminster. Presgrove's treatment was not very successful. 'After this, having another case of this kind under my care,' wrote Cheselden 'I thought of a much better bandage, which I had learned from Mr Cowper, a bone setter at Leicester, who set and cured a fracture of my own cubit when I was a boy at school.'

Because the two professions existed side by side and were in some part complementary to each other, it is difficult to fix an exact date for the emergence of an orthodox speciality. There is a train of events which leads back to Georg Friedrich Louis Stromeyer of Hanover and he is often named the father of orthopaedic surgery. His work was 'orthopaedic' in the correct sense of the word; he straightened or corrected the deformities of children. The tale starts with an operation.

In 1816 and again in 1823 Delpech of Montpellier attempted to cure the deformity of club-foot by the operation of tenotomy, cutting of a tendon. On both occasions he used an open operation; that is, he made a quite large incision in the skin, dissected out the tendon, and cut it. We must presume that on both occasions something went wrong, probably the wound became infected, for Delpech concluded that open tenotomy was an unjustifiable operation. Club-foot must be treated by irons or by repeated and very painful manipulations which rarely did any good.

Stromeyer, born the son of a surgeon at Hanover in 1804, set up in practice as a surgeon with a special interest in the treatment of deformities of joints and bones. In 1830 he started a small hospital at Hanover for the prolonged care that this type of work entailed. A few months before this he accepted as a patient a boy of fourteen who suffered from a club-foot; after eighteen months of unavailing manipulations, Stromeyer decided to perform tenotomy as a last resort. He used a quite different method from that of Delpech; instead of making a wide incision, he slid his knife under the skin and cut the tendon by sense of touch and not under vision. This was the first subcutaneous tenotomy, and the start of a number of different 'subcutaneous' operations. The disadvantage of such operations lay in the fact that they were blind and damage might easily be done to nerves or blood vessels; the advantage was the much lessened risk of infection, for the resilient skin acted as a cleaning rag to the knife as it passed through. Stromeyer was then able to manipulate the foot into a correct position; by doing this gradually he obtained not only straightening of the foot but also reunion of the cut tendon ends. The operation was successful; all trace of deformity had disappeared at the end of eight weeks. The happy outcome of this case led Stromeyer to believe that subcutaneous tenotomy would provide a surgical answer to many problems of misshapen or deformed limbs and even of curved spines, which the bone setters attempted to treat by forceful manipulation but so signally failed to cure.

We now turn to William John Little, who was born in 1810, qualified MRCS in 1832, set up in practice at Billiter Street, London, and applied for the post of surgeon to the London Hospital without success. Little then decided to forsake surgery for medicine and went to Germany to study for the doctorate of medicine of Berlin. He suffered from a club foot, probably the result of being attacked with poliomyelitis when two years old. His disability had been treated by bone setters with the usual rubbings and manipulations, but to no avail. Rather naturally he was particularly interested in this deformity; he made it the subject of his thesis for the doctorate and closely studied the anatomy of the foot. He came to the conclusion that clubbing of the feet was not caused by deformed growth of bone, as had previously been thought, but by disordered action of the muscles. It seemed to him that Stromeyer's reported operation, although opposed by the majority of surgeons in Germany, England, and France, had a rational basis.

In July 1836 Little entered Stromeyer's small hospital at Hanover. Stromeyer performed his operation of subcutaneous tenotomy on Little with complete success. Little stayed on in Hanover to familiarize himself with Stromeyer's technique, then went back to Berlin where he read his thesis on *The Nature and Treatment of Club Foot* and received his degree. He showed his straightened foot to the well-known surgeon Dieffenbach, who was so impressed that he performed the operation no less than one hundred and forty times in little over a year. Little returned to London in 1837 and did his first subcutaneous tenotomy on February 20. This was not the first time in England; Whipple, a Plymouth surgeon, had read of Stromeyer's work and had successfully tried his method in 1836. Like Stromeyer, Little became a firm advocate of tenotomy and published books on the subject in 1839 and 1844.

In 1838 Little founded the Orthopaedic Institution which, five years later, became the Royal Orthopaedic Hospital, and, in 1909, merged with the National Orthopaedic and the City Orthopaedic to form the Royal National Orthopaedic Hospital. W. J. Little's elder son, aptly named Louis Stromeyer Little, and his younger son E. Muirhead Little were both surgeons on the staff. But W. J. Little, although he may properly be called the father of English orthopaedic surgery, was not himself a surgeon; in 1840 he realized his ambition of being appointed to the staff of the London Hospital – as a physician.

The next character, and a strange one, in this tale of a developing speciality is John Hilton of Guy's Hospital, who was born in 1805 and died in 1878. Hilton delivered a course of eighteen lectures on *Rest and Pain* at the Royal College of Surgeons in 1860–2. These lectures, afterwards published in book form, are one of the classics of surgery and were to have a profound effect upon orthopaedic practice. The lectures are remarkable in themselves but become still more remarkable when the character of the man who wrote them is taken into account. John Hilton was outwardly a very ordinary type of man, a mid-Victorian scientific surgeon who accepted the evidence of experiment but had not the originality to devise experiments himself. He cannot have been a pleasant person; overbearing, rude, bitingly sarcastic. He had none of the appearance of a deep thinker, but looked more like a prosperous and self-satisfied shopkeeper or business man of the City. It seems that he departed from the strictly orthodox only in a liking for highly coloured waistcoats and vulgarly ostentatious gold watch chains. Yet his lectures reveal that beneath this very ordinary, somewhat repellent exterior there lived a creative spirit, an artist in words.

'Pain the monitor and Rest the cure.' This is the basis and the constantly recurring theme of Hilton's teaching. To take a simple example, a piece of grit in the eye will cause pain and spasm of the surrounding eye muscles. If the grit is removed, the

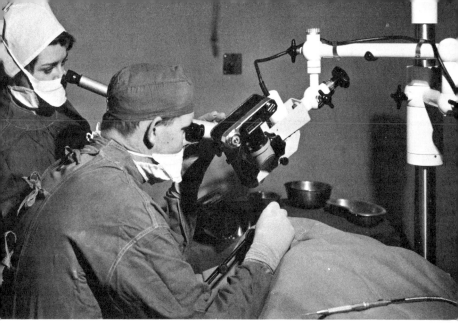

Operation on the ear under a Binocular Microscope (1967). The assistant can watch down the lens of the sidearm. Notice the drill in the foreground (used for cutting away bone) and the very simple instruments required.

A very early diagnostic X-ray apparatus (February 1896). The X-ray tube can be seen above the patient's ankle, and the screen, on which the bones will appear, beneath his leg.

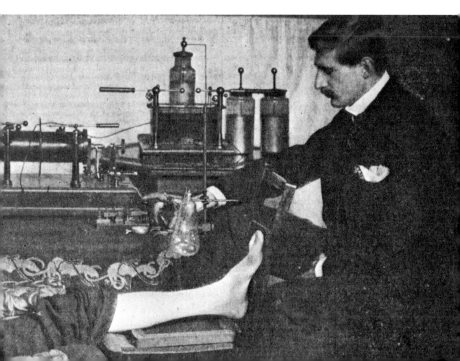

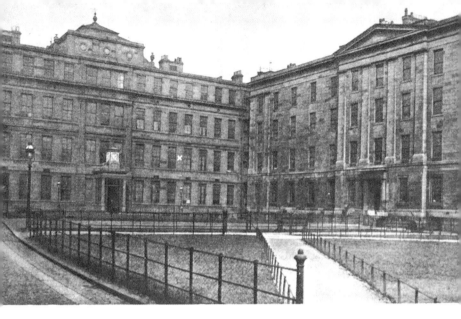

The New Surgical Hospital and the Fever Hospital of the Glasgow Royal Infirmary about 1890. Lister's wards are marked by white crosses. He first used his antiseptic method in the lower ward, Number 24. This historic building was demolished shortly after the First World War.

A culture-plate showing the dissolution of staphylococcal colonies in the neighbourhood of a penicillium colony. From Alexander Fleming's paper on Penicillin in the *British Journal of Experimental Pathology*, June 1929.

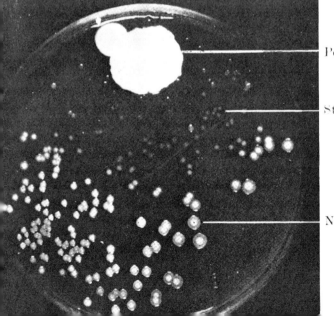

Penicillium colony.

Staphylococci undergoing lysis.

Normal staphylococca colony.

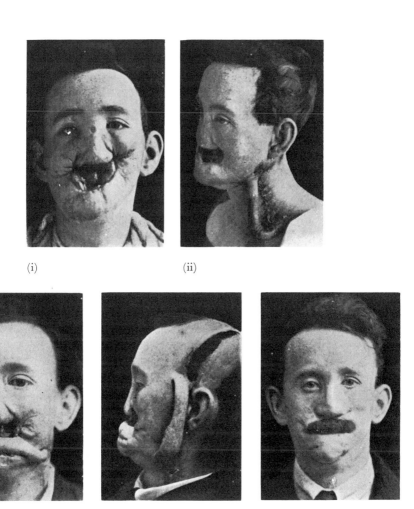

(i) (ii)

(iv) (v)

Skin grafting of a First World War casualty by means of tube flaps

  i   Total loss of the upper and lower lips 18 August 1917.
 ii   Tube flap formed from skin of the neck.
iii   Tube flap swung into position to restore the lower lip.
 iv   Remnant of the first flap has been joined to a second flap taken down
      from the scalp.
  v   The end result on 28 December 1919. The remnant of flap 1 forms
      the inner side of the upper lip. Flap 2 taken from the scalp forms the
      outer lip surface and enables the patient to grow a moustache.

The first Antiseptic Field Dressing (1878). The antiseptic used was salicylic acid, not carbolic. This dressing incorporates the famous triangular bandage, so commonly used in first aid.

A Listerian operation showing use of the Carbolic Spray. The surgeon and his assistant always work with their hands in the cloud of carbolic which is directed at the wound. The wound is surrounded with carbolic soaked towels. Instruments are taken from and returned to a bowl containing 1:20 carbolic lotion which also stands in the carbolized mist.

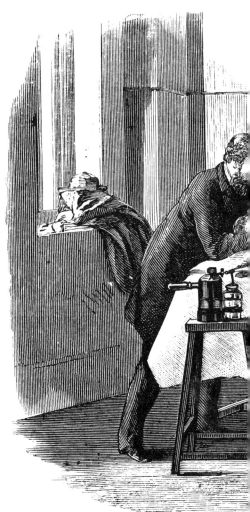

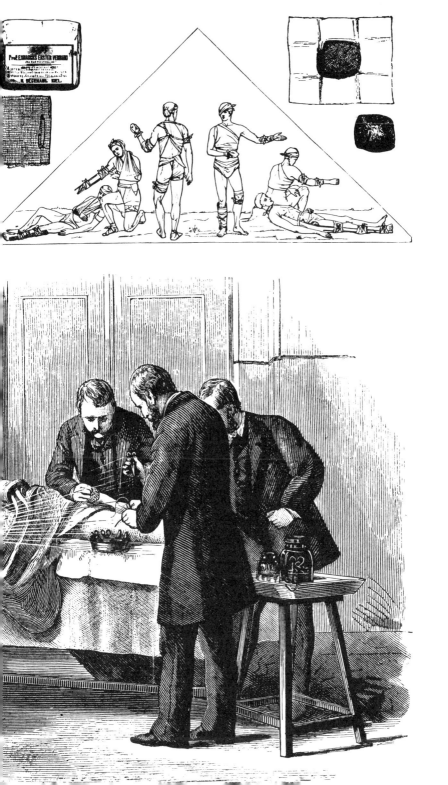

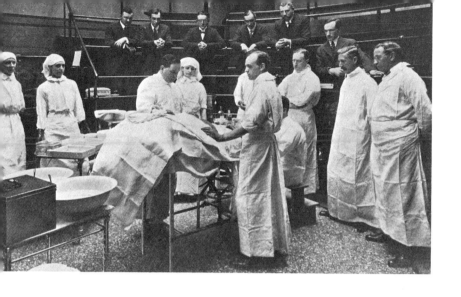

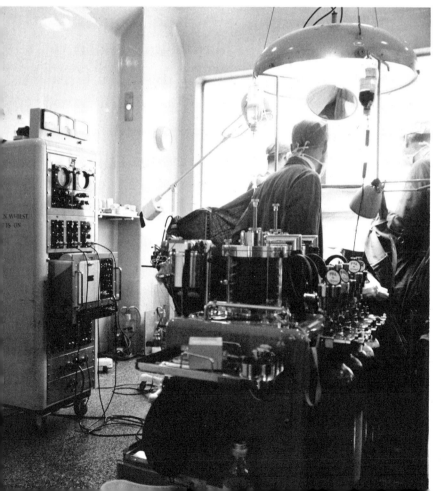

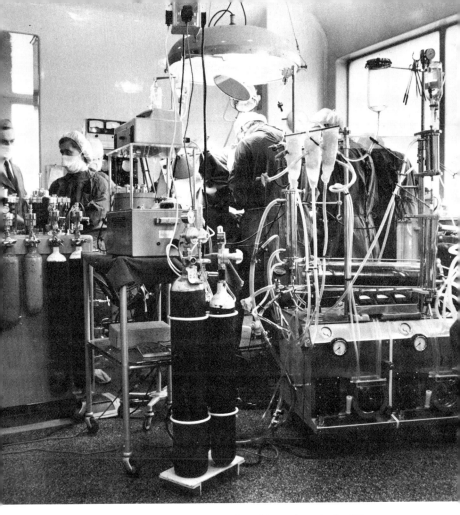

An operation upon the open heart under profound hypothermia (1966).
In the foreground is the Melrose pump which supplies oxygenated blood and thus allows the heart to be 'cut out of the circuit'. Oxygen supplied from the large cylinders. Behind the cylinders is the apparatus for cooling the supplied blood. The monitor for the patient's heart beat and blood pressure can be seen behind the cooling apparatus. Notice the anaesthetist (in spectacles) watching the operation in the mirror.

(*opposite above*) Sir John Bland Sutton (bending down to the patient) operating in the old theatre of the Middlesex Hospital in 1914. The theatre was built about 1890, with room for 100 spectators in the galleries. Notice the absence of masks and caps although an 'aseptic' technique is being used.

(*opposite below*) Modern theatre equipment. A shadowless lamp fitted with mirror to allow the anaesthetist to see the operation site. Under the mirror, a blood transfusion. Additional lights to left and right. In foreground, a respirator or ventilator for giving the anaesthetic and for automatically inflating the patient's lungs. Against the wall, a monitor which automatically records the patient's blood pressure and heart-beat. The trailing wires over the floor are a problem which will be solved one day!

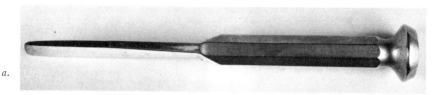

a.

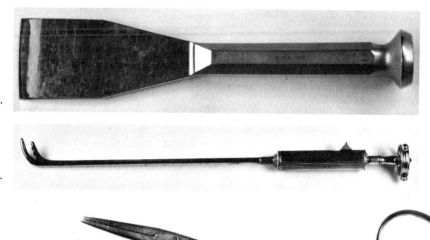

b.

c.

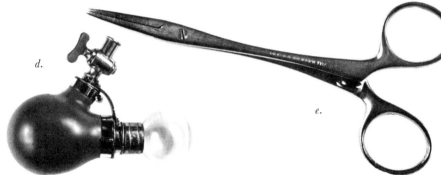

d.

e.

HISTORIC INSTRUMENTS STILL IN USE

a. and b. Osteotome. Devised by William Macewen of Glasgow in 1878. This is the first 'aseptic' instrument, made of polished steel so that bacteria could find no lodgement. The instrument shown has been slightly modified in shape, but the principle remains the same.

c. Lithotrite for crushing stones in the bladder. This instrument, used today, was devised by Sir Henry Thompson of University College Hospital in 1860. But the principle is the same as that of Civiale and Weiss, dating back to 1835 and 1820.

d. Evacuator for removing crushed fragments of stone from the bladder. Devised by H. J. Bigelow of Boston, U.S.A., in 1878. The instrument shown is a modification by Sir Peter Freyer.

e. Haemostat devised by Thomas Spencer Wells in 1872. Known as 'Wells forceps' or 'Spencers', these are the most commonly used instruments in surgery today. Indistinguishable from the original.

pain and spasm will cease; it is therefore the surgeon's duty to remove the grit. But the grit may have caused superficial damage; such damage is best cured by resting the eye with a pad and bandage. 'The surgeon will be compelled to admit that he has no power to repair directly any injury.' wrote Hilton. 'It will induce him to acknowledge, in all humility, that it is the prerogative of Nature alone to repair the waste of any injury. He will thus realize that his chief duty consists in ascertaining and removing those impediments which obstruct the reparative process or thwart the effort of Nature, and thus enable her to restore the parts to their normal condition.' Pain is therefore a pointer to the need for surgical intervention; by removing the cause, by maintaining a limb in a pain-free position, perhaps by tenotomy, even by cutting the nerves. The cause of pain having been removed, the cure can begin – and that cure consists of prolonged, absolute rest until Nature herself has treated the disability.

Hilton's teaching is important in itself but of still greater importance because it was put into practice by Hugh Owen Thomas, founder of the Liverpool school of orthopaedics. Thomas provides us with a direct, physical link with bone setting for, although medically qualified himself, he came of a line of bone setters. There is a story that his great grandfather, the first of the line, had been washed ashore from a wreck off the coast of Anglesey about the year 1730. Hugh's father, Evan Thomas, moved from Wales to Liverpool and, after near failure at the start, gained a reputation for his skill in treating fractures and dislocations. Although himself unqualified, Evan had the foresight – or the cunning – to apprentice all his sons to qualified practitioners. Hugh, born in 1834, was indentured to his maternal uncle, Dr Owen Roberts of St Asaph, studied at Edinburgh for three years and at University College Hospital, London, for one year, and qualified in 1858. He then became an assistant to his father, being later joined by his younger brother Evan. This strange partnership ended disastrously after only two years, when one of many notorious court actions opened the brothers' eyes to the fact that their primary duty was to act as respectably qualified cover for their unqualified father. They parted from him in anger; Hugh set up his plate two miles away in Hardy Street, Liverpool. In 1864 he married

Elizabeth, daughter of Robert Jones, and moved to a house in Nelson Street, retaining the Hardy Street house as a small hospital. 11 Nelson Street, occupied by three generations of orthopaedic surgeons, was destroyed, with all its relics and collections, during an air raid in May 1941.

Hugh Owen Thomas is best described as a character. Only five feet four inches in height, delicate looking but immensely strong, bearded, he wore at all times a seaman's peaked cap pulled at a rakish slant over his left eye, which had been injured in boyhood, and was never to be seen without a cigarette drooping from the corner of his mouth. An agnostic, a firm friend of Bradlaugh, brusque in speech, rude and often unnecessarily rough to his patients, he had no pleasure except in surgery; for thirty years he worked on seven days a week without a holiday. He paid no attention to his medical colleagues, save to decry their methods. Such was his withdrawal from orthodox medicine that the majority of his contemporaries, recalling his ancestry, thought him to be an unqualified bone setter, a mistake sometimes made today. He became immensely popular among the working classes of Liverpool, especially among the seamen, and at one time was medical officer to no less than twenty-eight trades unions and friendly societies.

Thomas had no use for the manipulations of bone setters and, we must remember, he possessed a greater knowledge of their practice than did most doctors. But equally he had little faith in the qualified surgeon. Excision of the joint aroused him to fury, despite the fact that he had studied under James Syme who, as we saw in the second chapter, was one of the first to advocate this type of surgery. Thomas argued that, if a diseased joint did not demand amputation of the limb, then that joint could be saved.

He treated fractures, dislocations, and many deformities with brute force. The fixed joints of a club foot were violently mobilized by means of a Thomas' wrench, a modification of an engineer's monkey wrench, still in common use. He dealt with old, badly-united fractures by a method of his own which he called 'damming, hammering, and dependence'. Dependence was simply extension by natural weight of the limb; hammering he carried out by percussion of the fracture site with a rubber covered mallet or sometimes by flagellation with a small leather whip; damming consisted of intermittent application of a narrow tourniquet so as to obstruct the venous and lymphatic circulation. He became particularly famed for his successful reduction of old dislocations; these affairs often developed into Homeric battles into which casual passers-by were drawn from the street to make counter-traction upon the patient while Thomas struggled with the dislocated limb.

So far his treatment has appeared the reverse of restful, but Thomas insisted that these violent manoeuvres were followed by a long period of complete rest. Like Hilton, Thomas claimed that no amount of rest could harm a joint, except for a transient muscular stiffness which would pass off as soon as the limb was freely used. Hilton advised splinting of the affected joint only, but Thomas went further; the entire limb must be placed at rest. He treated the tuberculous hip joint with a splint reaching from the arm pits to the foot, and his splint for a tuberculous knee stretched the full length of the leg. He never manipulated these or other infected joints but submitted them to prolonged rest alone.

Thomas devised his own splints, having them made in a workshop at Nelson Street by a saddler and blacksmith. He rarely used plaster of Paris, which had been introduced in 1851 by Mathijsen of Brussels, because he thought it interfered with healing by compressing the circulation at the site of fracture. He also discarded the old-fashioned wooden splint, finding that malleable wrought iron, covered if necessary with leather, could be shaped far more easily to the limb. Thomas had patterns of splints but no such thing as a 'standard' – he would have been the despair of a modern National Health Service bureaucrat – and he made or refashioned every appliance to the need of the individual patient, carefully attending to the fitting himself. He then sealed the straps of the splint with his signet ring, and woe betide the patient if his seal was not intact at the next attendance.

Thomas wrote a number of books dealing with the theme of rest. He expressed himself forcibly and in lucid English, but he had little influence upon his generation. Three reasons contributed to this immediate failure. Firstly, his bone setting background made him suspect; secondly, the violence of his attacks upon contemporary ideas of treatment aroused equally violent opposition and so diverted attention from the real usefulness of his teaching. The third reason is a curious one. He had all three of his books privately printed and he seems to have been at no pains to circulate any of them. They accumulated in one room of his house until they reached the ceiling, and were later destroyed.

Hugh Owen Thomas died in 1901. We have seen that he married Elizabeth, the daughter of Robert Jones. Elizabeth had a brother 'a feckless journalist' who begat a son named Robert. Hugh Thomas' nephew by marriage, Robert Jones, is the next link in the story. Born in 1857, he became his uncle's pupil and his disciple. Through Jones the medical profession learned of Thomas' methods.

Robert Jones, having been elected surgeon to the Stanley Hospital, Liverpool, in 1881, was appointed surgeon to the Manchester Ship Canal in the same year. The canal was in process of construction and the number of accidents gave Jones ample opportunity to test out his uncle's technique. More than that, he set up an organization for the treatment of injury which provided a small-scale plan for the much greater work that he was later called upon to do. In course of time the Manchester Ship Canal experiment evolved into the modern accident service.

Some twenty years later Jones became involved in an equally important experiment. Hospitals or institutions for cripples had existed for many years. Orbe in Switzerland was founded by J. A. Venel, well known for his work on curvature of the spine, in 1788; others were started in Germany, France, Holland, Italy, Denmark, and Russia; one of the oldest is the Orthopaedic Hospital, Birmingham, founded in 1817. These places were much like the chronic sick infirmaries of thirty years ago; the inmates received proper food, attendance, and nursing but little was done in the way of treatment or encouragement. In 1887 two nurses, who had trained at the Children's Hospital, Great Ormond Street, opened a small hospital, later called the Queen Alexandra, at Rhyl. The principles of treatment depended upon rest – naturally, since Hugh Owen Thomas became honorary consulting surgeon – fresh air, and happiness.

A very remarkable woman, Agnes Hunt, trained at Rhyl as a nurse; she found herself more than impressed with the treatment and with the happy atmosphere of the place. Herself a cripple from childhood, she had a particular sympathy with the crippled child. In October 1900 she opened her own small hospital at Baschurch in a derelict farm house with defective drainage, and a bank account chronically in the red. Four years later Agnes Hunt suffered from increasing pain in her hip joints and went to consult Robert Jones at Liverpool. That year Jones performed his first operation at Baschurch – in the dining room by candlelight – and from that time on he attended the hospital regularly until almost the day of his death. Here, too, Robert Jones first met G. R. Girdlestone, then a general practitioner at Oswestry, who acted as a kind of unofficial house surgeon to the hospital.

Working together in this curiously happy-go-lucky, haphazard experiment, Agnes Hunt and Robert Jones made a formidable partnership. The little cottage hospital expanded; from the Baschurch beginning there have derived nearly all the hospitals and homes for crippled children in England; Chailey in 1903, Pinner about 1907, Lord Mayor Treloar's Cripples Hospital at Alton (1908), Queen Mary's, Carshalton, in 1913 among others.

Until 1900 Robert Jones was quite unknown in Britain. Between 1881 and 1900 he published a number of papers, many of them translated into foreign languages, but his ideas commanded little attention at home. His colleagues at the Royal Southern Hospital, Liverpool, to which he had been appointed surgeon in 1889, regarded him simply as 'a good man with fractures', while in London the old taint 'someone related to bone setters' remained. For there was still no such thing as a speciality of orthopaedic surgery; St Bartholomew's Hospital had started the first orthopaedic department in 1864, but under the direction of a general surgeon; not until 1906 was an orthopaedic surgeon appointed as such to the staff of a teaching hospital; in that year Charing Cross elected H. A. Thomas Fairbank, the first purely orthopaedic specialist in Britain and one of the first in the world, who transferred to King's College Hospital after the First World War.

The First World War gave Robert Jones his chance. He was exactly the right age. Fifty-seven in 1914 and therefore too old for the exacting life of the front line, he was still young and active enough for service. He had, since 1900, acquired a considerable reputation in his limited field. Above all, he possessed a genial, patient, yet forceful character of the right type to make friends in high places and to get his ideas accepted. The retreat from Mons, the battles of the Marne and Aisne, made it clear within three months of the outbreak of war that casualties would be far higher than expected. Many of these men must be crippled or deformed for life unless lengthy treatment and rehabilitation could be instituted. Jones had the wit to see that here was not the simple tragedy of an individual but a massive social problem. Crippled soldiers were being discharged from the service 'unfitted either for military or civilian life,' he wrote, 'to become foci for seething discontent and a menace to successful recruiting'.

Early in 1915 the first orthopaedic centre was opened at Alder Hey, Liverpool, with Robert Jones in charge, assisted by T. Armour and T. P. McMurray. Jones was not content to remain in Liverpool but travelled widely, teaching, spreading his ideas, fighting for the enlargement of his scheme. In the front line he demonstrated that proper splinting at the earliest opportunity prevented shock and so saved lives. Compound fractures of the femur, which had previously been fatal in nearly 80 per cent of cases, now carried a mortality of some 20 per cent. Here Jones paid tribute to one of his uncle's most useful inventions. 'To what are we to ascribe this dramatic change?' he wrote. 'First and foremost to the recognition, too long delayed, of the value of the Thomas splint, and to its distribution to the regimental aid posts.'

Alder Hey proved immensely successful; as casualties increased, so new centres on the same lines were opened. The most famous of these started on its meteoric career in 1916. The Hammersmith workhouse at Shepherd's Bush (now the Royal Post-Graduate Medical School) became the Shepherd's Bush Military Orthopaedic Hospital with a complement of eight hundred beds, and is the ancestor of all present day rehabilitation centres. Here treatment and the primitive physiotherapy of the time was followed or varied by productive work at the lathe or in the carpenter's shop 'which fosters habits of diligence and self-respect, and converts indolent and often discontented patients into happy men who soon begin to feel that they are becoming useful members of society and not mere derelicts'. The occupational therapy of today depends upon exactly the same idea.

Some fifteen similar orthopaedic centres, providing over 30,000 beds, were opened in various parts of the country; the whole of this immense expansion was undoubtedly due to the genius of Robert Jones. They were training centres not only for the patient but also for the orthopaedic surgeon. Orthopaedic cases were segregated from all others; continuity of treatment by a single surgeon put a stop to indiscriminate surgery by casual practitioners accustomed to deal with the occasional accident in time of peace. So in these centres was born the science of orthopaedic surgery and the speciality matured in the urgency of war. Almost all of those who gained renown in the years after 1919 had been associated with Robert Jones during the years 1916–18. His influence spread to America, for twenty American surgeons came to serve under him in 1917. By the end of the war four hundred such had learned something of his methods.

The wartime orthopaedic centre developed into the peace-time fracture clinic and later, into the accident service. The first fracture clinic, or injury centre, is the organization set up by Jones for the workers on the Manchester Ship Canal in the years 1888–93. His very successful sowing did not bear an immediate harvest – few sowings do. Twenty years later, in 1912, a committee of the British Medical Association investigated the results of treatment of 3,000 fractures and found that there was malunion of the fracture in 40 per cent of cases. Even in the remaining 60 per cent of 'good' union, the functional results were often poor. It was an admission that treatment of fractures by relatively inexperienced doctors is unsatisfactory. During the war, Jones' system of carry-through supervision of each case by a single specialist proved its worth. Just after the war, Harry Platt persuaded his colleagues to allow him to hold fracture clinics at Ancoats Hospital, Manchester – certainly the first in Britain and probably the first in the world. His example was followed by Reginald Watson-Jones at the Liverpool Royal Infirmary; in 1922 Fairbank and St J. Dudley Buxton started the first fracture clinics in London. Other early examples are those of Leeds and Cardiff.

Accident services are a natural outcome of fracture clinics; though now extended to embrace the emergencies of poisoning, attempted suicide, and coronary thrombosis, the origin of these regional services lies in the specialized treatment of injury caused by accident in the home, in industry, or on the roads. Increase in horse-drawn traffic brought an increase of accidents; the motor-car, though probably no more lethal than the horse, produced a type of injury very similar to that inflicted by a high-explosive shell. But accident did not occur in the streets alone. As the Age of Steam progressed, more coal pits were opened and drove deeper underground; steam-powered factories sprang up almost daily in the industrial north and midlands; canals and railroads stretched a network across the country. All these brought an increasing toll of injury; from rock falls and explosion in the pits, from unguarded machinery in the factory, from the tragically common shunting accident or rarer collision on the railways. No organization existed to deal with these disasters and no attempt was made to re-habilitate the victims.

Just after the First World War, O'Neill Sherman, surgeon to the Carnegie (Illinois) Steel Trust in the United States, started a comprehensive accident service for the treatment and rehabilitation of employees who had sustained injuries at work. His scheme, based on the wartime organization of Robert Jones, included first-aid posts, casualty clearing stations, and hospital beds. In 1926 the Vienna Accident Insurance Company founded the first accident hospital for the treatment of injured workmen under the direction of Lorenz Böhler. In Britain the Delevigne committee, set up as the result of the successful fracture clinics in Manchester and Liverpool, made recommendations favouring the institution of special fracture services, but extending the scope to all injuries. 'We believe that the results of organized fracture treatment will lead to the adoption of similar measures for dealing with other disabling injuries,' said the report of 1937.

Experience gained in the Second World War, both at home and abroad, showed the need for organized treatment of all forms of injury. In 1943 the British Orthopaedic Association published a memorandum, prepared by its Fracture and Accident Services Committee under the chairmanship of

Watson-Jones, advising how such schemes should be put into practice. The opening of the Birmingham Accident Hospital in 1941 pointed the way for the development of a full accident service. This hospital came into being largely through the work of William Gissane, and may be regarded as the parent of the somewhat modified accident services now operating from hospitals throughout Britain.

Meanwhile, orthopaedic surgery had received academic recognition as a teaching speciality with the foundation of the Nuffield chair of orthopaedics at the University of Oxford in 1937. The first professor was G. R. Girdlestone who, as has been mentioned, came to know Robert Jones at Baschurch. Girdlestone was one of Jones' chief assistants during the 1914–18 war and, in 1917, became director of an orthopaedic centre at the Wingfield Hospital, Oxford. In June 1933 a new and enlarged Wingfield was opened through the generosity of Sir William Morris (Lord Nuffield). The Wingfield-Morris Orthopaedic Hospital is largely of Girdlestone's making and is the centre for the Nuffield professor. Girdlestone was followed in the chair by H. J. Seddon and by Joseph Trueta, whom we met in connection with the Spanish Civil War. Before the Second World War, chairs of orthopaedic surgery had been established at Manchester, where Harry Platt had formed an early department in association with Ancoats Hospital, and at Liverpool with T. P. McMurray as professor. McMurray was the last to live in that house which may justly be termed the home of orthopaedic surgery, 11 Nelson Street, previously occupied by Robert Jones and H. O. Thomas.

From the bone setter to the orthopaedic surgeon, the osteopath, and the physiotherapist; from Stromeyer's tiny venture at Hanover to the orthopaedic hospital; from Baschurch to the many homes for the education and treatment of crippled children; from wartime Hammersmith to the peacetime department of occupational therapy; from the Manchester Ship Canal to the fracture clinic and the accident service; here is a great expansion of social medicine rather than the development of a surgical technique.[17] Fractures, tuberculosis and osteoarthritis of the joints, loose bodies in the knee (originally described as 'joint-mice'), these and many more disabilities the orthopaedic surgeon treats by operation – and some of the operations have a long and fascinating history. But the development of the service is the most important part of the story and we must content ourselves with that.

CHAPTER 8

Surgery of Repair

All surgery is in part the surgery of repair, for the surgeon always repairs such damage as he has inevitably caused. In some types of operation the damage is trivial; if, for example, the simple fatty tumour known as a lipoma is excised, the removal of the tumour is the essential part and repair only consists of suturing the skin incision. In many procedures repair is the primary purpose and may be reinforcement of a weakened area or replacement of a deficient tissue. A parallel can be drawn between these techniques and the darning of a sock or mending of a broken window; in the former, the weakness is made good by suture with woollen thread; in the latter, a deficient tissue, the broken pane, is replaced by a new piece of the same material, a sheet of glass.

Many, but by no means all, of these operations are done by plastic surgeons, and here we shall first consider their art – for an art it truly is. 'Plastic' implies 'moulding', the rebuilding or remodelling of part of the damaged body to its undamaged contours. Plastic surgery does not mean skin grafting only; the surgeon rebuilds a structure with cartilage, fat, and bone as well as skin. There are many problems involved in the successful transplantation of these various tissues.

Plastic surgery in its present form is almost entirely derived from experience gained in the two world wars. The crux of that statement lies in the words 'its present form', for the art of plastic surgery has a very long tradition stretching back into the misty days of Chinese and Hindu medicine. One surmises that a great deal of the story – the successful replacement of a nose by a pig's snout or the Chinaman who kept a tame dwarf from whom he transplanted organs at will, for instance – belongs to the realm of mythology rather than to the serious history of medicine. There is, however, no doubt that Hindu practitioners successfully refashioned noses, the operation known as rhinoplasty. Disfigurement of the nose was commonly caused by disease or by punishment and, in both cases, the very obvious deformity called for repair. The Hindu surgeons dissected a flap of skin from the forehead, leaving it attached by the base above and between the eyes, and turned the free end down so as to cover the damaged area of the nose. This is known as a 'flap graft'.

In 1415 a different method of repairing noses was introduced by Antonio Branca which, over a century later, was taken up by Gasparo Tagliacozzi of Bologna, who wrote a treatise on the subject in 1597. Tagliacozzi did not take skin from the forehead; instead he raised a flap on the upper arm and sutured this to the nose, dividing the flap from the arm after union with the nose had taken place. It is interesting that he did not graft the nose at once; he raised the arm flap some time before the proposed grafting and sutured the cut sides. This was to ensure that the flap had time to develop an adequate blood supply before transposition. Tagliacozzi's method is known as a pedicle graft – a most important method of grafting today – and also as a delayed flap from the interval between preparation of the arm and transposition to the nose. Tagliacozzi formulated the law that a donor graft must never be detached until perfect union has taken place at the recipient site. He thus laid the foundation of modern skin grafting techniques and it is not surprising to find the term 'Tagliacotian' applied to this type of surgery in the nineteenth century.

Plastic operations on the face gained in popularity as a result of Tagliacozzi's work, but, because of the discomfort attending the prolonged period during which the arm was attached to the face, many surgeons returned to the method of taking a flap down from the forehead or else reversed the procedure, taking a flap up from the cheek. Flaps raised on the face entailed denuding one site to repair another or, as J. R. Wolfe of Glasgow later pointed out 'we cut the skin off the face to repair the face'. This objection, together with many disasters, due to failure of the skin to 'take' or to sepsis, brought plastic surgery into disrepute, so much so that it was altogether forbidden by the Paris faculty in 1788.

Despite this weighty decree, the art never fell wholly out of use. An Italian surgeon, Giuseppe Baronio, performed a quite large amount of experimental work upon animals, transplanting areas of skin from one site to another and from one animal to another. In 1804 he claimed to have successfully grafted a piece of sheep's skin on to man. Some type of grafting operation was also done by Eduard Zeis of Dresden, who is better remembered because he introduced the term 'plastic surgery' in 1838. Among many other surgical advances J. F. Dieffenbach of Berlin, mentioned in the last chapter, achieved good results when he grafted skin on to the injured lower eyelid, an operation also performed by another German, Karl von Graefe. Both these men worked in the first half of the nineteenth century. In his *Diary of a Medical Student* Shephard Taylor mentions that he saw skin grafted from the abdomen to a burned area on the wrist (1864). He calls this a 'Paliocotian' operation, an obvious mishearing of 'Tagliacotian', which suggests that the method used was the delayed pedicle graft.[1]

We cross the line from ancient to modern with the work of the Swiss surgeon Jacques Louis Reverdin in 1869. Reverdin avoided the use of large pieces of skin by what are called 'pinch' grafts. He picked up the surface of the skin with forceps and snipped the small area off with scissors; the pinch grafts were then pressed down at intervals over the site to be treated. Reverdin's method revived interest in skin grafting. The *Lancet* records that G. D. Pollock of St George's Hospital was the first to use the Reverdin graft in England (1871). Pollock's patient had suffered an extensive and deep burn of the right buttock and outer aspect of the right thigh; he made a good recovery after prolonged treatment.[2] In the same article it is reported that Cooper Forster of Guy's and Thomas Smith of St Bartholomew's Hospital had taken grafts of skin from newly amputated limbs and had transplanted them to other patients. Success here must have been a very lucky chance, for one of the difficulties of skin grafting is that only the autogenous graft, the patient's own skin, is reasonably certain of a successful 'take'.

Another difficulty in the treatment of surfaces denuded of skin, particularly burned areas, is that the fibrous tissue, by which the wound heals, is less elastic than is skin and also tends to contract. The small pinch grafts, sowed over the denuded site, took time to grow and to spread over the surface; where the surface was incompletely covered by the growing islands of graft, contracture by fibrous tissue usually occurred. In 1872 the French surgeon Louis Ollier, having noted that pinch grafts often failed to prevent contractures, modified the Reverdin graft by making it larger, hoping for more rapid spread. Ollier's modification was not appreciated at the time; it was left for an English surgeon, George Lawson of the Middlesex and London Ophthalmic Hospitals, to popularize the method by using Ollier grafts to cover large surfaces.[3] For this reason, Lawson is sometimes wrongly credited with this type of graft.

In 1875 J. R. Wolfe used a very similar graft to repair the eyelid. His patient, a twenty-five-year-old quarryman, had been involved in an explosion of blasting powder and had sustained injuries of the face, eyes, and eyelids. Wolfe successfully formed a new lower eyelid in three sections of a piece of skin, two inches long by one inch wide, taken from the forearm. The operation was done without anaesthesia and, so far as can be ascertained, without antiseptic precautions.[4] Wolfe repeated this type of operation on a number of occasions, but only around the eye. His technique came into more general use through the work of the German surgeon Fedor Krause, who successfully extended the method to other parts of the body in a large series of cases between the years 1893–6.

Reverdin's, Ollier's, and Wolfe's were all 'full thickness' skin grafts, that is, the donor area, however small in superficial size, was always entirely denuded of skin in depth. This is an obvious objection and, from the earliest days of the revival of plastic surgery, attempts were made to overcome it. In 1874 Karl Thiersch introduced his method of shaving sheets of skin, cut through only the superficial layer, so that the donor area would heal without scarring because the deeper, reproductive layer was left intact. The Thiersch graft at first met with little success; the paper-thin, wide sheets were awkward to manoeuvre and still more difficult to retain in place; they often failed to take because there was no effective method of holding them in firm contact with the recipient area; they had a fatal tendency to curl inwards so that portions were more often than not laid upside down. In addition to all this, the results were unsightly, for the deeper layers of skin were missing and the grafted area always appeared as more or less scarred. The Thiersch graft was, in fact, unsatisfactory for all but the most superficial injuries.

We now return to Louis Ollier. There is a certain doubt about the nature of his graft; he seems to have not appreciated that there is an essential difference between grafts of full thickness skin and grafts of only partial thickness. He undoubtedly used full thickness skin, but he also used grafts of partial thickness. As time went on and experience grew, surgeons tended to cut their 'Thiersch' grafts thicker, so that the deep regenerative layer remained in the donor area, but the donated graft was of sufficient thickness to be easily handled and to give a better cosmetic result. For this reason the modern 'Thiersch graft' is more properly known under the name 'Thiersch-Ollier'. In place of Thiersch's wide sheets, multiple grafts of postage stamp size are used, and the outer surfaces of these are fixed to paranet (tulle gras) which is open mesh fabric soaked in paraffin jelly. The true Thiersch graft, very thin and in small pieces, is used mainly to replace damaged mucous membrane at the lip edges and in the mouth, or to replace the fine skin of the eyelids. Thiersch grafts are also employed in the ingenious 'outlay' method devised by Gillies, Pickerill, and Waldron at Sidcup in 1918 to line cavities, such as wounds of the jaw inside the mouth. A mould of the cavity is first made with stent, a waxy material that can be softened in hot water but will retain its shape at body temperature; the mould is then covered with very thin skin, the inner surface facing outwards, and the covered mould inserted in the cavity. When the skin has taken, the mould is removed.

In 1914 the results of skin grafting were still by no means satisfactory and surgeons differed as to the best method. J. Staige Davis of Baltimore advocated a return to the Reverdin pinch graft in 1914 and again in 1929. Better methods of fixation and lessened risk of infection made a take more certain and the small Reverdin graft had the great advantage of rapid regeneration in the donor area. In 1930 Beverley Douglas of Nashville, USA, suggested that the greater area of skin should be transplanted to the recipient site and the lesser 'pinch grafts' left to regenerate skin at the donor area. This was the 'sieve graft' (the reverse of the Reverdin graft) in which small punched-out morsels of skin are left and the large perforated sheet transferred to the defect.

All the above methods, introduced since Reverdin first devised his pinch graft in 1869, suffered from one great disadvantage. They were all 'free' grafts, that is, pieces of skin cut from a leg or an arm and transferred to the damaged area. Their blood supply was interrupted and survival could not be certain until new blood vessels had grown in from the surrounding tissue. When it came to treating the gross injuries of the First World War, a more reliable type of graft became essential. This was found in a return to the Tagliacotian operation, but in a modified form, and resulted in the tubed pedicle graft, sometimes known as the bucket-handle or double-end graft. Here a rectangle of skin is raised, leaving both ends attached; the long free sides are then sewn together to form a solid tube of skin. The origin of this important graft is unknown. It was certainly used by Ceci and Putti in Italy at the beginning of the twentieth century, by W. Filatov of the Ukraine in 1917-18, and by Gillies at Sidcup from October 1917 onwards. Probably the form resulted from a general observation that skin will always curl inwards, which suggested the idea of making a tube. The tubed pedicle graft developed into the 'jump' graft, in which alternate ends are freed and reattached so that the blood supply is never wholly interrupted and grafts may be taken from a distance. The advantage of a tube or jump graft lies in its versatility; it may be turned on its long axis, attached to the recipient area by either end, and split to reform a single skin thickness. The disadvantage lies in the multiplicity of operations required; the simplest procedure entails at least two separate manoeuvres.

From the grafting of skin we pass to the grafting of bone. It is roughly true to say that skin will only take if donor and recipient are the same individual and it is certainly true that, whenever possible, all grafting material should be autogenous – from the person to be grafted. Skin cut at random from one human being and grafted into another – homogenous or homologous skin – will usually be treated by the recipient as a foreign body; it will be rejected and will die. Skin taken from another species of animal and grafted into a human being – heterogenous skin – will, practically speaking, always be rejected. In the case of bone this is not true. Heterogenous bone will not live; homologous bone may survive but with diminished viability; autogenous bone will live. But in no case will rejection be certain, for the bone, although dead, may act as a scaffolding along which the patient's own bone will grow to form new bone. It is therefore feasible to use bone grafts not only from other human beings but also from animals.

The possibility of grafting bone was first studied by Louis Ollier in 1858 and a certain amount of work was done on the subject in France and Germany during the next fifty years.[5] One of the more extraordinary operations in the history of surgery is that performed by William Macewen of Glasgow in 1879. Macewen was a remarkable man who added much to many departments of surgery. A disciple of Lister, a deep thinker, a brilliant operator, Macewen must at the same time have been one of the most difficult men ever born. He was the complete autocrat who lived his own life far above his fellow men.

Macewen was no specialist; we shall meet him again in other chapters. The operation of 1879 resulted from his interest in orthopaedic surgery. Osteotomy simply means the cutting of bone and is one of the basic techniques of orthopaedics; during the eighteen seventies osteotomy became a popular method of treating ankylosed joints, joints which have become fixed by growth of new bone. Macewen performed his first osteotomy in 1875, using a common mallet and chisel. Here it is necessary to make a short digression.

We must remember that, before 1878, the majority of bone surgery was done with ordinary carpenter's tools; chisels, mallets, gouges. When Lister first wired the broken patella, he used a carpenter's bradawl to bore the necessary holes in the bone. Macewen soon found that the straight edge of a chisel did not lend itself to accuracy in the cutting of bone; further, the wooden handle easily cracked, became contaminated, and caused infection. He had a special instrument made, bevelled on both sides, and marked in a scale of half inches. The whole of his 'osteotome' was of well-tempered, polished steel. 'They are finely polished,' wrote Macewen of his instruments, 'not for appearance, but because the finer the surface the less opportunity will organic matter have of becoming adherent and afterwards decomposing.'[6] The principle is of great importance in surgery. Macewen should be regarded as the first man to design a modern surgical instrument.

After this digression we can return to his operation. On 17 July 1878 a three-year-old boy named William Connell was admitted to the Glasgow Royal Infirmary suffering from osteomyelitis of the right humerus. On 17 August Macewen removed nearly the whole bone, including both the growing centres or diaphyses. The wound healed satisfactorily but the arm was, of course, quite useless. The boy's parents asked Macewen to amputate, but he persuaded them to allow him to attempt some improvement.

On 17 November 1879 Macewen performed osteotomy on a boy of six years old who suffered from bow legs. He removed two wedges of bone, cut them into small fragments with a chisel, and sowed these fragments along the groove or sulcus which had been formed by removing the humerus from the arm of the first boy. This first transplantation gave a new growth of bone one inch or so in length. On 1 February and 9 July 1880 Macewen made further transplants of bone which he had saved for the purpose from his osteotomy operations.

In March 1881 the bone chips had united to form a new mass stretching from the old upper end to the old lower end of the humerus and measuring six inches in length. The untouched left humerus measured six and a half inches. The child could lift his hand to his head and could make some use of his arm.

Macewen was able to follow up William Connell for over a quarter of a century. In 1909 he wrote: 'It is now thirty years since the humeral shaft was rebuilt and during the greater part of this period the man has depended upon his physical exertions for the earning of his livelihood. He worked as a joiner for many years and now is an engineer's pattern maker. His grafted arm has increased in length, but not proportionate to the increase of the sound one. The sound humerus is three inches longer than the other.'[7]

In 1912 Macewen successfully transplanted bone from dog to dog and believed that the grafted bone grew to form new bone. With this belief in mind, he used dog bone to fill a defect in the human skull. His idea worked, but the bone must have acted only as a scaffold, along which the patient's own bone could grow. Following on Macewen's work, Franz König of Göttingen used dead grafts of sterilized animal bone or ivory to repair defects. Specially prepared bone taken from a calf (a quite recent development) is now widely used in the United States.

In 1915 F. H. Albee of New York introduced his well-known Albee's graft, originally designed for the repair of damage caused to the vertebrae by tuberculosis. This is an autogenous graft taken from the shaft of the patient's tibia and sewn into a groove cut through several vertebrae above, below, and including the affected ones. At the beginning of the First World War, work on bone grafting was developed largely in Russia by three surgeons Nemiloff, Bashkirzeff, and Petroff, and in France where Mauclaire and Pierre Duval obtained good results. The successful repair of cranial injuries caused by shell-fire called for considerable ingenuity if a normal contour were to be retained. Autogenous grafts of living bone from the patient's own skull were out of the question. A. L. Ricard, following Macewen's example, tried heterogenous grafts, using the bone of a dog. Autogenous grafts were taken from the great trochanter of the femur by Mauclaire, from the curved surface of the tibia by H. Delagenière, and from the scapula by Leclerc. Another Frenchman, Kahle, made use of the natural curve of the rib by grafting portions across the defect.[8]

Cartilage grafts are a somewhat more difficult problem. They will 'take' but always tend to calcify and to form bone instead of cartilage. First attempted by the very distinguished Frenchman, Paul Bert, they were used by Franz König in 1896 as a purposive substitute for bone in repairing the skull. This largely experimental work was put to practical use by the French surgeon Morestin in February 1916 and by Villandre of Lyon in 1917. Morestin found that the best results were obtained with pieces of the patient's own rib cartilages.[9]

This has been a long and tedious explanation of the various methods tried out by surgeons in their attempt to repair damaged tissues. Until the First World War, plastic surgery was so rarely performed and so primitive that it can hardly be said to have entered its infancy. In the First World War, the need to repair gross injuries became acute; men survived their wounds but with features so shattered and distorted that a return to ordinary life was almost impossible. As so often happens, the need produced the man with the necessary vision and skill.

The name of Harold Delf Gillies is unquestionably that most renowned in the history of plastic surgery, not in Britain alone but in the world. He was born at Dunedin, New Zealand, in 1882 and came to London to study medicine, qualifying from St Bartholomew's Hospital in 1908. Until 1914 his special interest was in ear, nose, and throat surgery, but he joined the RAMC as an ordinary regimental medical officer shortly after the outbreak of war. The sight of the terrible facial mutilations caused by high explosive or bullet wounds quite appalled him; he realized that many of these men could never live a normal life again unless their faces were rebuilt, but he also realized that in the then state of surgery little or nothing could be done to repair the dreadful disfigurement resulting from the destruction, not of skin only, but of the underlying tissues and of bone.

Gillies heard of the work, chiefly grafting with bone, being attempted in Paris by Mauclaire and Pierre Duval among others. After considerable difficulty he obtained permission to study their technique; he saw that they were meeting with some success but that the endeavour was on far too small a scale. He found himself impressed not so much with what was being done as with what might be done. Gillies enlisted the help of William Arbuthnot Lane, then one of the most influential surgeons in England, and, largely through Lane, obtained official recognition as the first, indeed at that time the only, specialist in plastic surgery in the British Forces. As such, he was given charge of a few beds at the Cambridge Hospital, Aldershot, in January 1916.

It is, nowadays, difficult to appreciate that at this time there was no such thing as 'plastic surgery'; the speciality just did not exist. Nor could Gillies claim to be an expert; beyond the few operations that he had seen in Paris he had no knowledge of the subject whatsoever. In the words of his biographer, Gillies 'knew little of his subject, but surgical experience, his artistic temperament, his endless patience and boundless confidence carried him through'. He had, in fact, no very long surgical experience, for he had only been qualified six years in 1914, and perhaps the artistic temperament was the most important of the qualities mentioned by his biographer; Gillies had all the originality and the skill of an artist-craftsman, a creator, without which the essential improvisations of an entirely new technique could never have been transformed into established practice.

Neither sufficient space nor proper facilities existed at the Cambridge for the endless stream of facial injuries. Gillies realized that he could succeed only if provided with a special hospital. Treatment did not consist merely of repairing the damaged face; repair of the damaged mind was equally if not more essential. The morale of men who have suffered terrible disfigurement, who, for all the surgeon's skill, will never regain the facial contours that they have seen every morning in the shaving mirror, is at a very low ebb. Just as the crippled soldier must receive rehabilitation treatment before he can take his place in a civilian society, so the morale of the disfigured patient must be restored before he can face the outside world.

Once more Gillies turned to Arbuthnot Lane. Between them they persuaded the Red Cross to take over a large house and grounds at Sidcup, then in Kent but now in Greater London. Here was built the hutted hospital, first known as Queen's and later as Queen Mary's Hospital, Sidcup. Gillies set about gathering his helpers for, from the earliest days, he insisted upon team work in the true sense of the term; not 'Mr X and his team of surgeons' as in modern journalistic jargon – simply meaning the great Mr X and a train of assistants – but a team of specialists each having his own peculiar skill. As a large part of the repair of a face depends upon dental work, dental surgeons took their place beside the plastic surgeon, among them L. A. King and W. Kelsey Fry. Anaesthesia for facial injuries posed unusual difficulties, of which we shall have more to say later on; first R. Wade and then the two great anaesthetists E. S. Rowbotham and Ivan Magill solved the problems to the lasting benefit of the surgeon and his patient. Artists formed most important members of the team; Henry Tonks, Slade professor of fine art in the University of London and himself a fellow of the Royal College of Surgeons, sketched the various stages of re-construction to provide forecasts of the final result; models of the injury and of the restored contours were made by a sculptor, J. Edwards. Gillies himself undertook responsibility for the essential work of maintaining the patient's morale and preparing him for a return to civilian life. It is for this reason that so many of the patients at Sidcup became his devoted friends.

Injured soldiers came from all parts of the British Empire; probably because he was a New Zealander, Gillies tried to ensure that the wounded man was attended by someone from his own country; as the months went by an increasing number of Canadian, Australian, and New Zealand medical officers arrived at Sidcup to learn the methods of Gillies and to carry the art of plastic surgery over the world.

As practice and experience grew at Sidcup, so the principles underlying successful plastic surgery were evolved. The first of these was rigid asepsis, for infection is the cause of many failures. The second principle was the preliminary free exposure of all structures requiring repair; damaged tissue must be removed before new material can be grafted. The third principle was repeated operations. Each operation was carefully designed to attain a definite step towards the desired result, and no attempt was made to do more than one step at each operation.

The tubed pedicle flap was almost exclusively used for grafting skin. These flaps were made long and supple, generally some six inches in length by two and a half inches wide. Whenever possible they were taken from the chest or neck because fewer steps or 'jumps' are then required to bring the flap up to the face, but Gillies regarded it as essential that they should come from an unscarred area having a blood supply which had not been interrupted by injury. Only thus could a satisfactory take and clean healing be assured. Damage to the mucous membrane lined surfaces of the mouth and nose was repaired with Thiersch grafts, often by the 'outlay' method mentioned above, and Gillies took great care that the lip line, where thin mucous membrane meets the thicker skin, should be preserved. To repair damage to the jaws, autogenous grafts of bone were usually taken from the patient's iliac crest above the hip joint. Thus the injured face was rebuilt by tube grafting to restore loss of soft tissue, by outlays to line the mouth, and by transplants of iliac crest to repair bony defects. Destruction of areas of the body or limbs was, of course, also dealt with at Sidcup. By 1921 approximately ten thousand patients had passed through the hospital.[10]

Experience gained during the war ensured that plastic surgery emerged as an established speciality in the years of peace, with Harold Gillies as its chief exponent and greatest teacher. The men who had assisted him at Sidcup were also starting to make their names; of these one of the best known was T. Pomfret Kilner. After the war, Gillies was appointed plastic surgeon to St Bartholomew's and also to St James's Hospital, Balham; at the latter hospital he was joined by Rainsford Mowlem, who developed methods of bone grafting. In 1930 another New Zealander, Archibald McIndoe, who had taken up plastic surgery on Gillies' advice, was appointed to assist him at St Bartholomew's. The three men, Gillies, Mowlem, and McIndoe, made a team famous throughout the world.

If it be true that, during these inter-war years, the art of plastic surgery became slightly suspect – a suspicion that much of the work rightly belonged to the expensive beauty parlour rather than to the operating theatre – it is far truer that increasing experience, improved techniques, and widely spread teaching laid the foundations for the rapid expansion made necessary by the type of injury inflicted during the Second World War. On the outbreak of war in 1939 Gillies and Kelsey Fry organized a plastic surgical unit for treatment of jaw injuries at Park Prewitt Hospital, Basingstoke, while Archibald McIndoe took charge of a centre for the treatment of burns and injuries to the jaws and face at East Grinstead. Like Gillies in the First World War, McIndoe attached the greatest importance to restoration of morale as part of treatment, and, as with Gillies, many of his patients became devoted friends. The great success of McIndoe and his helpers made East Grinstead world famous as a centre of plastic surgery.

We mentioned above that tube grafts were used by two Italians named Ceci and Putti, and it is convenient to describe their work at this point. Hands, feet, and limbs are sometimes so mangled in accidents that they must be amputated, or they must be amputated because of disease. From the earliest times attempts have been made to provide some kind of a serviceable substitute for the member that has been lost. In the sixteenth century the great French surgeon Ambroise Paré employed armourers to make artificial limbs, because they were particularly well skilled in the fashioning of flexible articulations at the knee, elbow, and even the fingers in order that their armour should combine protection with the freest possible movement. On at least one occasion Paré fitted one of his patients with a 'mechanical' hand made to his design by a Paris armourer. This was, no doubt, a similar prosthesis to that worn by the German soldier of fortune, Götz von Berlichingen or Götz of the Iron Hand. Hieronymus Fabricius ab Aquapendente of Padua, better known as the teacher of William Harvey who discovered the circulation of the blood, described various substitutes for amputated limbs at the end of the sixteenth century. But the most common type of replacement remained the simple wooden peg-leg, which figures in so many pictures of ancient warriors, and the metal hook, perhaps more useful as an offensive weapon than as an artificial hand. Such 'artificial limbs' were attached to the amputation stumps by leather collars and straps; although better than nothing, they did not provide a very useful range of movement.

In the Italo-Abyssinian campaign of 1896, the victorious Abyssinians captured many Italian prisoners and, besides other less seemly amputations, frequently cut off their right hands. Such of these as survived the operation faced a grim future in their poverty-stricken country. The muscles of the forearm and the long tendons were still there, but they ended at the wrist; the muscles were still capable of activating the tendons, but the latter could be put to no useful purpose.

Quite a lot of work had already been done on tendons. If a muscle is damaged, it may be possible to free it from its tendon, to attach the tendon to another muscle, and to educate that muscle to do the work previously done by the damaged one, the operation known as tenoplasty. In 1881 Karl Nicoladoni, then of Vienna and afterwards professor of surgery at Innsbruck, tried to transplant the tendons of a patient who suffered from a paralysed foot after being attacked by poliomyelitis, but without success. Eleven years later B. F. Parrish of New York successfully performed much the same operation. Tenoplasty became the recognized means of treating some kinds of paralysis and, from 1897 onwards, was used by a number of surgeons, including Robert Jones and an American orthopaedist E. H. Bradford of Boston.

Meanwhile, in 1896, Professor Giuliano Vanghetti of Florence, anxious to do something for the unfortunate ex-prisoners of war of the Abyssinians, conceived the idea of using the muscles and tendon ends of the stump to activate the fingers of an artificial hand. It may be that he had read of the work of Nicoladoni or Parrish, or it may be that he developed the idea of his own accord. But the principle was the same as that of tenoplasty; to employ a useful tendon and to reeducate the muscle to perform an unaccustomed function. Vanghetti proposed to form 'clavae', as he named them, tendon ends dissected out and covered with tubes of skin. Two clavae would then be joined together to form a loop from which a cord passed to a finger of the artificial hand.

Professor Vanghetti, a physician, was unable to put his plan into practice himself, although he published details of his proposed operation in 1899, calling it 'cinematic prosthesis'. At the time he failed to interest any surgeon, but he continued with his experiments. In 1905 Antonio Ceci published his first case of a Vanghetti operation, in which he had made use of tube grafts of skin to form the clavae. The work was taken up by Professor Vittorio Putti of Bologna in 1911; by the end of 1914 about twenty Vanghetti operations had been done, most of them in Italy. In 1918 the German surgeon Ferdinand Sauerbruch of Greifswald greatly improved the operation by introducing a glove type of artificial hand, depending for its movements upon the Vanghetti principle, which became known as the 'Sauerbruch arm' and was instrumental in returning many wounded soldiers to an active and useful life. 'Cineplastic prosthesis', as it is now called, reached a high standard of perfection in the Second World War through the work of R. Nisser and E. Bergmann of New York (1942) and has been carried on by H. H. Kessler of Newark, New Jersey, among others.

So far we have dealt only with the reconstruction of injured tissues, but operations of repair are commonly performed upon congenital malformations or defects. One of these is the cleft palate and hare lip, which often occur together. The point of interest here is that in both these congenital deformities the type of repair of today is based on an operation introduced more than a century ago. Karl von Graefe of Warsaw devised his method for the hare lip in 1825 and Germanicus Mirault repaired by a plastic flap in 1844, though it seems that he only operated on two patients. Mirault's flap operation was modified by William Rose of London at the end of the nineteenth century and by the American surgeons V. P. Blair and J. B. Brown in 1930.

It was comparatively easy to perform a plastic operation on the hare lip, but the closure of a cleft palate was more difficult; until fifty years ago people 'who had no roof to their mouths' often went through life unable to talk clearly and suffering from other disabilities. If the cleft was only in the back part of the palate, composed of soft tissue, it might be possible to pare the edges and sew the two parts together so that they would heal into one. But a cleft extending into the anterior, bony, hard palate demanded a more complicated operation. The first successful closure of a defect in both the hard and soft palate was by J. F. Dieffenbach in 1834; he made lateral incisions in the palate and brought the two halves together. Another German surgeon, Langenbeck, performed much the same operation in 1861, and it is still in use. William Fergusson introduced a number of improvements and became renowned for his success; he invented a special instrument, a gag to keep the mouth open, which is now a standard piece of equipment on the anaesthetic trolley or in the dentist's surgery. Another surgeon, Jonathan Mason Warren of Boston, devised his own operation in 1842. All these different methods added up to what has come to be known as the 'classical operation', usually given the name of Dieffenbach–Langenbeck–Warren in America and of Langenbeck–Fergusson in Britain.

William Arbuthnot Lane of Guy's introduced a somewhat different technique in 1897, but the operation itself is of less importance than the age at which it was done. Earlier surgeons delayed operation until the child had reached ten or twelve years; they taught that a co-operative patient, eager for repair, is essential to success. Lane preferred repair at the earliest possible age. In order to keep his very small patients quiet he prescribed brandy as a sedative after operation. It is told that his ward Sister managed with great skill to maintain the babies in a state of alcoholic euphoria, with the happy result that they never cried and the wound healed in peace.

Another important repair is that of hypospadias, the defect in the penis and urethra caused by failure of the two edges of the foetal urethral groove to fuse together. This has exercised the ingenuity of surgeons for over a century, but no certainly

176

successful method was evolved until that true artist, Arthur Edmunds of King's College Hospital, described his three-stage operation in 1913. Various forms of plastic repair had already been attempted by Dieffenbach, Thiersch, and Charles Mayo but none of these had met with much success. Edmunds' operation was really a combination of one devised by Thiersch with another used by the French surgeon L. Ombrédanne in 1911; he cleverly manipulated the spare skin so as to form both a floor and a roof to a new urethra which ran from the old, inconvenient opening at the hinder end of the penis to the new opening at the tip.

Edmunds' operation was modified by Denis Browne of Great Ormond Street in 1936, but more recently Browne has introduced an entirely new principle, based on the observation that a strap of epithelium or mucous membrane buried beneath the skin of the penis will form a tube. The Denis Browne operation (1949) has been generally adopted for young children. Other methods that have been tried are the grafting of 'tubes', such as portions of vein; G. Axhausen actually removed the patient's appendix and transplanted it! All such methods have failed, but there has been some success with grafts of skin. A French surgeon, G. Nové-Josserand of Lyon, tried covering stent moulds with skin and burying them beneath the skin of the penis, but he met with no success. In 1937 Archibald McIndoe modified the technique of outlay grafting by attaching Thiersch grafts to a length of gum elastic catheter, tunnelling the penis, and inserting the skin covered catheter in the tunnel. McIndoe's operation has proved successful in adult patients when previous attempts at correction have failed.

Sometimes the testis fails to descend into the scrotal sac – undescended testis – and remains just beneath the skin at the junction of the thigh with the abdomen. In this position it is very liable to damage and, for this reason, boys are not accepted as midshipmen in the navy or for some other careers unless the testis has been successfully transposed to the correct position. It sounds quite simple to free the testis and push or pull it down into the scrotal sac, but the problem is quite a difficult one. If the testis is not freely mobilized and is not firmly fastened in the scrotum, the pull of the structure to which the shortened spermatic cord is attached will cause it to reascend to its original position in the abdominal wall; if the fastening is too tight or too much tension is put upon the attached structure, atrophy will result.

Fixation of the undescended testis into the scrotum was first attempted by J. F. Rosenmerkel of Munich in 1820 and by another German, M. J. von Chelius, in 1837. These were mere experiments and unjustified experiments at that; no further operations were attempted until 1881. In 1899 the American A. D. Bevan pointed out that the testis will always reascend unless freely mobilized; a review of 573 subjects of the Bevan operation in 1926 showed that about fifty per cent were successful. In 1910 L. Ombrédanne devised a method of making a hole in the scrotal septum and passing the testis through into the sac on the opposite side. The hole in the septum could then be sutured around the cord to provide a stay. Ombrédanne's operation is often used at the present time. Sixteen years before Ombrédanne, the English surgeon C. B. Keetley published in the *Lancet* his operation of first fixing the testis to the fascia underlying the skin of the inside of the thigh and, at a second operation, of freeing it from the fascia and closing the scrotal sac.[11] Keetley's operation was taken up by Franz Torek who wrote a full and well-illustrated paper on the subject in the *New York Medical Times* of 1909. The method, popular until quite recently, is commonly known as the Torek two-stage operation, but should properly be given the name of Keetley. In 1933 a survey showed that about ninety per cent of these operations had been successful. But the Ombrédanne can be done in one stage and gives equally good if not better results.

One of the finest examples of a surgeon's perseverance, or perhaps of a patient's fortitude, is to be found in the attempts made by the American J. Marion Sims to close a vesico-vaginal fistula. A vesico-vaginal fistula is a defect between the walls of the vagina and bladder causing incontinence of urine, usually the result of a tear during childbirth. About the year 1847 or 1848 Sims was consulted by a lady whose life was made miserable by this most unpleasant disability. He attempted to close the fistula and failed; again he tried, and again he failed. In 1849 at the *fourteenth* attempt, he succeeded in closing the hole with silver wire sutures. He did the operation through the vagina, using a specially designed instrument, a speculum, to obtain a view. Sims' speculum is a commonly used instrument today. He became well-known for his skill in this form of repair; in 1873 the American surgeon D. H. Agnew described sixty cases of Sims' operation with three deaths and five failures. In the next twenty years various improvements were introduced, but in 1893 von Dittel suggested that the vaginal approach should be given up in favour of operation through the abdomen, and this is the method now used for the larger defects.

Another repair operation with a rather curious history is that for congenital absence of the vagina. We saw in the first chapter that this was one of the thirty-nine operations recorded by William Fergusson in his case book for the years 1830–7. The date was 1836, when similar attempts had already been made by three French surgeons, Dupuytren (1817), Villaume (1823), and Amussat (1832); in all four cases the method was simply that of cutting a passage through the tissues and had no lasting effect. There was no further advance until 1904 when J. F. Baldwin of Ohio excised a short length of the small intestine and grafted this into a prepared tunnel, which required several operations and carried a high mortality. In 1914 G. Schubert simplified this technique by transplanting the lower part of the rectum, bringing down the upper part of the rectum and joining it to the anus so as to secure continuity of the bowel. His operation also carried a high mortality and often resulted in incontinence of faeces.

In 1872 a German surgeon named Heppner had attempted to form a vagina with skin, taken from the upper and inner part of the thigh. His attempt failed utterly, but the idea was revived by an American, Graves, in 1917. This stimulated research into various operations of plastic repair with skin. Gillies suggested a method which was taken up by two surgeons, R. T. Frank and S. H. Geist, who reported four successes in 1932. Then, in 1936, three French surgeons, Monod, Iselin, and Nové-Josserand, tried making an artificial passage and lining it by the outlay method, Thiersch grafts on a stent mould. The drawback of both operations was that the passage very rarely remained patent. In 1937 McIndoe suggested to V. S. Counsellor of the Mayo Clinic that somewhat thicker grafts might give a better 'take' and prevent later contracture. The grafts were mounted on a mould which was kept in place until all danger of con-traction was over. In 1939 Counsellor reported sixteen successes with McIndoe's operation in two years. It is the generally used method today.

Lastly the repair of hernia. A hernia may be congenital or acquired; a child may be born with a hernia or a sudden strain may cause a hernia to appear in later life, although when this happens there is probably a congenital weakness present. The hernia itself is a protrusion, or sac, of peritoneum (the abdominal lining membrane) which contains some part of the abdominal contents, usually a length of gut or part of the fatty tissue called omentum. But practially every organ in the abdominal cavity has been found at some time or another in a hernial sac; we shall see in the next chapter that one of the historic surgical operations resulted from the presence of an appendix. The principle of repair is to remove the sac and to strengthen the wall through which the sac has protruded.

The repair of hernia is, without doubt, one of the more important operations in surgery. Indeed, it may be questioned whether the comparatively simple procedures of the cure of hernia, piles, and varicose veins, so often consigned to a junior member of the surgical department, are not of considerably more benefit to the community than any of the epoch-making operations devised by the great. This is not to suggest that great names are not attached to hernia; in fact a full eponymous list of all the many modifications of the operation for inguinal hernia alone (the type which appears at the groin and the only one we shall here consider) would incorporate many of the best known names in surgery. Nearly one hundred variations of the Bassini operation, the most commonly performed operation today, have been introduced since 1889; Harold Edwards, briefly describing in the *British Journal of Surgery* only those modifications which contain a new idea, gives details of no less than twenty-two.[12]

The hernia operation is described by the Roman Celsus in his *De Re Medicina* written about AD 30 and the type of instruments used, found at Pompeii (which was destroyed half a century later), can still be seen in the Naples Museum. But, as we saw in the second chapter, the operation was not often attempted until after the introduction of anaesthesia, except as a life saving measure for strangulation. When these early surgeons tried to deal with the ordinary hernia (which they called 'reducible' hernia because the contents of the sac could be easily pushed back into the abdominal cavity) they used the method known as herniotomy, the simple removal of the sac without reinforcement or strengthening of the overlying wall. This operation is still done in the case of infants, but is useless for the adult because the hernia will recur if the wall is not strengthened.

The weak point in the wall through which the hernial sac protrudes is known as the internal abdominal ring; the first attempts to strengthen the wall were by plugging the ring. In 1836 the French surgeon Amedée Bonnet advised that inflammation should purposely be allowed to occur in the wound; this resulted in the formation of inflammatory adhesions and was known as the 'cure by sepsis', obviously a very dangerous and uncertain method. The same reasoning lay behind the 'seton treatment', introduced by the German Wurzer in 1840; here the ring was plugged with a piece of glass or porcelain rod, and success depended upon the formation of adhesions. In 1886 William Macewen actually used the hernial sac to plug the ring; instead of removing it, he pushed the contents back into the abdominal cavity and stitched the rolled-up sac into the ring. A very successful combined operation of plugging the ring with both the rolled-up sac and a porcelain seton had already been devised by John Wood of London in 1857.

It was the adhesions, and not the seton or the sac, which strengthened the edges of the ring; this gave rise to an entirely different technique but still based on the formation of adhesions. In 1844 the American Pancoast injected a solution of iodine into the sac, which caused strong adhesions to form between the walls of the sac and so turned it into a kind of plug or seton. Seven years later the French surgeon Velpeau dissected out the sac, opened it, and painted the inner surface with iodine. This 'sclerosing' or injection treatment of a hernia has been resurrected from time to time, and was advocated by A. E. Porritt of St Mary's Hospital as recently as 1938.

From 1860 Wood and a few other surgeons started to use various methods of strengthening the tissues overlying the hernial site.[13] They reinforced the muscles with hemp string or wire sutures, materials which are not absorbed by the tissues, or they fastened pins through the muscles and interwove thread or wire from pin to pin. A simpler operation was introduced by Vincenz Czerny in 1877, and this was made safer in 1881 when H. O. Marcy started to use antiseptic suture material. Three years later there comes the most important date in the history of hernia, when Edoardo Bassini of Padua performed the operation bearing his name for the first time on 23 December 1884.

Edoardo Bassini was a remarkable man. Born of an aristocratic Italian family at Pavia on 14 April 1844, he graduated from the University of Pavia in 1866. For the next eleven years he spent part of his time serving in the army and the remainder in study under Langenbeck in Berlin, Billroth in Vienna, and Lister in Edinburgh. On his way back from Scotland to Italy he stayed for some weeks in London, working with Thomas Spencer Wells at the Samaritan Hospital. In 1877 he was appointed professor of surgery in the University of Padua, where he remained until his retirement at the age of seventy-five in 1909. He died in 1924. Besides his work on hernia, Bassini is credited with the first attempt to by-pass a stone impacted in the bile duct by joining the gall bladder to the duodenum (1882) and he was one of the earliest surgeons to perform a gastro-enterostomy. All his life he remained a simple, hard-working man who cared little for money or honours. The story is related that, when Bassini was made a Senator of Italy, his students chose a convenient pause between operations to present him with an instrument fashioned in gold accompanied by a flowery speech of congratulation. 'Thanks, thanks,' replied Bassini. 'But let's get back to work.'

Bassini published a long and interesting paper on hernia in 1890. He said that all methods then in use were variants of the operations introduced by Wood and Czerny. Of Wood's results he wrote 'The last publication by Wood (1886) shows he repaired 339 reducible hernias; 17 with a hemp string; 49 with straight pins and an intertwining suture; 273 with subcutaneous wire sutures, the latter nine times bilaterally. Re-operation was necessary in eleven instances. Of these 339 cases, if we subtract 91 unknown results and 7 deaths, there remain 189 cures and 52 recurrences. I have used this operation twice in medium-sized reducible hernias. Both recurred after one year.'

This is the point; until Bassini introduced his method, the

number of recurrences after operation was very high; about 20 per cent in the figures given above. At the time of writing his paper, Bassini had operated on 262 cases, using his own method exclusively. There was only one death, from pneumonia on the fifteenth day after operation. Bassini had followed up his cases for a length of time ranging from one month to four and a half years, and there had been only seven recurrences in the 250 cases, a recurrence rate of less than $2\frac{1}{2}$ per cent.

Bassini's operation has stood the test of time. Despite all the ink that has been spilt – and the tempers lost – upon 'new' procedures, it is doubtful whether any of these are an improvement upon the original. The more important modifications are those of the German Anton Wölfler (1892) and of W. S. Halsted (1889). A modified Halsted operation, though not commonly performed in Britain, is popular in the United States.

Various attempts have been made to strengthen the repair by mechanical means; this was the idea which lay behind the use of silver wire sutures or hemp string. In 1909 L. McGavin of the Dreadnought Seamens' Hospital, Greenwich, invented a silver wire filigree to reinforce the hernial area. This method was used continuously at the Seamen's Hospital for over forty years by McGavin and P. P. Cole. Only twelve recurrences could be traced in 448 cases. Another mechanical support was the 'darn and stay lace' introduced by Sampson Handley in 1918, a lattice repair with ordinary stout silk. Floss silk, more easily sterilized by boiling, gave better results; another popular reinforcement material was kangaroo tendon, which may be looked on as a very strong catgut.

Reinforcement by transplants of living tissue has also been suggested. Martin Kirschner of Greifswald described a method of grafting the whole area with sheets of fascia taken from below the skin in 1910. Kirschner is better remembered for his 'wire', used for applying traction to fractured bones. A more widely employed method was that of the 'living suture' advocated by W. E. Gallie and A. B. LeMesurier of Toronto in 1921. These living sutures are strips, about ten inches long and a quarter of an inch wide, cut from the fascia of the thigh (the fascia lata) and threaded by means of a special needle in a crisscross or shoelace pattern when repairing the muscles. The idea was that the material would remain alive and would reinforce the area with strong fascial bands. Excellent results have been obtained, particularly in recurrent or abnormally large hernias. In 1930 Gallie and LeMesurier reported on ten years' experience during which they had operated on two hundred patients with only six known failures. Among the first fifty were soldiers who had suffered a recurrence after one, two, or three previous attempts at repair by other methods. 'There were also ventral and inguinal hernias so enormous as to be almost unbelievable, and several were in patients suffering from chronic bronchitis and asthma, in whom the hernia had recurred because of uncontrollable cough.' wrote Grey Turner in his *Modern Operative Surgery* (1956).

A drawback of this method is the long wound left in the thigh; it is of no danger, but the absence of a strip of fascia makes it possible for the underlying muscle to herniate through the defect. Harold Edwards, in the article referred to above, pointed out that this disability can be a real problem in the services, for the malingering type soon learns to make good use of it; some patients are genuinely frightened by what they think must be a serious disability and it is difficult to reassure them that the 'bulge' is of no importance.

Coughing or 'the post-operative chest' is one of the dangers of surgery. The patient may be afraid to cough because his wound is painful, in which case he will not get rid of sputum, or the coughing may cause a weakening of the wound. In the case of a hernia operation, weakening of the wound will result in recurrence of the hernia. The problem is not nearly so great as it was; better methods of anaesthesia, the antibiotic drugs, and encouragement of the patient to get out of bed sooner after operation, have all contributed to improvement. But, above all, physiotherapy, breathing exercises before and after operation and controlled movements of the limbs, have decreased the frequency of post-operative chests and so diminished the recurrence rate of hernia. Experience among young, fit soldiers in the Second World War showed that stopping smoking for even a few days before operation had a very good effect upon the rate of recurrence. It is these apparently small things which add up to make surgery safer.

The hernia operation is commonly done by a 'general' surgeon. From here we will pass on to a type of surgery which can hardly be regarded as a speciality; the general surgeon also looks upon abdominal surgery as his province, although there are some who have a greater interest in this type of work than have others.

CHAPTER 9

Abdominal Surgery

The continuing history of abdominal surgery stems from two operations, that of colostomy and that for the removal of an ovarian cyst. Colostomy is the making of a false anus when the lower part of the large bowel is obstructed, particularly when the rectum is obstructed by a growth which cannot be excised. An ovarian cyst is often of very large size, containing several pints of fluid; it is a cause of great discomfort and potential danger, but, being attached by only a narrow pedicle, can be easily removed.

The earlier colostomy operations were performed, not for bowel obstruction in elderly patients, but for the congenital absence of the anus in new-born children. We saw in the first chapter that Fergusson considered this procedure but decided against it and in favour of trying to make a passage into the bowel from below. No doubt he was aware of the great danger of all pre-Listerian abdominal sections; opening of the abdominal cavity brought the grave risk of peritonitis, infection of the lining membrane. This, in addition to the fact that abdominal operation without anaesthesia is extremely painful and productive of shock, deterred the surgeon from taking any action except in the most acute emergency.

But the congenital absence of an anus is an acute emergency, which will inevitably result in death if it is not treated. Nor is there any hopeful method but by surgery, for only an opening into the bowel can relieve the obstruction. In other cases of obstructed bowel the surgeon was left to choose between two dangers. Age-old attempts to relieve the distension resulting from obstruction by passing a sharp-pointed trochar into the gut invariably resulted in disaster; for this reason, the seemingly obvious method of bringing the cut bowel to the surface above the obstruction had been advocated from very early times. But, because of the ever present risk of sepsis, it soon became apparent that such an operation rarely succeeded in saving life or even in producing a less painful form of death.

Alexis Littre (or Littré) of Paris may be called the father of colostomy. In 1710 he was consulted about an infant who suffered from congenital malformation of the rectum, probably an imperforate anus. The child died on the sixth day after birth; Littre took the opportunity at autopsy of investigating possible means of dealing with similar defects in life. Having practised on the infant's body, he declared it possible to 'make an incision in the belly, and open the two ends of the closed bowel and stitch them together, or at least to bring the upper part of the bowel to the surface of the belly wall where it would never close but perform the function of an anus.' This was ventral or abdominal colostomy, performed through the abdominal wall and traversing the peritoneum with consequent danger of infective peritonitis; although very rarely performed in these early years, it became known as Littre's operation.

In 1776 H. Pillore, a surgeon of Rouen, performed caecostomy which is much the same as colostomy, except that the large bowel is entered at a higher point. The reason for his operation was an obstruction due to cancer of the rectum – or perhaps the cause was two pounds of mercury which had been given by mouth in an endeavour to cure the obstruction – but, whatever the cause, his patient died twenty-eight days after operation. In 1793 C. Duret of Brest, having been called to attend a child of three days old suffering from imperforate anus, made an incision in the left groin and brought the large bowel to the abdominal surface; he then cut into the bowel and allowed it to act as an artificial anus. This is the first successful colostomy, for Duret's patient lived until the age of forty-five. An interesting little note on this operation reminds us that 1793 was the year of Terror. 'Citizen Massac, Chief of the Administration, and Citizen Coulon, Physician in Chief, were charged to provide the necessary dressings.'

P. J. Desault of Paris also performed Littre's operation for imperforate anus in 1794, but the child died four days later. In

187

1797 C. L. Dumas of Montpellier, the leading French surgeon of his time but quite forgotten today, advised that colostomy should be used for the relief of intestinal obstruction and claimed to have devised the operation. In fact, Dumas never did a colostomy in his life, but his weighty approval served to arouse interest. Three years later, Professor Fine of Geneva performed colostomy in the case of a woman of sixty-three suffering from cancer of the rectum, giving credit to Dumas for the original idea. Fine's patient survived for three months. Freer of Birmingham was the first to attempt Littre's operation for imperforate anus in Britain (1815), but his patient died four days later; his second patient, attempted in 1817, was a man of forty-five, apparently suffering from a stricture of the anus; he died on the ninth day. The first successful case in England was that of Daniel Pring, a surgeon of Bath; in 1817 he performed a colostomy for cancer of the rectum and his patient lived. Four years later R. Martland of Blackburn also achieved success; his patient lived for at least seventeen years.

About the year 1839 J. Z. Amussat of Paris attended his colleague, Professor Broussais, who was dying from intestinal obstruction due to a cancer of the rectum. Amussat declared that he would never again stand idly by while a patient of his died so terrible a death. He collected particulars of all known colostomies since Pillore had first performed the operation on the living subject in 1776. Of twenty-nine cases, twenty-one of whom were infants suffering from imperforate anus, twenty had died within a matter of hours or days. Only four of the infants had survived, and it is curious that all four were treated at Brest, where Duret had first succeeded with the operation, but that Duret had attended none of the other three cases. Of eight adult patients, five had survived.

Amussat concluded that the twenty deaths were all due to peritonitis, as we should call it today, and that Littre's abdominal approach through the peritoneum must be held to blame. After experimenting in the post-mortem room, he advised opening the large bowel by an incision in the back, close to the spine, an approach which had already been practised on the dead body by Duret and by Callisen of Copenhagen in 1800. This is the lumbar colostomy or Amussat's operation, a great advance because it did not entail approaching the bowel via the peritoneal cavity and so tended to avoid peritonitis. Amussat himself performed his operation nine times successfully between 1839 and 1856; the number of his failures is unknown.

Lumbar colostomy became the operation of choice, and retained its popularity for over thirty years. In England it was first performed by W. J. Clement of Shrewsbury for a stricture of the colon in 1841; Clement's patient lived for three years. John Erichsen of University College Hospital, who had been a pupil of Amussat and present at his first operation, became the leading exponent of this method. Another who regularly practised the Amussat technique was Caesar Hawkins of St George's; in 1852 he collected all known cases of colostomy, performed for 'stricture of the colon' but not for imperforate anus in infants, and found that in forty-eight patients the mortality was exactly fifty per cent. He advised that there was little difference in the result whether Amussat's or Littre's approach was used.

In 1850 three surgeons at the London Hospital returned to the abdominal method of Littre. The London Hospital became noted for successful operations; in 1865 one of their surgeons, Nathaniel Ward, made the very important pronouncement that when a cancer of the rectum is diagnosed, colostomy should always be performed without waiting for signs of obstruction; this made the operation safer because the patients were in better general health. With the introduction of antisepsis, operations on the abdomen could be performed with less risk of peritonitis; from 1880 onwards there was an increasing tendency to give up the Amussat method, although we occasionally find mention of lumbar colostomy in the case notes during the eighteen nineties.[1]

A colostomy is not a curative operation; it will relieve obstruction of the bowel but, if that obstruction is caused by a cancer, the cancer remains to imperil the patient's life. One of the objections put forward by the London Hospital surgeons to the lumbar colostomy was that the abdominal cavity cannot be explored through the incision; a doubtful diagnosis must remain in doubt. In 1887 C. B. Ball of Dublin recommended abdominal colostomy with exploration of the abdomen (laparotomy) in all cases. A few years later W. Ernest Miles started to explore the abdomen through a midline incision and to make the colostomy through a separate opening. This is the method generally used today. Attempts to hack a way through a rectal growth had often been made, but it was not until 1868 that Billroth removed a cancer of the rectum for the first time; by 1876 he had done thirty-three cases. Billroth's operation was improved by the Swiss surgeon Theodor Kocher and by the German Paul Kraske. Kraske's operation remained the method of choice from 1885 until 1908; in that year W. E. Miles introduced the abdomino-perineal approach, which is still used in suitable cases.[2] In all previous methods the operation had been done only from below; the Miles operation is commonly performed by two surgeons working together, one from below (the perineal approach) and one from above, through the abdomen.

With the exception of colostomy and the removal of rectal growths, all abdominal operations derive, directly or indirectly, from the first removal of an ovarian cyst; for this reason many of the more successful abdominal surgeons of the earlier years were particularly interested in diseases of women. The course of events is easy to follow: the discomfort, not to mention the risk to life, of a very large ovarian cyst tempted the pre-Listerian 'gynaecologist' into his first assault upon the abdomen and, despite the high mortality, the simplicity of removal lured him on to attempt more difficult operations.

Ovariotomy, as it was called, was suggested as a feasible method by both John Hunter and John Bell. Neither of these performed the operation, but Bell may quite probably have directly influenced Ephraim McDowell, who had been his pupil at Edinburgh. After qualifying from Edinburgh, McDowell returned to the United States and settled as a general practitioner in the backwoods village of Danville, Kentucky. In 1809 he successfully removed an ovarian cyst or tumour from a patient named Mrs Crawford without, of course, either anaesthesia or antisepsis. This historic operation has some of the qualities of drama; an ominous crowd hovered outside the house to await the result, while the stout-hearted Mrs Crawford sang hymns to support herself during her ordeal. She lived for thirty-two years.[3]

This first operation would be unknown but for the fact that McDowell published an account of it with two more cases in 1817. He sent his paper to John Bell and it came into the hands of John Lizars, also of Edinburgh. Shortly afterwards Lizars attempted operation on a woman named Janet Ireland, but he did not succeed in removing the whole tumour 'notwithstanding, the patient got well, gathered flesh, and was relieved of her central pains'. Three further attempts by Lizars all resulted in death. In 1821 Nathan Smith of Yale performed a successful ovariotomy for a cyst 'containing a few pints only', seemingly without being aware of McDowell's cases. During the next ten years McDowell, who must have been outstandingly skilful, unusually lucky, or working in a relatively bacteria-free district, operated on a further eleven patients with at least eight recoveries.

Ovariotomy was not again attempted in Britain until 1840 when Benjamin Phillips of the St Marylebone Infirmary and later of the Westminster Hospital performed one operation with a fatal result. Two years later Charles Clay of Manchester, who became the leading advocate of ovariotomy in England, did his first case. Within a few weeks D. H. Walne, surgeon to the German Hospital in London, successfully removed a large ovarian tumour (probably not a simple cyst) from a patient of fifty-eight.[4] He was assisted by Blundell of Guy's, whom we met in connection with blood tranfusion; here is a short description of the operation:

'The woman was seated propped up on a couch, and Walne's finger was passed into the peritoneum through an incision one and a half inches long; this was then enlarged to rather more than thirteen inches by means of a probe-pointed bistoury guided by two fingers. As the tumour prolapsed, one assistant pressed the abdominal wound margin together to prevent prolapse of intestines; another held up the tumour, weighing $16\frac{3}{4}$ lbs, while the pedicle was transfixed and tied. An additional ligature round the pedicle stopped all bleeding. The other ovary was examined by Blundell's finger and found normal; the wound was closed by a dozen interrupted sutures.'

The ligatures, left with their long ends hanging from the wound, came away ten weeks after operation. This and two more cases survived; Walne's fourth patient died from peritonitis nine days later. Within a few months Robert Liston stigmatized all ovariotomists as 'belly rippers'.

In France Nélaton and Eugene Koeberlé performed ovariotomy but, on the whole, opinion in the country was against it
and few were done until after 1862. The history of ovariotomy
in Germany is of some importance, for the German and
Austrian schools did more to advance abdominal surgery than
those of any other nation. A surgeon named Chrysman is
credited with the first operation as early as 1819 and his
example was followed by Dieffenbach, Nussbaum, Langenbeck,
and F. A. Kiwisch von Rotterau, but results were poor. In
1852 Kiwisch von Rotterau collected reports of fifty-four cases;
of these no less than fifty-one had died. He came to the conclusion that the operative mortality throughout the world must be
well over fifty per cent. Four years later, in 1856, F. W. Scanzoni
von Lichtenfels denounced ovariotomy as an unjustifiable
operation and strongly recommended that it be abandoned.

By this time ovariotomy had fallen into universal disfavour;
indeed, most hospitals forbade the operation to be performed
within their walls, a ban which the surgeon sometimes circum-
vented by removing his patient to a room in the near neighbourhood. The committee of management minutes of King's
College Hospital show that ovariotomy was forbidden until
1878, when Lister deliberately broke the rule in order to
demonstrate that antisepsis had made the operation a reasonably safe one. But, meanwhile, a certain interest had been
aroused by the work of Thomas Spencer Wells of the Samaritan
Free Hospital for Women and Children, then a small hospital
of only twenty beds in Portman Square.

Thomas Spencer Wells was born in 1818 and entered the
Royal Navy after qualifying. In 1853 he started to practise in
Brook Street, London, but volunteered for service in the Crimea
a year later; at the end of the war he returned to London,
lectured on surgery and anatomy at a school attached to St
George's Hospital and was elected surgeon to the Samaritan in
1856. He first became interested in ovariotomy in 1848, while
on a visit to Paris, but he dismissed the operation as too dangerous. In 1854 he assisted a London surgeon, Baker Brown, with
his eighth case; this died as also did the ninth; Baker Brown,
threatened with an inquest, gave up the operation.[5] Meanwhile
Wells had left for the Crimea; here he saw a number of soldiers
who had been wounded in the abdomen and the fact that some

of these recovered without much trouble suggested to him that the abdomen was more tolerant of injury than had been supposed; he did not, of course, understand that these recoveries occurred simply because the wound was lucky enough to escape infection. His findings encouraged him to give ovariotomy a trial when he returned to England; he performed his first operation in December 1857 and was not unduly dispirited when the patient died.

His first success came in February 1858 and, by 1864, Wells had achieved sufficiently good results to encourage a fairly general revival of interest. His success undoubtedly resulted from attention to strict cleanliness. Wells is commonly stated to have opposed antisepsis; he was certainly a member of the cleanliness and cold water school, but he was also one of the very earliest surgeons to understand the importance of Pasteur's germ theory. Indeed, an article by Wells in the *British Medical Journal* of 1864 suggests that he realized the importance of Pasteur's work before Lister.[6] Nor did he oppose antisepsis. He persisted with 'cleanliness' until 1878, when Lister's example in London made him think that he might be able to improve his own figures. He publicly declared that, after adopting antisepsis in 1878, the improvement in his results was 'startling to himself'.[7] Of his first five hundred cases of ovariotomy, 373 recovered and 127 died, a mortality of 25·4 per cent. Of his next three hundred, 223 recovered and 77 died, a mortality of 25·6 per cent, but he was now tackling more difficult tumours. Eighty-three recovered out of his next hundred, a 17 per cent mortality. It was during this penultimate series that Wells changed over to antisepsis. Of the final hundred, all treated with full antiseptic precautions, only eleven died.[8] This fall to less than half the previous mortality is a good instance of the increased safety of surgery resulting from Lister's work.

Wells was very particular about his instruments, choosing each type with great care, and trusting no one except himself to clean and dry them after operation. No book on the development of surgery could neglect mention of the Wells' haemostat for securing blood vessels. A disgruntled anaesthetist has been heard to say that he can detect only one difference between a first-, second-, and third-class surgeon: a first-class surgeon asks for Wells; a second-class surgeon demands Spencer Wells; and a third-class surgeon shouts for Spencers. So great is the present-day popularity of this instrument and so varied the name given to its inventor.

Ambroise Paré probably introduced the ligature for tying blood vessels, and he also invented a 'crows beak' 'fit for to draw the vessels forth of the flesh wherein they lie hid, that they may be tied or bound fast'. Three hundred years later, Liston originated the idea of 'forcipressure', twisting the cut end of a small blood vessel so that the walls adhered together and bleeding was stopped without ligature.

Liston's method seems never to have become popular; Wells wrote that he greatly admired the dexterity with which Fergusson's assistants seized a spouting vessel with their fingers and tied it 'at a glance from the great operator'; but he also saw William Bowman use 'bulldogs' which were probably the forceps introduced by Liston. In 1858 a surgeon named Webber of Yarmouth and Norwich suggested 'anti-ligature' forceps, strong crushing instruments not meant to be used with ligatures at all, for the reason that he regarded them as a potent cause of infection. In 1867 Koeberlé invented an instrument for 'forcipressure', a modification of a well-known type of dressing forceps introduced by the French surgeon Charrière in 1858; ten years later Péan devised a somewhat better model which became very widely used.

Both Koeberlé's and Péan's instruments suffered from the defect that the shanks were widely curved and so left spaces in which tissue could easily be entangled. Wells introduced his first model in 1872; this also had shanks that were too much curved. In 1879 he modified his instrument into the present form with straight shanks.[9] The modern surgeon either 'twists off' a vessel with Wells' forceps or catches the vessel with them and passes a ligature around it; they are the most commonly used of all instruments in surgery today.

Ovariotomy led on to other abdominal operations. Konrad Langenbeck, uncle of the more famous Bernhard and one of the earliest ovariotomists, was probably the first man to remove the uterus successfully. Wells and another famous ovariotomist, Lawson Tait of Birmingham, became well known for their skill in this operation. Quittenbaum of Rostock, another German ovariotomist, was the first man to remove a spleen in 1826, but the patient died six hours later. In 1865 Wells removed the spleen for the first time in Britain and the fifth time in the world; his patient also failed to survive. The mortality of splenectomy remained very high and the operation for disease, as opposed to emergency splenectomy necessitated by injury, was hardly done at all until W. J. Mayo published a series of 243 cases with only 26 deaths in 1920.[10]

Another operation which has descended directly from ovariotomy is that for gallstones. In 1869 Lawson Tait, who did his first ovariotomy at the age of twenty-three when still a house surgeon, was consulted by a patient about a discharging sinus in her abdominal wall; he followed up the track of the sinus and removed a few small stones, which must have ulcerated through from the gall bladder. In 1878 Marion Sims, the famous American 'gynaecologist', attempted to remove gall stones by opening the abdomen and slitting up the gall bladder, the operation of cholecystotomy, but his patient died; in the same year Theodor Kocher of Berne drained an abscess of the gall bladder. The first successful removal of stones from the gall bladder was by Lawson Tait in 1879.[11] Another interesting cholecystotomy is that performed by Joseph Lister in 1883, for it is often stated wrongly that Lister never opened the abdomen. Unfortunately we cannot credit him with a successful operation; he removed several stones, but the patient, a man named Laurence Trancovitch, was suffering from cancer of the pancreas and liver. He died in April 1884.

The operation which Lawson Tait performed successfully for the first time in history was that of removing stones from the gall bladder. He is sometimes credited with the first cholecystectomy, removal of the gall bladder itself, but this is a mistake for he never did the operation. Cholecystectomy was first performed in 1882 by the German C. J. A. Langenbuch,[12] who is often confused with the more famous Langenbeck. This was an isolated case, but in 1896 Hans Kehr, another German, started to do the operation as a routine procedure for removal of stones and had performed over a thousand cholecystectomies by the time of his death in 1916. Berkeley Moynihan in England and Mayo in America were well known for their success in cholecystectomy. After 1921 it became the operation of choice and has now entirely replaced cholecystotomy.

Next for the stomach. This group of operations does not start with ovariotomy nor with an ovariotomist, but with an animal experiment. Cancer of the pylorus, the opening at the lower end of the stomach into the duodenum, had often been shown to be present at post-mortem, but nothing could be done for the sufferer. In 1810 a young German physician named Karl Theodor Merrem showed that the pylorus of a dog might be excised and the stomach joined by suture to the duodenum; he suggested that the operation might be a feasible method of dealing with pyloric cancer in the human, but his idea lay dormant for sixty years.

Another very distressing disease is cancer of the oesophagus, for the growth obstructs the oesophagus and the patient is unable to swallow, with the result that he slowly starves to death. This suggested the making of an opening into the stomach through which the patient could be fed – a gastrostomy. Gastrostomy is the earliest operation to be performed upon the human stomach. In 1846 Charles Emmanuel Sédillot informed the Academy of Sciences of Paris that he had attempted gastrostomy for the relief of oesophageal cancer, but that his patient had died a few days later. Similar attempts were made by Cooper Forster of Guy's Hospital in 1858 and 1859, but neither patient survived. Although some twenty-five of these operations were done in the next fifteen years it was not until 1875 that Sydney Jones of St Thomas' performed a gastrostomy with success, and then only with partial success.[13, 14] His patient, a man of sixty-seven, lived for forty days, dying of a massive haemorrhage from an oesophageal cancer.

Meanwhile, in 1871, Theodor Billroth of Vienna had studied Merrem's work and had performed animal experiments himself. Billroth did not excise a dog's pylorus, but a section of the oesophagus; he then sutured the two cut ends together and found that they healed well, leaving only a slight constriction which could be easily dilated. In the same year Vincenz Czerny applied Billroth's experiments to the human, excising a cancer of the oesophagus and joining the two ends together, an operation also done by Billroth in 1872.

This work suggested a number of operations upon different parts of the digestive tract. About 1875 Alexander von Winiwarter and C. Gussenbauer, Billroth's assistants, started a series of animal experiments, designed to show that one part of the gut might be readily excised and the cut ends anastomosed by suture. Gussenbauer successfully excised a part of the human sigmoid colon in 1877; in the same year, Billroth performed a small local excision of a wound or sinus of the human stomach, joining the cut surfaces together. In 1879 Jules Péan attempted to remove the pylorus in a case of cancer. Despite transfusion with 130 grammes of blood, his patient died on the fourth day after operation.

At the end of January 1881 Billroth's assistant, Anton Wölfer, showed him a woman of forty-three who suffered from an un-doubted cancer of the pylorus. Examination by palpation with the hand made it clear that the tumour was not fixed to any surrounding organs. Billroth decided to attempt removal on 30 January 1881. He made an incision through the abdominal wall about eight centimetres long transversely over the tumour, which he found to be of large size, involving more than one third of the lower portion of the stomach. He brought the tumour to the surface (with some difficulty because of the small incision), made openings into the stomach and duodenum above and below the tumour; then cut it away. Next he stitched up the major part of the hole in the stomach so that it exactly fitted the hole in the duodenum and sewed the two together with about fifty sutures of carbolized silk. The portion of stomach removed measured fourteen centimetres along its greatest length. 'The operation lasted, including the slowly induced anaesthesia, about 1½ hours,' wrote Billroth 'No weak-ness, no vomiting, no pain after the operation. Within the first 24 hours only ice by mouth, then peptone enema with wine. The following day, first every hour, then every half hour, 1 table-spoon of sour milk. Patient, a very understanding woman, feels well, lies extremely quiet, sleeps most of the night with the help of small injections of morphia. No pain in the operative area, subfebrile reaction. The dressing has not been changed.'[15]

This is the first successful removal of part of the stomach, the operation of partial gastrectomy which is so often and so successfully performed today. But the early results were by no means good and the method soon fell out of favour. The first operation in Britain was by F. A. Southam of the Manchester Royal Infirmary in 1882; six months later Sydney Jones did one at St Thomas', but both patients died within a matter of hours. By this time twelve gastrectomies had been done in Germany and France, eleven for cancer and one either for or following a perforated gastric ulcer. The latter patient is said to have recovered, but only four of the cancer cases survived operation; one of these died within four months. In 1885, when fifty-six partial gastrectomies for cancer had been recorded, the mortality worked out at 76 per cent.[16] In 1888 an English surgeon, H. T. Butlin wrote that the operation could not be considered justifiable: he produced evidence that, of thirteen patients who had survived operation, no less than ten died of recurrence of the cancer within twelve months.[17]

The high operative mortality of partial gastrectomy and the disappointing number of recurrences, which were chiefly due to the fact that operation was delayed until too late because of its danger, caused many surgeons to despair of removing the growth and to turn to a palliative operation which would relieve the obstruction at the pylorus and so give the patient some prolongation of life and a more comfortable end. In 1881, the same year that Billroth had performed the first partial gastrectomy, Anton Wölfler successfully made a gastro-enterostomy, short circuiting of the stomach to the small bowel without removal of the pyloric growth. This became the method of choice, particularly after Courvoisier of Basle introduced an improved operation known as posterior gastro-enterostomy in 1883. The stomach and selected portion of bowel were opened and sewn together; so afraid of disastrous leakage of bowel contents (which would result in peritonitis) were the early operators that they often put in as many as two hundred sutures when performing an ordinary gastro-enterostomy; this not infrequently defeated its own purpose by weakening the walls of the gut. In 1888 Nicholas Senn of the Rush Medical College, USA, introduced perforated plates of bone, which could be inserted into the lumen of the two cut ends of bowel. These were largely replaced by the American J. B. Murphy's 'buttons' in 1892 and the 'bobbins' devised by Mayo-Robson of Leeds in 1893. The principle was the same; the divided discs or buttons were inserted in the lumen of the two cut bowel ends, anchored by a purse-string suture, clamped together, and oversewn; a simple contrivance which restored continuity of the bowel without multitudinous stitches. Better methods of suture have rendered these aids of historical interest only, but they were of great value at the time.

Mention has been made above of a partial gastrectomy performed for or after a perforated gastric ulcer – the disaster that occurs when the wall of the stomach, weakened and eroded by an ulcer, gives way and allows the contents to flow into the peritoneal cavity. Suture of the perforation was first suggested by Bernhard von Langenbeck; he never performed the operation which was first attempted by Mikulicz-Radecki in 1880, but his patient died three hours later. A certain mystery attached to the operation mentioned above, for it may perhaps have been done by Ludwig Rydygier before Mikulicz. Rydygier attempted some form of stomach resection in 1880, but his patient is said to have died, whereas our mysterious case is said to have lived.

The first man certainly to have sutured a perforation with survival of the patient is Ludwig Heusner of Germany in 1892; this operation is sometimes attributed to another German surgeon, Kriege, who reported it. The first attempt in Britain was by Hastings Gilford of Reading in 1893, but his patient died. In the following year T. H. Morse of Norwich succeeded; the patient, a woman of twenty who had perforated five hours before operation, made a good recovery.[18] All these were simple closures of the perforation by suture, an emergency treatment in common use until quite recently.

In 1897 a surgeon named Braun suggested that suture of the perforation ought always to be accompanied by gastro-enterostomy, which was beginning to be used as the surgical treatment of gastric ulcer. His advice received little or no attention at the time, but was resurrected as an original idea by Moynihan in Britain and by Deaver in America; this was in 1929, thirty years after Braun. Another method of treating the perforation was by excising the ulcer area and then suturing the incision; first performed by J. W. Dowden in 1909, it was suggested as a routine method by H. von Haberen of Vienna in 1919. Excision of the ulcer led naturally to excision of a larger portion of the stomach combined with gastro-enterostomy: in other words to the partial gastrectomy. First suggested by A. Odelberg of Stockholm in 1927, the 'emergency gastrectomy for perforation' was popularized by Doberauer of Carlsbad and Sergei Yudin of Moscow.

We have said that gastro-enterostomy was used as a palliative measure in gastric cancer and also as a treatment of gastric or peptic ulcer. In 1900 Mayo-Robson of Leeds declared that all peptic ulcers which did not respond to a medical regimen within a reasonable time should be treated surgically. Five years later over five hundred gastro-enterostomies for peptic ulcer had been performed at the Mayo Clinic alone. In 1905 Berkeley Moynihan published his important first book on gastric ulcer, which had a great influence upon methods of treatment. From then until 1925 gastro-enterostomy for simple ulceration took its place as one of the more common operations in surgery; by 1925 doubt was beginning to creep in and there were a few surgeons who had started to speak of gastro-enterostomy as a 'surgically produced disease'. Results were sometimes good, but all too often the operation only gave temporary relief because a new ulcer formed at the point of anastomosis of the stomach with the small bowel. Braun first described the 'anastomotic ulcer' in 1899; Mayo-Robson wrote a paper on the subject in 1905, but he still regarded it as a rare complication. As doubt increased a number of substitute procedures were suggested; these are of little interest for none of them provided the answer.

Very few partial gastrectomies were performed, because of the high mortality. In 1900 W. J. Mayo started to preach the dogma that gastro-enterostomy can only prolong life for a short time in a case of cancer; cancer of the stomach, he said, is a surgical disease and can only be treated by excision of the cancer. He started to perform routine partial gastrectomy and, by 1906, had done over one hundred and fifty gastrectomies for cancer with a small immediate mortality and quite good end results. The method was taken up by Hans Finsterer of Vienna, who became a master of gastric surgery between the two world wars, and by Eugene Pólya of Budapest, who in 1911 modified the original Billroth operation into the type which is commonly done today. In England, partial gastrectomy did not become anything like popular until the late nineteen thirties, possibly because of Moynihan's preference for gastro-enterostomy, but after 1935 gastro-enterostomy gradually started to give place to gastrectomy, largely through the insistence of W. H. Ogilvie of Guy's Hospital.

Gastrectomy became the operation of choice not only for cancer, but for such peptic ulcers as did not respond to medical treatment. Better anaesthesia, better pre- and post-operative care, use of blood transfusions, earlier and more accurate diagnosis, have contributed to the increased success of this operation. It has stood the test of time although, because it is a destructive operation, attempts have been made to avoid it in cases of simple ulceration; two of these, which are of no practical importance but of some historical interest, are freezing of the stomach, advocated by the American Professor Wangensteen, and cutting off the stomach blood supply to a point just short of gangrene, suggested by Wilson Hey of Manchester in 1937.[19] A simpler and more successful operation, at one time hailed as the answer to excision but now regarded as suitable only in selected cases, is the cutting of the stomach's nerve supply, vagotomy, which was first used by L. R. Dragstedt of Chicago in 1943–4 after prolonged animal experiment.[20]

It is partly by the aid of two instruments, the X-ray machine and the gastroscope, that the dismal picture of late nineteenth century gastric surgery has been changed into the brighter one of the mid-twentieth.[21] The first attempts to see into the stomach via the mouth and oesophagus were by Kussmaul of Freiburg in 1868 and by Nitze in 1876; Nitze used the 'cystoscope' which he had devised with the help of Joseph Leiter; Kussmaul tried the Desormeaux instrument, and it is not altogether surprising to learn that he employed a professional sword swallower as his demonstration subject. In 1881 Mikulicz-Radecki examined several patients successfully with his own instrument and even detected an unsuspected cancer of the stomach in one. But his gastroscope could not be rotated and so he was unable to obtain a complete view of the stomach. Mickulicz came to the conclusion that exploratory operation was nearly as safe and a more certain method.

Other early workers who tried to obtain a view of the stomach are Theodor Rosenheim, who experimented with a straight, rigid tube in 1895, and Rewidzoff, who made the patients swallow a flexible tube first and then passed a rigid tube through the lumen. Neither of these attempts was successful. In 1900

Georg Kelling of Dresden devised a gastroscope consisting of a number of hinge-jointed sections, which could be introduced through a large-bore rubber tube, and then braced straight by longitudinal tension wires. This had the essential addition of a rotating eyepiece, so that the whole stomach could be examined, and it was lit by a filament bulb. It was an ingenious invention which should have marked a great advance, but proved to be much too complicated and too fragile. On the first occasion of use, the fully-conscious patient bit through the whole thing, causing irreparable damage. Kelling did not repeat his experiment.

Meanwhile X-rays had entered surgery and the importance of attempted gastroscopy receded, particularly after Cannon demonstrated the radiopacity of bismuth given as a meal. Even with the aid of bismuth, early X-ray examinations revealed only gross defects. Reich, a German radiologist, first clearly showed the presence of a gastric ulcer by means of a bismuth meal in 1909. (It is of some interest that a quite different Reich, Adolph Reich of New York, first obtained X-rays of the gall bladder and bile ducts accidentally while experimenting with a mixture of bismuth and petrolatum in 1912.) The bismuth meal technique was much improved by R. D. Carman of the Mayo Clinic; in 1910 Martin Handek described his 'niche, sign or syndrome', a residue of bismuth or barium remaining and filling the ulcer crater after the stomach has emptied.[22] This is a diagnostic X-ray sign today.

A mild interest in gastroscopy revived in 1908 when H. S. Souttar and Theodore Thompson of London produced an instrument much like that of Kelling, but considerably stronger. Kelling's unfortunate accident occurred because he did not pass his instrument under anaesthesia. Souttar realized that the ordeal could not be tolerated by the conscious patient – unless he was a professional sword swallower. Although fairly successful, he soon abandoned his experiments, partly because the need for anaesthesia suggested that exploratory operation might be no more dangerous than gastroscopy, and partly because better X-ray methods were giving good results. No further attempt was made until 1932 when Schindler of Berlin devised a gastroscope with the help of Wolf, an instrument maker. The Wolf-Schindler gastroscope, parent of the instrument used today, was a much thinner and more flexible tube fitted with a system of lenses. Schindler and Henning of Leipzig showed that it was not only safe but efficient and, unlike the bulky Souttar model, could be tolerated by the unanaesthetized subject. Thus gastroscopy became a routine examination, often requiring only outpatient attendance. In 1935 Henning had gastroscoped over two thousand patients.[23]

The last disease and operation that we shall consider in this chapter is appendicitis and appendicectomy, inflammation of the vestigial vermiform appendix and its removal. We start with 'the iliac passion', a favourite diagnosis of medieval practitioners, which could occur on the left or right side in the lower part of the abdomen. Most of these cases of iliac passion resulted from a perforated typhoid ulcer in the large bowel, a common cause of death in those insanitary times. William the Conqueror and the Black Prince are two who died from the delayed effects of typhoid; so probably did King John, although his surfeit of peaches and new cider may have been the immediate cause of a diarrhoea that ruptured the ulcer.

Sometimes iliac passion must have been the old-time diagnosis of a modern appendicitis. Jean Fernel, professor of medicine in Paris, gave an account of right-sided iliac passion with a description of the post-mortem appearances in 1567; this is the earliest clear record of an appendix abscess. Nearly two hundred years later Claudius Amyand of St George's, while operating on a boy of eleven for a strangulated hernia, discovered the appendix lying in the hernial sac. He not only dealt with the hernia but also removed the appendix; this is the first appendicectomy (1736). The wound healed up well and the boy recovered but Amyand described the operation, which lasted upwards of half an hour, as being equally distressing to himself and to his patient.

In 1755 a German surgeon, Lawrence Heister, described the clinical signs and symptoms of acute appendicitis. Four years later, in 1759, the Parisian surgeon Mestivier diagnosed that an abscess had formed in the right iliac fossa – the right lower quadrant of the abdomen in which the appendix normally lies – and made an incision through the abdominal wall. He drew off a pint of foul pus, but his patient died. Mestivier's operation, although unsuccessful, is the first deliberate attempt to deal

with an abscess resulting from perforation of an acutely inflamed appendix. Three more drainages of the appendix
abscess were performed in France before 1827; in England
James Parkinson of London tried to drain an abscess in 1812.
His patient died and this is the first occasion on which perforation of the appendix is described as the cause of death.

The important work of François Melier, another Frenchman,
followed in 1827, when he published his observations on 'certain
maladies of the caecal appendix'. He clearly stated that an
abscess in the right iliac fossa is derived from the appendix, and
he strongly advocated operation when such an abscess was
diagnosed. Unfortunately Melier's views were hotly opposed by
the great French surgeon Dupuytren. Dupuytren held that the
fact that pain and an abscess occurred more frequently on the
right side than on the left had nothing to do with the appendix
at all, but was connected with the existence of a valve in the
portion of large gut, the caecum, to which the appendix is
attached. He also declared that no structure so insignificant as
the appendix could possibly cause such disastrous and wide-
spreading effects. Dupuytren therefore supported the terms
'typhlitis' and 'perityphlitis', inflammation of and around the
caecum (typhlon being the Greek variant of the Latin
caecum). Dupuytren's weighty opinion did much to confuse
the issue and to hold back advance.

Not everyone believed in the existence of typhlitis. Between
1820 and 1840 thirty-three attempted operations on the
appendix abscess were reported, but it was not until 1843 that
Willard Parker of New York successfully performed drainage
and saved his patient's life; five years later Henry Hancock of
Charing Cross Hospital succeeded for the first time in Britain.[24]
Between 1843 and 1867 Parker achieved three more successes,
but the number of failures is unknown. He advised waiting until
an abscess had definitely formed, even though a diagnosis of
appendicitis had been made. Drainage became more popular as
the result of Parker's work; one hundred and two attempts
were recorded between 1840 and 1860.

Little further progress was made until May 1880 when
Lawson Tait operated on a diagnosed appendix abscess and,
for the first time since Amyand, successfully removed the
appendix. Amyand's operation had not been planned; Tait is

therefore the first man to perform a deliberate appendicectomy. Charters J. Symonds of Guy's Hospital did the same three years later. In 1884 Mickulicz-Radecki, who had been investigating treatment of bowel perforations, reversed the teaching of Parker by recommending that operation should not be deferred until the formation of an abscess but should be performed immediately in all cases of diagnosed appendicitis. His advice was bereft of some authority when he followed it himself and lost his patient. J. H. Webb of Melbourne was another who advised that the abdomen should always be opened, but he never had the audacity to do it himself. This teaching was followed by Lawson Tait in 1886; having diagnosed inflammation of the appendix before the formation of an abscess, he opened the abdomen and performed a successful appendicectomy.

These and a few others were all isolated incidents, for opinion was very divided on the best form of treatment. The contradictory views of Melier and Dupuytren, of Mikulicz and Parker, had thoroughly confused the issue. The majority of physicians and surgeons supported Dupuytren in his belief that a vestigial structure like the appendix could not possibly be the cause of such grave trouble. This, the orthodox school, regarded typhlitis and its more dangerous relative perityphlitis as a physicians' disease, to be treated by hot fomentations, turpentine enemas, or any other nostrum in temporary favour. Lawson Tait probably performed his operations because the orthodox school regarded operation as contra-indicated: he was that type of man. A second but very small school of thought held that the appendix must have some function and that removal must therefore not be lightly undertaken, although they preached that it should be treated surgically if inflamed or perforated. Their teaching resulted in some very peculiar and rather delightful operations at which one would like to have been present.

In 1885 Henry Sands of New York, having correctly diagnosed a perforation of the appendix, stitched up the hole and returned the repaired appendix to the abdomen; his patient recovered. So did that of Morton of Philadelphia, who in the same year, finding only part of the appendix to be unhealthy, carefully excised the diseased tip. Tait, finding an inflamed appendix but no sign of abscess formation, made a small incision in the end, inserted a thin celluloid catheter, and so drained it. The best one of all is in 1887 when that famous abdominal surgeon, Frederick Treves, having diagnosed inflammation, discovered on operation that the appendix appeared innocent though grossly kinked by adhesions to the caecum. Treves solemnly cut the adhesions, straightened out the kinked appendix, and returned it to the abdomen. Afterwards he admitted that it might have been simpler to perform appendicectomy.

This muddled thinking was largely ended by the work of Reginald Heber Fitz, professor of pathology at Harvard, who had studied under Rokitansky and Virchow. Fitz examined the records of 466 cases, comparing the signs and symptoms of 209 living patients, diagnosed as suffering from typhlitis, with the post-mortem appearances of 257 patients, in whom the presence of an abscess or an inflamed appendix had not been revealed until after death. He showed that the symptoms of the second series, as noted in life, were similar to those in whom a diagnosis of typhlitis had been made and who had survived. Typhlitis and an inflamed appendix, perityphlitis and an appendix abscess, were the same thing; he suggested that the old terms should be dropped in favour of 'appendicitis'. Fitz published his findings in 1886.

Three years later J. B. Murphy of Chicago wrote a classical description of the signs and symptoms of appendicitis; in the same year, 1889, Charles McBurney of the Roosevelt Hospital, New York, published the results of a large investigation into the disease. In the course of his paper he enunciated one of the best-known 'signs' in surgery, still called 'McBurney's Point'. This is the point of maximum tenderness when the abdominal wall is pressed with one finger and is a good localizing sign in appendicitis. McBurney also described a technique of operation in 1894, but the so-called McBurney or gridiron incision was, in fact, devised by L. L. McArthur of Chicago. Another commonly used incision or approach for the appendicectomy operation was introduced by W. H. Battle of St Thomas' Hospital in 1895.[25,26,27]

Noteworthy as these various dates are, it is doubtful whether any of them are of so great importance in the history of the appendix operation as is 24 June 1902. The coronation of King Edward VII had been arranged to take place on 26 June, but the king fell ill with abdominal pain and fever only a few days before. At a consultation of some of the most distinguished surgeons in the land, including Lord Lister, it was decided that the only chance to save his life lay in urgent operation. Frederick Treves, who had performed his first successful appendicectomy in 1887, opened the abdomen and drained an appendix abscess on 24 June; he did not, as is sometimes stated, remove the appendix. The king made a good recovery and the operation was entirely successful, a success that becomes more remarkable when one considers the advanced age (for those days) and not altogether ascetic habits of the patient. After the postponed coronation on 9 August, Treves received a knighthood and Lister was made a Privy Councillor and one of the twelve original members of the Order of Merit. When welcoming Lister to his Council, the king is supposed to have said: 'I know that if it had not been for you and your work, I would not have been here today.' No king in history has ever spoken truer words.

We can easily see the immediate effect of Treves' operation by consulting the case notes of William Watson Cheyne. In 1901 Cheyne operated for appendicitis seven times; in 1903 he operated on twenty-two cases. Appendicitis had become a fashionable disease, but there were some surgeons who now advised that operation should not be lightly undertaken. A. J. Ochsner of Chicago advocated 'expectant' treatment and did much to popularize what is now known as the 'interval appendicectomy' operation at a time when the appendix is quiescent after an acute attack. His treatment embodied bed rest in a sitting-up position (to minimize the risk of spreading infection in the abdominal cavity), nothing by mouth, gastric lavage, nutrient enemas, and, most important of all, constant medical supervision. Expectant treatment became widely practised during the years 1934–9, particularly in America, and gave quite good results. The use of first bacteristatic and then antibiotic drugs, by diminishing the risk of general peritonitis, has made the 'interval' or 'cold' appendicectomy the operation of choice, but these drugs have by no means provided a substitute for surgery.[28]

At the end of the nineteenth century abdominal surgery was viewed with considerable suspicion by surgeon and patient alike. By listing the operations performed and the successes scored, a wrong impression of eager acceptance can be given. Only the groundwork had been done; it required some quite small but widely publicized 'miracle of surgery' to alter the whole attitude. Just as Lister's wiring of the broken kneecap in 1877 served to convert London to antisepsis, so Treves' operation on King Edward inspired confidence in the surgeon's ability to deal with abdominal catastrophe. As experience increased, so operation became safer. When a surgeon is in doubt today, it is far less dangerous for him to explore the abdomen than to take the chance that there is nothing seriously wrong.

CHAPTER 10

The More Recent Specialities

Brain, Lung and Heart

1. BRAIN

Surgery of the head is of comparatively recent origin but contains one operation which is probably the oldest in history. Trephining or 'trepanning', the making of an opening in the skull, has been practised since the New Stone Age. These antique 'surgeons' used a flint scraper with which a circular portion of bone could be laboriously removed. Strangely enough some of their patients recovered, for skulls have been found which show the formation of new bone around the rim of the trephine hole, a clear proof of survival. The object of the operation was no doubt to allow escape of the imprisoned demon, who made his presence known by the convulsive movements of epilepsy or by intolerable headache. Demoniac possession is part of all primitive religions; for this reason trephining has continued to be practised among primitive peoples until almost the present day. As medicine became divorced from religion, so the doctor took over the curative function of the priest. The persistent folk-memory of miraculous cures of men who had been possessed by the devil after suffering a fall or an injury in battle entered surgery as an indication for purposeful trephining to relieve the pressure headache and convulsive twitchings that follow a depressed fracture of the skull.

Trephining for 'traumatic epilepsy' resulting from a head injury remained one of the commoner operations until the middle of the nineteenth century. According to Samuel Pepys, Prince Rupert was 'trepanned' at Whitehall by the French surgeon Moulins on 3 February 1677. 'Having cut the outer table, as they call it, they find the inner all corrupted, so that it come out without any force; and their fear is, that the whole inside of the head is corrupted like that.' Pepys must have been misinformed, for Prince Rupert recovered from the operation. Then there is the case of Philip of Nassau who 'having been thrown from his horse, fractured his skull by striking his head against the stump of a tree. He was trepanned twenty-seven times by a surgeon of Neomagen. He gave a certificate of this signed by himself; and as a proof of his complete recovery drank three of his companions to death.' Percivall Pott of Bart's trephined in the eighteenth century with instruments hardly distinguishable from those of the ancient Greek and Roman surgeons; he considered that any fracture of the skull warranted operation. John Hunter, Astley Cooper, Henry Cline of Guy's all frequently operated; Cooper, however, advised against trephining unless the fracture of the skull was a compound one.

As experience and knowledge grew, so the surgeon started to lay down indications for operation. The Frenchman Jean Louis Petit declared these to be 'obvious fracture, unconsciousness, haemorrhage from the nose, mouth, and ears, paralysis and convulsions'. Baron Larrey, working on the wealth of material provided by Napoleonic battles, regarded trephining as indispensable in depressed fractures (when the skull is driven in upon the brain) and for removal of foreign bodies such as bullets from the brain substance. G. J. Guthrie, who was present at the battle of Waterloo, laid down the rule 'when operation is necessary in a fractured skull it should be done at once – delay is fatal.' Guthrie also made the very pertinent observation: 'Injuries of the head affecting the brain are difficult of distinction, doubtful in their character, treacherous in their course, and for the most part fatal in their results.'[1]

Quite suddenly trephining went out of fashion – there are fashions in surgery as much as in dress or the equipment of feminine kitchens – but the reason for this almost universal unpopularity is a little difficult to unmask. Perhaps the death rate, high even by pre-Listerian standards, daunted the majority of surgeons. The figures from various centres show an astonishing variation. In the American Civil War trephining for gunshot wounds of the head resulted in only 95 recoveries out of 220 operations; at Guy's thirty-nine out of fifty-one died, at University College Hospital eleven out of seventeen, and at St George's sixteen operations resulted in thirteen deaths.[2] On the other hand J. S. Billings of Cincinatti analysed the figures for trephining in 1867 and found that, of 72 cases, 42 were cured, ten improved, four unchanged and sixteen had died. The state of brain surgery at that time is revealed in the comment of Callender of St Bartholomew's that no patient had been trephined in the hospital during the years 1860–7.[3]

Interest in this type of brain surgery reawoke during the years 1877–80, and the initial stimulus was given in a most curious manner. In July 1877 Robert S. Hudson, a quite unknown surgeon of Redruth in Cornwall, read a short paper to the South Western branch of the British Medical Association. He was careful to tell his audience: 'I am well aware that you have come for a holiday, so I do not propose inflicting on you a dry narration of cases.' Hudson then went on to say that, in the tin mining districts of Cornwall, Percivall Pott's belief in the necessity of trephining for any injury of the skull had persisted despite the fact that the operation was generally out of favour. 'Around Redruth and Camborne Pott's principles still prevail,' he said, 'taught by Pott himself to the great-grandfathers of the present generation of surgeons. Talleyrand, it is said, observed that the philosophy of a previous generation might be gathered from the common people of the existing one, and it is so in this case.'

Hudson remarked that the majority of trephinings in Cornwall gave no trouble but healed without infection; he believed this success to be due to the purity of the Cornish air. He then pointed the way; sepsis, he said, need no longer be dreaded in 1877 'if the antiseptic system be carried out in the spirit of its apostle'.[4] This, of course, was the answer; general acceptance of the antiseptic method made the outlook for brain surgery more hopeful. In 1880 James West of Birmingham brought Hudson's views to the notice of the influential Royal Medical and Chirurgical Society of London, the predecessor of the present day Royal Society of Medicine.[5]

Trephining over the site of a fracture was simple, but it was quite a different matter when it came to trephining for an abscess or a tumour. As the brain is contained in the rigid skull, the site of an abscess or tumour will not be apparent on the surface; successful surgery depended upon diagnostic signs which would enable the surgeon to localize the lesion. The rather ugly word 'localize' is here used purposely, for these are known as localizing signs. As far back as the days of Hippocrates, attempts had been made to correlate the various movements and functions of the body with parts of the brain; in more modern times Larrey was the first to describe such signs: loss of speech, loss of memory, and paralysis occurring on the side of the body opposite to the injury of the head. In 1829 the Frenchman Jean Cruveilhier had under his care a woman of forty-five who suffered from frontal headache, weakness of the left leg, slow speech, mental impairment, and incontinence of urine. Cruveilhier first saw this case on 3 September; after studying her signs and symptoms he tentatively diagnosed that a tumour was pressing on or growing in the right frontal lobe of the brain. The patient died on October 3; autopsy revealed that a tumour, of the type now called a meningioma, had formed a cup-like depression in the right frontal lobe.

In 1861 the French neurologist and surgeon Paul Broca showed to a meeting of the Anthropological Society of Paris the brain of a man who had lost the faculty of speech twenty-one years before death.[6] There was obvious softening of an area, the third frontal convolution on the left side. Broca therefore believed this ('Broca's area') to be the centre in the brain which controls speech. Three years later John Hughlings Jackson of the London and National Hospitals confirmed Broca's findings and forecast that it would soon be possible to map the brain into limited areas each having its distinct function. His forecast was partly confirmed the next year by two Germans, Gustav Theodor Fritsch and E. Hitzig, who in animal experiment stimulated areas of the brain with the galvanic current and obtained movements of groups of muscles on the opposite side of the body.

This work was carried on and brought to the point at which Jackson's prophecy was proved correct by the physician David Ferrier of the National and King's College Hospitals. In 1873 Ferrier mapped out definite areas for the face, arms, and legs by faradic stimulation and by actual operation on the brains of higher apes. He published a book *The Functions of the Brain* in 1876 and showed specimens of his animals at the International Congress of Medicine in 1881. It is related that the great French neurologist Jean Martin Charcot, on first seeing one of Ferrier's monkeys, paralysed down one side after operation on certain areas of the brain, gave vent to the startled exclamation 'It is a patient!'

Broca was the first man to trephine for a lesion of the brain which he had already diagnosed by localizing signs. The patient died, but in 1861 Broca showed to the Surgical Society of Paris a child whom he had successfully trephined for an abscess, having defined the position of the abscess before operation. Knowledge of localization was sufficiently far advanced in 1878 for Lucas-Championnière to publish a book *La Trépanation Guidée par les Localisations Cérébrale* which applied the theoretical work of Broca, Hughlings Jackson, and Ferrier to the practice of surgery.

Meanwhile, in July 1876, William Macewen had successfully diagnosed an abscess of the brain by localizing signs. The patient died before operation but at post-mortem Macewen's diagnosis was proved correct. Three years later he removed blood clot, lying between the brain substance and the covering membrane, the dura mater, from the skull of a boy of fourteen, with recovery of his patient. In the same year (1879) he studied the signs and symptoms of a girl of fourteen and concluded that something must be pressing upon the anterior part of the left frontal lobe of the brain. Macewen operated and found a tumour, a meningioma, exactly where he had prophesied that it would lie. He removed it and the patient recovered with complete relief of all symptoms. It is strange that this, the first successful removal of a cerebral tumour, is almost unnoticed in the histories of medicine.[7]

As knowledge of localizing signs spread, reports of operations came from many parts of the world. Francesco Durante of Rome and Rickman Godlee of University College Hospital and the National Hospital, Queen Square, both removed meningiomas in 1884.[8] A much less well-known operation is that of Godlee's uncle, Joseph Lister, six months later. In both Lister's and Godlee's cases the presence of a tumour was diagnosed by David Ferrier, who marked out the site for trephining on the skull. Sad to say, neither patient survived for long and the operations cannot be counted successful, but here is an early example of the co-operation between specialities which is so marked a feature of modern practice. The American William Williams

Keen successfully removed a large meningioma in 1887 and published details of this and two more cases in 1888. In Germany progress was delayed, owing to the opposition of Stromeyer, but von Bergmann described operations for brain abscess, for tumours of the brain, and for traumatic epilepsy in 1889.

The first 'neurosurgical specialist' worthy of the name is Victor Horsley of University College Hospital. He did not confine himself to neurosurgery, as would a modern specialist, but his particular interest was in surgery of the brain, the spinal cord, and the nerves. Horsley read his first paper on the subject to the British Medical Association meeting at Brighton in 1886.[9] He described three operations on the brain and, six months later, reported seven more. His first case was one of traumatic epilepsy; the patient suffered from over three thousand fits within a fortnight and was cured by operation. The second proved at operation to be a tuberculous growth or abscess – a tuberculoma – occupying the exact site postulated.

Horsley was the first to operate successfully for an accurately localized tumour of the spinal cord. Over twenty years before Horsley's operation, in 1865, a Dublin surgeon named McDonnell had 'trephined or decompressed' the spinal cord by removing part of one vertebra which had been fractured, an operation also performed by Astley Cooper. It is interesting that the experiment – for it was no more – was undertaken on the advice of the famous physiologist C. E. Brown-Séquard of Harvard and Paris, who happened to be visiting Dublin at the time. McDonnell's operation was partially successful, in that he cured the patient's urinary incontinence, but death occurred within a few weeks.[10] The first man to perform this operation, known as laminectomy, with success seems to have been the great William Macewen. In 1883 he removed part of three vertebrae of a nine-year-old boy who suffered from a severe curvature of the spine, causing partial paralysis and incontinence of urine; five years later the lad was able to play football.[11] By 1888 Macewen had done six laminectomies with two deaths.

Victor Horsley was a true scientist who planned every operation on the localizing signs shown by the patient and, if in doubt, by animal experiment. His example started a vogue for neurosurgery, but the results proved to be so bad that most surgeons gave up in despair. The difficulties were not sufficiently well understood. Localization of the lesion was still unsatisfactory; tumours were removed by tearing them out with the fingers; wounds often became infected despite rigid antisepsis; haemorrhage killed many patients because the brain tended to ooze blood (although Horsley introduced a lasting contribution, Horsley's wax, an effective means of sealing or plugging the troublesome vessels in the bone of the skull). As a result, mortality was very high; some writers have estimated the overall death rate to be as much as fifty per cent. The death rate from attempts to remove tumours varied between thirty and eighty per cent according to the type of tumour and the surgeon's skill – and so late as 1932 a well known surgical text book stated that only 7 per cent of brain tumours were removable.[12] In the more generally popular trephining for traumatic epilepsy a mortality of 7 per cent was regarded as remarkably low. Neurosurgery may be said to have been established by 1900, almost entirely through the work of Macewen and Horsley, but the number of surgeons who operated, or who believed operation to be justifiable, was very small.

Macewen and Horsley may be honoured as the pioneers of neurosurgery, but they founded no school. That honour must willingly be conceded to Harvey (Williams) Cushing of Harvard, from whose work the modern practice is derived. Born at Cleveland, Ohio, on 8 April 1869, Cushing graduated MD Harvard in 1895 and spent the next year as house officer to the Massachusetts General Hospital. Here, in the fashion of the day, he learned that speed was the first essential in successful operating. In 1896 he removed to the Johns Hopkins as assistant to William Halsted who, although himself a quick operator, taught the modern doctrine that surgical safety lies in avoidance of blood loss, meticulous care, and gentle handling of the tissues. This combined experience gave Cushing the ability to work brilliantly and rapidly in cases of urgency, but also the knowledge that speed for the sake of speed is no surgical virtue.

During his time at the Johns Hopkins, Cushing took the first X-ray picture in the history of the hospital, using 'a decrepit and perverse static machine, as big as a hurdy-gurdy and operated in the same way – by turning a crank'. This unimportant work with an early X-ray machine had the unexpected outcome of introducing Cushing to neurosurgery. Quite by chance a patient who had been shot through the spine was sent to him for examination. Cushing located the bullet by X-rays and was interested enough to follow up the case, noting the gradual disappearance of paralysis as the patient recovered.

Shortly after this, Cushing met William Osler, the brilliant physician who became equally if not better known as a historian, a writer, and a bibliophile. Their intimate, lifelong friendship had a profound effect upon the development of Cushing's mind and interests. In 1900 the two came to Europe, first to Berne where Cushing worked with the famous Theodor Kocher, and then to London, where he had hoped to study the methods of Victor Horsley. But Horsley, immensely busy and a very poor teacher, proved to be unsympathetic; Cushing went up to Liverpool to work on the brain functions of the higher apes with the great physiologist Charles Sherrington, who became another lifelong friend.

Cushing returned to the Johns Hopkins in 1901 and was appointed associate professor of surgery in 1903. He had decided to specialize in neurosurgery, against the advice of his professor who saw no future in what was by now almost a dead subject. But a limited fame had already come to Cushing for his work on trigeminal neuralgia, the distressing condition sometimes known as tic douloureux. He had started to operate with some success; this operation is so important in the history of neurosurgery that we must enter into a little explanation.

Trigeminal neuralgia results from a disease process occurring in the largest of the cerebral nerves, the trigeminal, which is the sensory nerve of the face and a large part of the scalp; it is also the motor nerve of the muscles of mastication. One of the points to remember is that the sensory fibres, that is the part which is responsible for the feelings of touch and pain, arise from a ganglion situated just behind the temple of the skull. This is known as the Gasserian ganglion or the semilunar ganglion. Affection of the trigeminal will produce quite agonising pain as well as a 'tic', spasmodic contraction of the muscles supplied.

On 2 April 1890 William Rose of King's College Hospital removed the Gasserian ganglion for the first time in a case of obstinate trigeminal neuralgia. The patient recovered but lost the sight of his right eye, presumably because the optic nerve, which lies close to the ganglion, had been damaged at operation. In the course of a discussion of this procedure, David Ferrier gave his opinion that it would be better and safer to cut the nerve rather than to remove the ganglion.[13]

A year later Victor Horsley took Ferrier's advice and cut the nerve, but his patient died of surgical shock seven hours later and Horsley never attempted operation again. In 1892 another British surgeon, Frank Hartley, returned to the method of removing the ganglion. A similar operation was done by Fedor Krause of Berlin only a few months later; Krause seems to have been unaware of Hartley's work and is often given credit for prior operation. Cushing improved the Hartley-Krause technique and, in a large series of cases, encountered a mortality of only 5 per cent, or about half the then accepted mortality of this dangerous operation. In 1901 C. H. Frazier of Philadelphia returned to the method of nerve section, but Cushing persisted with the Hartley-Krause operation for six more years. In 1907 he turned over to the Frazier technique because, it is said, he found the ganglion impossible to remove in one case and was forced to divide the nerve with equally good after results. Here is the start of modern neurosurgery.

Meanwhile Cushing had been attempting other operations on the brain. It must be understood that, at the beginning of the twentieth century, Horsley was almost the only man to practise this type of surgery with any frequency – and his mortality was in the region of forty per cent. Cushing's results were at first no less disastrous but, unlike many surgeons, he persisted with his attempts. He soon learned that rough surgery, tearing out of a brain tumour with the fingers, was a potent cause of death, and he introduced a gentle method of dissection, pushing of the brain substance away with swabs. He learned that blood loss is no less dangerous and he made a special clamp with which he could apply small silver clips to bleeding points in the brain. He learned that faulty methods of localization often made search for a tumour more disastrous than non-intervention, and he introduced the operation of palliative decompression, which was really a return to simple trephining, to relieve the headache and other symptoms caused by the pressure of the tumour. By 1905 he had become the first full time neurosurgeon and his results had started to improve.

In 1912 Cushing moved to Boston as professor of surgery and surgeon-in-chief to the Peter Bent Brigham, that small hospital of only two hundred and fifty beds which has had so profound an influence upon medicine. Cushing had made himself into a complete diagnostic and operating team – a one man team; he had become a skilled neurologist, ophthalmologist, and general physician, a laboratory scientist, a statistician, and a morbid anatomist, all this in addition to his work as a neurosurgeon. From 1912 onwards he tended more and more to specialize in the localization and subsequent removal of brain tumours. In 1915 he published his results; he had removed 130 tumours with a mortality of only 8 per cent; Horsley could still claim a survival rate of only 60 per cent.

Cushing's work on tumours, though not on surgery of the brain, was interrupted by the First World War, for he joined an ambulance unit while America was still neutral and served with distinction in France from 1915 until 1919. Wide experience of head injuries taught the surgeon that the brain is more tolerant of surgery than had been previously supposed. Cushing's great pioneer work became recognized; on his return to Boston in 1919 he found that younger men were eager to learn his methods and he gathered a team around him to continue and to improve his technique. By 1932 his mortality in the surgery of brain tumours had fallen to as little as 5 per cent. Another well-known neurosurgeon has recorded: 'His mortality indeed appeared so fantastically low to some that they openly refused to credit it. There can be no doubt whatever that it was strictly accurate.'

Cushing's name is particularly associated with disorders of the pituitary gland, situated at the base of the brain. He commenced his study of the pituitary about 1906, performed his first operation in 1909, and published *The Pituitary Body and Its Disorders* in 1912. In this book he recorded an operative death rate of 14 per cent; by 1927 it had been reduced to 4 per cent. He described Cushing's Syndrome, a type of pituitary tumour which produces gross obesity, sexual changes, and infertility or impotence, in 1932.

In 1932 Harvey Cushing retired from active surgery to become professor of neurology at Yale University. From 1937 until 1939 he also filled the post of director of studies in the history of medicine – a reminder of his friendship with William Osler. Cushing died from coronary thrombosis on 10 August 1939. A difficult man of great character, he aroused devotion among his followers who spread his teaching all over the world. He had a lively personality, a sense of humour, and an impish sense of fun – he once disguised his house surgeon and introduced him to a distinguished company in place of an important guest who had failed to turn up – but he was a hard taskmaster who did not spare his assistants or hestitate to lash them with a bitingly sarcastic tongue. His capacity for warm friendship made him as much at home in Britain as in America. He instituted a scheme whereby the director or senior surgeon of a London teaching hospital took temporary charge of the surgical beds at the Peter Bent Brigham, while Cushing himself deputized at the hospital in London; he believed that international exchange of ideas could best be fostered by a knowledge of actual working conditions.

During and after Cushing's lifetime the progress of neurosurgery was assisted by advances in diagnostic and operative methods. Cushing himself introduced the use of diathermy (1928) which did much to reduce blood loss; strict asepsis, followed by the sulphonamides and penicillin, lessened the danger of infection. In 1918 Walter E. Dandy of Baltimore showed that it is possible to obtain X-ray photographs of the brain cavities by aspirating some of the fluid normally present and replacing it with air. He gave his new method, now known as ventriculography, the name of 'cerebral pneumography'. In Britain ventriculography was first used by A. A. McConnell of Dublin in April 1921[14] and the following year by John Fraser of London. The examination could not be regarded as a safe one; Fraser lost two patients out of his first series of fourteen cases.[15]

Walter Dandy also introduced the examination known as encephalography, which is much the same as ventriculography except that the air is introduced into the spinal canal. Both these examinations are used for the localization of brain lesions today. Dandy devised operations for removal of tumours and is particularly renowned for his work on the pineal gland. After Cushing, he was perhaps the greatest of neurological surgeons. Another method of localization, particularly for the spinal cord, was the injection of a contrast medium, lipiodol; this was first used by Professor J. A. Sicard of Paris and was largely popularized by Percy Sargent of St Thomas' and the National Hospitals, who had been present at Sicard's early experiments. Lipiodol, a toxic substance, was not without risk; in 1935 two workers in Manchester introduced a safer contrast medium known as Thorotrast.

In 1929 H. Berger showed that it is possible to demonstrate the presence of some diseases of the brain by the variation in electrical activity which they cause, and that these variations can be detected from outside the skull. He named this very important examination the 'Elektrenkephalogram' a name now commonly shortened to EEG. In 1935 it was shown that a distinctive pattern is produced by epilepsy, and in 1936 the method was adopted to the localization of cerebral tumours. Another often used method of localization is arteriography or angiography, in which the brain blood vessels are shown up by means of a contrast medium. First introduced by Antonio Egas Moniz of Lisbon in 1927, the X-rays are now obtained with an iodine derivative.

Egaz Moniz also devised the somewhat controversial operation of prefrontal leucotomy, section of an area at the front of the brain, in 1935; this may have the effect of changing the patient's personality and has been used for the relief of obsessional or melancholic states. In 1947 an analysis of one thousand prefrontal leucotomies in Britain showed that just under a quarter of the subjects had been discharged from hospital 'recovered' and a further 10 per cent 'improved'. 32 per cent were 'improved' but still required in-patient hospital treatment, 1 per cent were worse after operation, 25 per cent in hospital 'unchanged' and 6 per cent had died, half of the deaths being directly attributable to operation.[16]

An operation which has given very good results is that for hydrocephalus or water on the brain. Walter Dandy was one of the pioneers; he and others attempted to deflect the hydrocephalic fluid into the bowel, the peritoneal cavity, or the ureter. None of these methods proved successful, but in 1956 Dr E. Spitz of Philadelphia devised a special valve which was modified and improved by J. Holter, an engineer, whose son suffered from hydrocephalus. Holter's child was one of the first patients to be so treated. The Spitz-Holter valve, used today, drains the fluid into the internal jugular vein; it is a non-return valve, so that blood cannot pass upwards from the vein, and incorporates an ingenious pumping device in the wall.

We must end with mention of a rather more 'difficult' procedure – difficult to explain – that is probably going to be of very great importance in the future. Stereotactic surgery, first practised by Horsley in 1908, is localization of a lesion in all three dimensions, the positioning of an electrode in the substance of the brain, the finding of the lesion by means of the reaction to the electrical stimulus given by the electrode, followed by the destruction of the minute area at fault. The uncontrollable tremor of Parkinson's disease or paralysis agitans has been successfully treated by this method, but it has not yet proved entirely successful for the cure of other symptoms.

2. LUNG

During the nineteenth century tuberculosis accounted for nearly a quarter of all hospital admissions and many of these patients suffered from the pulmonary form, often called consumption or phthisis. Considering the appalling mortality of pulmonary tuberculosis, it is perhaps surprising that attempts at surgical treatment were so long delayed. The first man to suggest that a lung might be rested by filling the thoracic cavity on the affected side with air (artificial pneumothorax) was an English physician James Carson in 1821, but there is no record of this comparatively simple operation being performed until over sixty years later.

In 1882 the Italian physician Carlo Fornanini discussed artificial pneumothorax as a theoretical treatment, but he did not make a clinical trial until 1888. Meanwhile J. W. Hulke, a surgeon, and W. Cayley, a physician, both of the Middlesex Hospital, had inserted a double rubber catheter into one side of the chest of a twenty-one-year-old man who had been admitted to the hospital after suffering a very large haemorrhage (haemoptysis) from the lung. The operation took place on 10 March 1885, but the patient died five days later from the effects of another haemoptysis.[17]

Not many of these operations were performed before the First

World War. Between 1888 and 1911 Fornanini did eighty-six; he found that air was absorbed too quickly and started to use nitrogen instead. J. B. Murphy in America and Ludolph Brauer in Germany took up the method; Brauer was a physician who persuaded a surgeon, P. L. Friedrich to operate but, after a few experiences, Friedrich refused to do any more because of the high mortality, and Brauer was forced to operate himself. In Britain interest was aroused by Parry Morgan and Leonard Colebrook of St Mary's, where the first successful injection of nitrogen was carried out on 11 August 1910. But only four hundred cases could be traced in the world literature in 1910; this is a minute number when related to the terrible prevalence of tuberculosis.[18]

Another method of resting the lung is by destroying the nerve supply of the diaphragm, the large respiratory muscle separating the chest cavity from the abdomen. Ferdinand Sauerbruch of Griefswald, having experimented on animals, first suggested simple cutting of the nerve in 1905; another German, Carl Sturtz, applied Sauerbruch's idea to the human patient in 1911. Four years later P. L. Friedrich, whom we have already met, suggested that the nerve should not be cut but crushed; the temporary damage would allow a period of rest, but the nerve would be capable of recovering and of taking up its function again. The 'phrenic crush' was often used as a preliminary to more extensive operations upon the chest between the world wars.

We must now pass to another operation, the drainage of an empyema. An empyema is a collection of pus contained in a cavity; in this case the cavity between the lung and the chest wall. In 1852 Henry Ingersoll Bowditch of Boston pointed out the need to make an incision so that the pus could escape. He performed this operation 270 times between 1852 and 1873, with no immediate death, but his method cannot have been effective, for he only made a stab incision low down in the back of the chest, which could have allowed only very limited drainage. In 1870 Georges Dieulafoy, a Paris physician, invented an aspirator by means of which it was possible to draw off pus and other fluids and this came into use for draining the chest in 1873. But free drainage could not be instituted without the insertion of a tube through the chest wall, first advocated by J. L. Béhier, and unless the negative pressure in the potential space between the lung and the chest wall was maintained. Without that negative pressure, an opening through the chest wall would cause the lung to collapse under atmospheric pressure; the result would be a large space from which the pus could not be removed. In 1876 the latter problem was partially solved by Gotthard Bulau of Hamburg who introduced the method of under-water drainage: when the patient breathed out, pus was forced down the tube; when he breathed in, the water rose in the tube and maintained the seal.

In 1879 J. A. Estlander drew attention to the fact that a narrow bore tube, inserted through a small stab wound, will almost invariably be blocked by thick pus, and suggested the essential modification that a portion of rib should always be resected; this would allow a larger drainage space and prevent early closure of the wound. Although Estlander usually receives credit for this advance, William Thomas of the Birmingham and Midland Free Hospital had already performed the operation in 1876 and was able to report the results of nine cases in May 1880. Four children had entirely recovered; the wound had healed, the cut ends of the rib had grown together again and the collapsed lung had re-expanded; three children were 'much improved', one 'doing well', and one had died.[19] In England this technique is particularly associated with the name of William Arbuthnot Lane. Surgeons had previously tried a simple stab incision first and had only resorted to resection of the rib when this failed to establish satisfactory drainage. Lane, while he was still a house surgeon at the Victoria Hospital, Tite Street, started to resect the rib as a first operation; between January and October 1882 he treated five children by primary rib resection; four of the five were successful and one died.

Resection of a small length of one rib led naturally to the more drastic operation of thoracoplasty, the resection of a number of ribs over a diseased area of lung. The operation was not for drainage but to rest the lung; the skin of the chest wall was closed over the excised ribs and, since the rigid cage had been removed, the lung could no longer fully expand. The method was first used for resting the tuberculous lung by Edouard de Cerenville of Lausanne in 1885, but did not become at all popular until the work of Julien Gourdet of Paris ten years later. Carl Semb and John Alexander advocated thoracoplasty in America; the first of these operations in Britain was by Morriston Davies at the Brompton Hospital in 1912. Thoracoplasty was popular until quite recently.[20]

So far we have dealt only with surgery of the chest wall and not of the lung proper. Attempts to close wounds, not only of the chest but in the lung substance, were certainly made by Larrey and probably by earlier military surgeons. The first well-documented case is in 1873, when William Macewen removed part of the broken-off blade of a knife from the lung of a boy aged twelve. Two years later Macewen resected part of the rib from a man who had been wounded in the chest, and sutured the injured lung. The first attempt to remove a diseased portion of a lung is open to considerable doubt. The operation may have been attempted in 1884 when a German surgeon named Block tried to resect part of the lung of a female relation supposed to be suffering from tuberculosis. The patient died on the operating table, post-mortem examination revealed no sign of tuberculosis, and Block committed suicide.

There is, however, no doubt that Theodore Tuffier of Paris successfully resected the apex of a tuberculous lung in 1891. Two years later a similar operation was performed by D. Lowson of Hull. Lowson was not aware of Tuffier's case at the time, but learned of it soon after. He performed a number of operations on animals before applying his idea to the human, and he states that he had been influenced by the work of a Russian scientist, Zakharevitch, who had also done many experimental resections in animals. Lowson's patient, a thirty-four-year-old woman suffering from tuberculosis, underwent operation on 14 February 1893; Lowson excised a piece of the upper lobe of the right lung 'the size of half a fist and containing a dense tuberculous mass'. She made a good recovery after a somewhat stormy convalescence and was discharged from hospital on 4 May.[21]

An interesting man, who performed an early lung resection, was the brilliant but intolerably self-advertising E. L. Doyen of Paris. The date of his operation is about 1894; among his other feats, Doyen introduced the cinematograph camera into surgery as early as 1898, and separated the Siamese twins Radica and Doodica, amid a blaze of publicity that puts any recent attempts into the shade. He is said to have written his own account of the operation for publication in the French popular press. William Macewen performed a very extensive lung resection, or clearance of the left side of the chest, in 1895. There is much controversy among surgical historians about Macewen's operation; it is sometimes stated that he removed the whole lung for the first time in history, but Macewen's own account makes it clear that the lung had been almost totally destroyed by tuberculosis before operation. The patient must have been desperately ill but made a good recovery. Eleven years later Macewen wrote 'since his convalescence he has been able to engage in light work, supporting his wife and family thereby. He can walk about easily while taking time, and enjoys good health'.[22] Another surgeon, J. T. Morrison, met the man in 1926 – that is thirty years after operation – and found him well and still doing light work.[23]

These early resections were described by the surgeons concerned as 'pneumonectomies', a term now applied to the removal of the whole of one lung. For this reason Tuffier, Lowson, Doyen and Macewen are often credited with the 'first' pneumonectomy. Setting aside Macewen's controversial operation, the remainder would nowadays be called 'lobectomies' or 'partial lobectomies', the removal of only a portion of the lung. All were done on account of tuberculosis. In 1910 a German, Hermann Kümmell, removed the lung of a patient suffering from cancer. This is thought to be not only the first operation for cancer of the lung, a rarely diagnosed disease in those days, but also the first true pneumonectomy. It was not, however, successful, for the patient died on the sixth day after operation. In 1912 Hugh Morriston Davies of University College Hospital, the earliest specialist in chest surgery, resected a lobe of the lung for cancer with survival of the patient; this is thought to be the first successful operation for cancer of the lung.

We must look upon this type of surgery as a series of isolated experiments; open surgery of the lung cannot be said to have any continuing history until after the First World War. As in surgery of the head or of the abdomen, a number of different discoveries and improvements in general operating technique made advance possible; surgery of the lung in particular owes a debt to better methods of anaesthesia. It will be convenient to consider at this point how the many problems of anaesthesia for operations on the lung were solved.

Until well into the twentieth century the vast majority of anaesthetics were given by a mask over the nose and mouth or by a lead tube tucked into a corner of the mouth. The anaesthetic drug was either dripped directly on to the mask or vaporized by means of a hand bellows; the one gas used, nitrous oxide, was given through a rubber mask, sometimes mixed with the vapour of ether or chloroform. These crude methods made operation on the head, mouth, throat, nose, and neck both difficult and dangerous; and, whatever the type or site of operation, there was always the hazard of obstructed respiration because relaxation of the muscles, a result of anaesthesia, caused the tongue to fall back into the throat.

In order to avoid the danger of an obstructed airway in some specially difficult operations, a few early surgeons performed a preliminary tracheostomy, cutting a small hole through the skin and the cartilaginous rings of the trachea, and inserting a tube through which the anaesthetic might be given. Although this greatly lessened the risk of respiratory obstruction, the method was by no means a safe one because of the risk of pneumonia following tracheostomy. In 1878 Macewen had the idea of passing a tube through the mouth, between the vocal cords, into the trachea; thus the anaesthetic could be fed directly into the trachea without fear of obstruction from the tongue falling back into the throat. His tubes, made of silver or gum elastic, were at once rigid and flexible; they could be bent to the desired angle but would retain their shape when inserted. His first intubation was for an operation upon the tongue; Macewen practised passing the tube upon the unfortunate patient several times, by sense of touch alone, before deciding that his method was a safe one. 'It was found that, with the exception of the cough which ensued immediately upon its insertion, he bore the tube sufficiently well to warrant the success of the procedure.'[24] Everything went well on 5 July 1878, the first operation at which the anaesthetic was given by the endotracheal method.

Macewen's second experiment ended in disaster, but the tube cannot be blamed. After several preliminary trials 'next morning, in the ward adjoining the theatre, the tube was introduced into the trachea, the patient as usual holding the outer end; he remained there for a quarter of an hour, breathing easily. He then walked into the theatre and lay down on the table. Chloroform was just commenced to be given him, when he rose up, withdrew the tube, handed it to the surgeon, said he would prefer to take the chloroform without it, and that it could be introduced afterwards. He then lay down to inhale the anaesthetic.'[25] It is interesting but not surprising that this, the first suggestion that the tube should be passed after and not before the commencement of anaesthesia, came from the patient. He died from the effects of chloroform shortly after the administration had been renewed.

At the International Medical Congress of 1881, Macewen described his tube, not only for anaesthesia, but as a substitute for tracheostomy in the treatment of respiratory obstruction caused by croup or diphtheria.[26] Credit for the introduction of intubation in these diseases is usually assigned to Joseph O'Dwyer of America, but he did not invent his tubes until 1885. Combined with a bellows attachment suggested by another American, G. E. Fell, the O'Dwyer tube became the Fell–O'Dwyer apparatus for artificial respiration. With this it was possible to reinflate a lung that had collapsed as the result of opening the chest. In 1899 Rudolf Matas of New Orleans adopted the Fell-O'Dwyer apparatus for this purpose and to maintain anaesthesia while the opening in the chest wall was repaired. Macewen and O'Dwyer had both passed the tube by sense of touch; passage of the endotracheal tube became much easier with the invention of the direct vision laryngoscope, by means of which a view of the opening between the vocal cords into the trachea could be obtained. The first practical instrument was devised by a German, Alfred Kirstein, in 1894.

Fell's bellows could only blow air impregnated with ether or chloroform down O'Dwyer's tube. In 1887 the London anaesthetist, Frederic Hewitt, designed the first practical nitrous oxide-oxygen apparatus. The pressure of the gases, packed in iron cylinders, was reduced to a safe level by means of valves, and a known quantity of oxygen could be added to the nitrous oxide. Thus it became possible to cut the patient's respiratory system entirely off from the air, and to maintain both anaesthesia and expansion of the lung under a positive pressure. Hewitt's apparatus, or some modification of it, was used by Ferdinand Sauerbruch to maintain expansion of the lung in the opened chest; he did not pass an endotracheal tube but applied a tightly-fitting mask to the face. In 1904 Sauerbruch suggested the exact reverse of this method; he maintained expansion of the lung by placing the patient in a negative-pressure cabinet (this, incidentally, is the prototype of the iron lung) and allowing the atmospheric pressure to exert its effect through the trachea. Both of Sauerbruch's innovations, although theoretical advances, proved unsuitable for practical surgery; positive pressure by means of a face mask inflated the stomach as well as the lungs, and the negative pressure cabinet produced almost impossible operating conditions.

Part of the answer was to blow the anaesthetic vapour down an endotracheal tube under positive pressure; two Frenchmen, Barthélemy and Dufour, introduced 'endotracheal insufflation anaesthesia' in 1907. A. L. Meltzer and J. Auer of the Rockefeller Institute experimented on animals with positive pressure insufflation methods in 1909; they built an apparatus which was first applied to chest surgery by A. Schachner of Kentucky in 1909 and by C. A. Elsberg of Philadelphia in 1910; the British anaesthetist Robert Kelly devised a somewhat complicated positive pressure insufflation apparatus in 1912. But positive pressure had to be used with great care or the lung would become over-distended; further there was no means of removing that troublesome product of the body, carbon dioxide, which stimulates the respiration and so causes increased movement of the lung.

Positive pressure insufflation was maintained through a narrow-bore rigid tube. E. S. Rowbotham and Ivan Magill, the two famous anaesthetists who worked at Queen Mary's Hospital, Sidcup, found by experience of facial injuries that a specially shaped, wide bore, soft rubber tube will not become obstructed by kinking if passed through the nose or mouth into the trachea. They came to the conclusion that to-and-fro respiration at only a slight positive pressure is preferable to insufflation. By 1921 they were able to report almost trouble-free anaesthetics in some three thousand cases. Pressure could be varied by opening or closing a simple valve; if open, the patient would breathe out through the valve; if closed, a positive pressure could be maintained for short periods. In 1932 Ralph Waters of Wisconsin modified the Magill tube by making it longer and adding an inflatable cuff just over the lower end. This could be passed down the trachea into one or other of the main bronchi; by inflating the cuff, the lung into which the anaesthetic was being fed could be sealed off from the lung which was being operated on. A no less important advance was made in 1936, when Magill modified his tube by adding a removable cap; when the cap is taken off, a fine tube connected to a sucker can be passed down the endotracheal or endobronchial tube and any secretion removed.

There still remained the troublesome problem of the patient's carbon dioxide which could not be removed if an adequate positive pressure was to be maintained; it is interesting that John Snow understood the importance of this problem as early as 1851. In 1915 Dennis E. Jackson designed an anaesthetic apparatus incorporating a carbon dioxide absorber. Jackson never applied his invention to the human, but three American doctors made trial of it in minor surgery and, on one occasion, when removing the thyroid gland. In 1924 Ralph Waters much improved the Jackson apparatus and introduced it into routine use; the carbon dioxide is removed by breathing through granules of soda lime.

A most important advance in anaesthesia for operations on the lung came in 1933 with the introduction of the gas cyclopropane. This gas is not irritant to the lungs and can produce deep anaesthesia when mixed with 90 per cent of oxygen. These two advantages largely solved the problem of anaesthetising the patient with pulmonary tuberculosis. Cyclopropane is 'inert', breathed out unchanged by the patient, and is also very expensive; the only economic method of using it is by allowing the patient to breathe the same gas over and over again, adding the requisite amount of oxygen and removing carbon dioxide by means of soda lime.

The removal of carbon dioxide added to the anaesthetic effect of cyclopropane causes the breathing to become depressed, sometimes so depressed that, even with the high percentage of oxygen used, the patient may show signs of oxygen-lack. In 1941 M. D. Nosworthy of St Thomas' and the Westminster Hospitals drew attention to the fact that this could be altered by squeezing the breathing bag of the anaesthetic apparatus with the hand – in fact, performing a slight degree of artificial respiration, 'assisted respiration'. Nosworthy used assisted respiration in chest surgery, because it allowed lung movement to be brought largely under the anaesthetist's control.

The outstanding importance of Nosworthy's simple and curiously 'unscientific' contribution has gone almost unremarked, but it forms the basis of most modern anaesthetic methods. In 1942 there came what is probably the greatest advance in anaesthesia since 1846, when H. R. Griffith and G. E. Johnson of Montreal introduced the active principle of the South American arrow poison curare. Tubocurarine, the derivative in commonest use today, produces relaxation or actual paralysis of the muscles. Thus, by means of 'curarization' and 'squeezing the bag', lung movement can be brought under complete control; the patient's own respiratory movements can be assisted or the movements can be ended entirely – but temporarily – and life be maintained by artificial respiration. Today 'squeezing the bag' in chest surgery and prolonged operations of all kinds has largely given place to rhythmical inflation of the lung by mechanical respirators, of which there are many models. The first practical respirator was the 'spiropulsator' invented by Clarence Crafoord of Stockholm in 1938.

This diversion into methods of anaesthesia has caused us to jump ahead of advances in chest or thoracic surgery. During the First World War experience in dealing with chest and lung injuries encouraged a number of surgeons to embark on procedures which they would not have contemplated in July 1914. Notable among these surgeons are Pierre Duval of Paris and George Ernest Gask of St Bartholomew's Hospital, the first professor of surgery in the University of London. In the early nineteen twenties the surgeon operated more frequently upon the chest, but the range of his operations was still very limited. Only those for the induction of artificial pneumothorax and for the drainage of an empyema were commonly performed; the latter carried a high mortality.

In 1922 Howard Lilienthal of New York declared that, just as the abdominal cavity is explored by the operation of laparotomy, so the interior of the chest should be explored by a wide incision between the ribs. In cases of bronchiectasis, the multiple abscesses usually caused by secondary infection of a tuberculous lung, Lilienthal explored the chest and, if he found the trouble confined to one lobe of the lung, removed that lobe by a two-stage operation. His results were not encouraging; in 31 cases his mortality was 42 per cent. In ten cases where he had tried to remove more than one lobe of the lung, his mortality was as high as 70 per cent.[27]

Increasing experience led to better results. In 1923 Evarts Graham of Washington adopted Lilienthal's technique of two stage lobectomy but, instead of cutting the lobe away, he burned it off with the actual cautery. In a series of 54 cases, spread over several years, he experienced only six deaths. The two-stage operation, designed with the idea that the first stage would produce adhesions between the lung and the chest wall and so prevent collapse of the remainder of the lung, was never a satisfactory one. In 1929 H. Brunn of San Francisco devised a special tourniquet to prevent bleeding from the large vessels at the root of the lung; three years later he published a series of eight one-stage lobectomies with only one death. Brunn's tourniquet operation, improved by Shenstone and Janes of Canada in 1931, was adopted by Clement Price Thomas and Tudor Edwards of the Brompton Hospital in 1934.

Tudor Edwards had already performed a one-stage lobectomy. He nearly succeeded in 1926 but his patient died within twenty-four hours. On 5 December 1928 he resected the lower lobe of the left lung, affected with cancer, from a woman of forty-eight. Recovery from operation was uneventful and the patient lived for nearly thirty years, dying on 21 May 1957 from another, and very large, cancer in the *right* lung. Lord Brock, well known as a thoracic surgeon and a medical historian, states that this is the first successful one-stage lobectomy in the history of surgery. Tudor Edwards also performed the first successful one-stage lobectomy for bronchiectasis in Britain (1929).[28] By 1939 he had recorded 199 lung resections for this disease alone.[29]

Meanwhile attempts were being made to remove the whole

lung. We have seen that, except for Kümmell's case in 1910, all previous 'pneumonectomies' are open to question. In 1919 Lilienthal definitely performed a total pneumonectomy for bronchiectasis, but his patient died six hours later. Willi Meyer, a German, also removed a lung in 1920, but again the patient died very soon afterwards. Sauerbruch tried doing the operation by several stages in 1923; he did not actually remove the lung but depended on sloughing of the lung tissue and it is probable that some tissue remained.

The disastrous outcome of these operations resulted in no further attempt being made for eight years. Then, in 1931, the German R. Nissen successfully used much the same technique as Sauerbruch's on a twelve-year-old girl who had suffered a crushing injury of the chest. As Kümmell's patient had died, Nissen's case may be regarded as the first successful pneumonectomy, but for injury and not for disease. E. Windsberg, C. Haight, and E. Archibald, all of America, performed multistage operations in 1932. Windsberg's operation (for bronchiectasis) was for three years considered to be the first successful pneumonectomy in the United States. At the end of that time the patient died, and post-mortem revealed that the removal had been incomplete, the lower lobe of the lung having been left.

In April 1933 Evarts A. Graham of Washington performed his historic operation. Fourteen years later he described his experience to the Royal College of Surgeons of England; the essentials of his account will here be given in his own words. He said that he 'was fortunate in having an ideal patient present himself with a squamous carcinoma (type of cancer) involving the bronchus of the left upper lobe. He was a physician, forty-eight years old. The condition was complicated by several abscesses in the lobe. It was my intention before operation to remove the left upper lobe, but at the operation it seemed to me that this procedure would allow some of the cancer to remain. If all the tumour was to be removed a total pneumonectomy would therefore be necessary, and it seemed to me desirable to perform the operation in one stage . . . Knowing the patient as well as I did I felt even more justified in taking the risk because I was certain that he would rather die of the operation than after a prolonged illness from his cancer. After the lung was out the empty pleural space seemed so enormous that seven ribs (the third to the ninth inclusive) were removed in order to accomplish a partial obliteration of it. The immediate post-operative course was uneventful and on the tenth day the patient for three hours attended a meeting of the Clinical Surgery Society which was held at the Barnes Hospital. Later he developed a small empyema at the upper part of the pleural cavity. The removal of the first and second ribs resulted in the complete obliteration and healing of the cavity ... He is now (1947) in his sixtieth year, free from any symptoms, and he carries on an extremely large obstetrical practice in Pittsburgh.'[30]

Evarts Graham's operation at the Barnes Hospital is the first one-stage pneumonectomy and the first successful pneumonectomy for cancer. By 1947 229 one-stage total pneumonectomies had been done at the Barnes Hospital, 161 of them for tumours of various kinds. In the first years the mortality was as high as 53 per cent, but it had fallen to 6·2 per cent by September 1947, largely due to increased experience, better anaesthesia, use of blood transfusion, and the bacteristatic and antibiotic drugs. The first successful one-stage pneumonectomies to be performed in Britain were at the Brompton Hospital by Tudor Edwards and his rival, J. E. H. Roberts, who both performed the operation in the same week in 1935.

Today operations for lung cancer are increasing in number, and those for tuberculosis have shown a decrease. In the latter disease especially, a more limited operation has become possible since E. D. Churchill showed that the lung can be anatomically divided into segments and not, as was previously thought, into three relatively large lobes. A very important drug, streptomycin, exerted a profound effect upon the surgery of tuberculosis and has made it possible to defer operation until the disease is quiescent. Streptomycin was the first important antibiotic discovered in the deliberate search for other drugs having an action on bacteria similar to that of penicillin. It was obtained from a mould, *Streptomyces griseus*, by Waksman in 1944 and was introduced into medicine in 1948. Waksman obtained his cultures from a heavily manured field and from the throat of a chicken!

3. HEART

Modern surgery of the heart has been born partly of an increased familiarity with the open chest and partly of the age-old compulsion to save the victim of imminent death. As with surgery of the lung, so the early surgery of the heart was not upon the heart itself but upon the surrounding structures, the pericardium which covers the heart, and the chest wall. The pericardial sac is a covering of two layers which are normally in close apposition save for a thin film of 'lubricating fluid'; in disease the sac may become distended with fluid or frank pus and, if the pressure rises sufficiently high, the heart will be stopped by the simple fact that it is unable to continue pumping against the distended sac.

The first attempt to deal with a pericardial effusion came in 1649 when John Riolan (who opposed William Harvey's views upon the circulation) recommended that the heart should be approached by making a trephine hole through the sternum or breast bone, and tapping the distended sac with a trochar and cannula. Riolan's operation, though rarely attempted, persisted until as late as 1871, when a surgeon named Malle is known to have performed it. In 1870 Georges Dieulafoy suggested that his aspirator, mentioned in the last section, might be used for drawing off a pericardial effusion and, some years before this, Armand Trousseau of Paris advocated that the heart should be approached by an incision between the ribs, rather than by trephining the sternum. In 1866 the great physician Clifford Allbutt, who had studied under Trousseau, persuaded the surgeon Wheelhouse of Leeds to tap a much distended pericardium by Trousseau's method, and the patient recovered. So far as is known, this was the first 'operation on the heart' in Britain. Wheelhouse's successful example was followed by Bowditch in Boston and by William Roberts, a physician of Manchester. In 1883 Lister conceived the idea of irrigating the sac with a solution of mercuric chloride in the case of a patient suffering from purulent pericarditis. The very scrappy notes give no indication of the incision which Lister used to approach the heart, but he cannot have obtained an adequate view, for the exit tube became blocked with flakes of pus, resulting in over distension of the pericardium by the stream of mercuric chloride, and the patient died.

In 1895 the French surgeon Délorme suggested the possibility of dividing adhesions which had formed after an infective disease. He called his operation 'decortication' and advised it for both the lungs and the heart; with another French surgeon, Alfred Mignon, he devised a method of approaching and of opening the pericardial sac in order to divide adhesions. The operation was also advocated by Edmond Weill of Lyon in the same year and by Alexander Morison in 1897. Morison wrote that the severing of cardiac adhesions would be 'an ideal triumph of modern surgery'. It would, however, seem from an article written in 1909 that the operation had never been done on the human subject.

The next procedure also derived from an operation originally suggested for the lung. We saw that thoracoplasty, the removal of several ribs, was one of the methods used to rest the lung. In 1902 Ludolph Brauer, a physician of Heidelberg, persuaded his surgical colleagues Petersen and Simon to resect the ribs over the heart of a patient suffering from adherent pericarditis; the idea being not to rest the heart but to allow greater freedom of movement. In the following year Brauer showed three successful cases at the German Congress of Surgery. Koch of Groningen performed this operation in 1904 with great benefit to his patient, the young son of a colleague. The first case of this kind in Britain, also successful, was by E. C. Stabb of the Great Northern Central Hospital in 1908; another was performed at about the same time by Wilfred Trotter of University College Hospital. In 1910 William Thorburn of Manchester discussed fifteen cases known to him, five by Petersen and Simon, and said of the operation that 'it has been conclusively shown not only that it can be performed with reasonable safety, but that in suitable cases it may prove of great value'. This is the first 'operation on the heart' to have attained any popularity, but it was not very successful in its object.

Attempts had occasionally been made to deal with injuries to the heart itself. A stab wound of the heart may not cause quick death; the hole in the pericardium may become closed by bloodclot when the heart will continue to pump blood through its own wound into the pericardium; death will then be delayed until the pressure in the pericardium is sufficient to stop the heart's action. Baron Larrey tried to deal with such a case in 1810 by incising and draining the pericardium; it seems that operation was delayed until no less than forty days after the self-inflicted injury, for the patient is described as having died sixty-eight days after wounding and twenty-eight days after drainage. In 1871 Thomas Watson, a physician of the Middlesex Hospital, advised 'tapping' of the pericardium as a last resort in the treatment of stab wounds. Surgeons also tried to remove sharp-pointed instruments which had become embedded in the heart. Two attempts of this kind were made in 1835 and 1845, but the first successful operation took place on 28 October 1872 when G. W. Callender of Bart's extracted a long needle which had pierced the heart.[31] The state of cardiac surgery at that time can be gauged by Billroth's remark in 1875 that aspiration of the pericardium or any attempted operation on the heart was 'nothing short of madness'. The possibility of repairing an injury of the heart itself had already been mooted, for in 1888 a surgeon named Riedinger dismissed the suggestion of suturing a wound as scarcely deserving mention.[32]

Within ten years Riedinger's opinion was proved incorrect. In 1895 the Italian del Vecchio made an experimental wound in an animal's heart and succeeded in closing it by suture. Del Vecchio's experiments were repeated in Italy by Salomini and Messina. But, by this time, the Norwegian Axel Cappelen had tried to repair a rent in the human heart. In 1895 a man of twenty-four was admitted to hospital having suffered a stab wound of the left side of the chest some hours before. He was unconscious; his pulse could not be felt; but the heart sounds could still be very faintly heard. Cappelen enlarged the wound and found the left side of the chest to contain nearly one and a half litres of blood. He cleared out the blood and saw a wound in the pericardium about one centimetre in length. He incised the pericardium, cleared out the blood clot contained therein, and found a wound, two centimetres long, in the left ventricle of the heart. This he sutured, at the same time ligaturing a bleeding vessel in the wall of the heart. The patient died from sepsis sixteen hours later.[33]

In the following year the Italian surgeon Guido Farina made the attempt. We must be careful here. Medical historians have recorded that Farina was not successful, but a letter from Farina to the English surgeon Sir John Bland Sutton, written in 1909, makes it plain that his *operation* was successful although he lost his patient.[34] The man, aged twenty, had been stabbed in the left side of the chest with a fine and sharp dagger which had penetrated the heart. Farina opened the left side of the chest by removing a piece of the fifth rib and found a wound in the heart seven millimetres long, which he sutured with three silk stitches and 'two others of less importance'. The patient recovered from the immediate effects of operation, but developed a pneumonia of the *right* lung and died three days later. The point is that the pneumonia was on the right side, whereas Farina had, naturally, operated on the left side of the chest; obviously he lost his patient by sheer bad luck. Farina was annoyed, for his letter to Bland Sutton ends 'at the autopsy the wound in the heart was found perfectly healed. The heart was not allowed to be preserved for further study. It was precisely because of my irritation at this fact that I have not published any communication on this very interesting case.'

Farina should probably be credited with the first successful suture of a wound in the heart, but his fame is overshadowed by that of Ludwig Rehn of Frankfurt who, six months later, achieved an undeniable triumph. Rehn's patient, a twenty-two-year-old gardener (who had been discharged from the army a few days previously with 'advanced heart disease'), received a stab wound from a table knife in a drunken brawl. On the next day, 9 September 1896, Rehn opened the left side of the chest by an incision much like that of Farina, removed blood clots from the chest cavity and pericardium, and found a one-inch wound in the lower part of the left ventricle. This he sutured with two silk stitches and a third through the pericardium. By the fourteenth day his patient was able to walk about the ward; in the following year Rehn showed him alive and well at the International Surgical Congress in Berlin.[35]

By 1906 seventy-eight suturings of heart wounds had been listed, with thirty-nine survivals and thirty-nine deaths, twenty of which were due to sepsis. In 1909 one hundred and fifty operations were known, but the mortality had risen from exactly 50 per cent to about 60 per cent; again, sepsis was the greatest killer. Sir John Ballance, who was interested in surgery of the heart, reckoned that just over three hundred suturings had been done by 1914; he thought the mortality had fallen to 45 per cent. During the First World War there were many attempts to suture wounds in the heart and to remove foreign bodies; Ballance had notes of fifty-eight suturings of which forty-four recovered, and fourteen died; indeed, as Ballance remarks, a wonderful record.[36]

In the First World War sepsis was still the most potent cause of death; the introduction of bacteristatic and antibiotic drugs made the operation much safer during the Second. In 1946 Dwight E. Harken of Boston, working at the time in the south of England, published a series of one hundred and thirty-four patients, wounded by missiles which had lodged in or near the heart and the great blood vessels, without a single death. This magnificent series included the actual removal of thirteen foreign bodies from the chambers of the heart.[37]

The curious point may have been noted that all three of the 'first' suturings occurred within two years but in three different countries. It is doubtful if any of the three surgeons knew of the operations performed by the others. The probable explanation is that experimental work on the heart and operative treatment of the chest had drawn general attention to the possibility of including the heart in the scope of surgery. Some evidence in favour of this view is to be found in the story of the first suggestions for the relief of mitral stenosis, the narrowing of the valvular orifice by vegetations often caused by rheumatic fever, which results in both heart and lungs working at a mechanical disadvantage.

The first man to have the idea of enlarging or dilating the constricted valve was William Arbuthnot Lane. In 1890 he discussed the matter with Lauriston E. Shaw, a physician at Guy's; Shaw wrote that Lane 'satisfied me that he could without any harmful result temporarily enlarge, by surgical means, the orifice of a constricted mitral valve' but that he 'deliberately decided against regarding it as a justifiable therapeutic measure.'[38] In 1898 D. W. Samways, an English physician practising in Mentone, ended an article in the *Lancet* with the words: 'I anticipate that with the progress of cardiac surgery some of the severest cases of mitral stenosis will be relieved by slightly notching the mitral orifice.'[39]

The most direct suggestion came from another well-known physician, H. Lauder Brunton of St Bartholomew's who did a certain amount of experimental work, cutting the valve in healthy hearts removed from cats and practising operations upon the stenosed mitral valves of hearts removed in the post-mortem room. He described a technique of operation, suggested that the valve might be cut with a tenotomy knife have a cutting edge of a half to one inch in length, and made sensible proposals to avoid excessive bleeding and to prevent the pericardium becoming distended with leaked blood.[40] But he never performed the operation nor persuaded any surgeon to do so.

A certain amount of animal experiment continued during the next twenty years. Harvey Cushing and a colleague named Branch performed animal experiments at Johns Hopkins Hospital in 1908; Bernheim, also of Johns Hopkins, produced artificial mitral stenosis in dogs which he successfully relieved by surgery (1909). In 1914 the two French surgeons Alexis Carrell and Tuffier carried out successful section of heart valves in animals. There is a not very well authenticated story that Doyen attempted to divide a stenosed valve with a small tenotomy knife in 1913, but that the patient died; in this case the valve was not the mitral but the pulmonary. In the same year Tuffier tried to dilate the third valve, the aortic, with his finger. He did not open the aorta or the heart but simply made pressure with the tip of his finger through the aortic wall.

On 20 May 1923 E. C. Cutler and S. A. Levine of the Peter Bent Brigham Hospital performed the first successful surgical treatment of the stenosed mitral valve in a human patient.[41] A girl of twelve suffered from severe mitral stenosis and was steadily going down-hill with recurrent bouts of heart failure and congestion of the lungs. Cutler and Levine had been experimenting on animals for nearly two years; they decided that operation was justified because the girl was clearly going to die within a very short time. They exposed the heart by cutting through the mid line of the sternum, surrounded a small site in the wall of the left ventricle with sutures, then plunged a thin, curved tenotomy knife through the site and pushed it upwards for about two and a half inches until it encountered the mitral valve; they then cut the valve on one side, turned the knife round, and made a cut on the opposite side. The knife was quickly withdrawn while the sutures were pulled tight so as to seal the hole in the ventricular wall. The surgeons encountered little or no trouble; the whole operation took about one and a quarter hours. Convalescence was uneventful and the girl lived in much improved health for four and a half years.

Cutler's operation was a blind one; he could only judge that the knife had made contact with the valve and that the cut was being made in a suitable place. Blind 'valvotomies' were repeated at intervals during the next six years but, as can be readily appreciated, they proved to be somewhat dangerous procedures. Meanwhile an entirely different method had been used by Henry Sessions Souttar of the London Hospital.

Souttar's patient was a girl named Lily Hine who was first admitted to the London Hospital in January 1921 when she was eleven years old, suffering from chorea which has a close affinity with rheumatic fever. She developed mitral stenosis and during the next four years was continually in and out of hospital; in March 1925 it became obvious that nothing more could be done for her. By May her state was hopeless and Souttar decided that there was nothing to be lost by attempting operation.

On 6 May 1925 Souttar exposed the heart; he did not use Cutler's incision but made a flap or window by cutting through the ribs on the left side close to their attachments to the sternum and then making longitudinal incisions above and below the cut ends, almost exactly the same approach suggested by Lauder Brunton. John Challis, the anaesthetist, kept up a positive pressure via an endotracheal tube so as to maintain partial expansion of the lung. Souttar did not attack the valve through the left ventricle, in which the blood pressure is high but through the thinner walled left auricle and he chose the part of the auricle known as the auricular appendage, because the walls are 'floppy' and the blood pressure low. This is the essential difference between the Cutler and Souttar operations; Cutler attacked the valve from below and Souttar from above. He drew the auricular appendage out of the pericardial sac by two sutures, applied a soft curved clamp to the base and made an incision. Souttar then inserted his left forefinger into the appendage, the clamp was removed, and the appendage was drawn over his finger like a glove by means of the sutures, so that the finger acted as a plug and stopped all bleeding. He had intended to slip a thin knife down beside his finger and to cut the valve, but when he had fully explored the valve with the tip of his finger he found that there was less stenosis than he had thought, and he decided that it would be enough to break down the adhesions and to dilate the valve with his fingertip. Having dilated the valve, Souttar withdrew his finger while the two purse string sutures were drawn together so that the hole in the appendage gradually closed after it. Then the sutures were tied, closing off the hole. The patient made an uneventful recovery; at the end of three months she said she felt perfectly well although still a little breathless on exertion.[42] She lived until 1930.

Perhaps the most extraordinary part of this story is that Souttar, in spite of his success, never again performed an operation on the heart. In 1961, when eighty-six years of age, he remarked that he must be the only cardiac surgeon in the world who had never experienced a death.

The next major advance did not come until thirteen years after Souttar's operation. The ductus arteriosus is peculiar to the arterial system of the foetus; it connects the pulmonary artery to the aorta and closes after birth. Very occasionally it fails to close, when it is spoken of as a persistent or patent ductus arteriosus. The prognosis of this congenital defect is not good, chiefly because the heart is unusually susceptible to infection, the very dangerous disease known as bacterial endocarditis. On the face of it, treatment would seem to be simple; if a suture is tied round the patent duct it will be effectually closed. This simple manoeuvre was first suggested by J. C. Munro in 1907, but was not carried out until 1937, when John Strieder of Boston ligated the duct, but his patient died five days later. In the same year Laurence O'Shaugnessy – who lost his life at the evacuation of Dunkirk – set out with the intention of closing the duct, but at operation the diagnosis proved to be incorrect. On 26 August 1938 Robert E. Gross of Harvard successfully ligated the patent ductus arteriosus of a seven-and-a-half-year-old child. 'The child underwent the operation exceedingly well and showed no signs of shock. Prior to operation blood had been taken from a donor in order to have it ready whenever needed, but the patient's condition was so good that it was not given.

There was only mild discomfort on the afternoon of the day of operation, and on the following morning the child was allowed to sit up in a chair. By the third day she was walking about the ward ... Because of the interest in the case the child was detained in the hospital until the thirteenth day.'[43] In 1940 Gross reported another three successes and during the next twenty years one thousand five hundred cases of patent ductus were treated by ligation at Harvard with a mortality of only 3 per cent. In his 1940 report, Gross was doubtful whether patients already affected by bacterial endocarditis could be regarded as suitable for operation. O. S. Tubbs of St Bartholomew's, making use of the bacteristatic drug sulphapyridine, first ligated the ductus of a patient suffering from bacterial endocarditis in December 1939.[44]

Treatment of coarctation of the aorta, stenosis or narrowing of the main artery of the body, was the next step. In 1944 Clarence Crafoord of Stockholm excised the narrowed segment in two cases, one a boy of twelve and the other a middle-aged man, reuniting the cut ends with sutures. Less than a year later Gross also performed this operation successfully. In 1946 Crafoord reported five more cases without a single failure.

The next major attack came upon Fallot's tetralogy, the much publicized 'blue baby' operation. Congenital heart defects rarely occur singly; Fallot's tetralogy, first described by Etienne Fallot of Marseilles in 1888, consists of four such defects. For our purpose, the only important one is stenosis of the pulmonary artery. The pulmonary artery arises from the venous or right side of the heart and the blood is pumped through it to the lungs; here carbon dioxide is released into and oxygen absorbed from the atmosphere; the oxygenated blood then travels by way of the pulmonary vein to the left or arterial side of the heart and is pumped through the aorta to the various parts of the body. Stenosis of the pulmonary artery will obviously result in inefficient oxygenation of the blood and in back pressure upon the right side of the heart.

The original 'blue baby' operation was suggested by the patent ductus arteriosus. In 1942 Dr Helen B. Taussig of Baltimore noticed that a child with a patent ductus in addition to Fallot's tetralogy did not suffer to the same degree as a child with Fallot's tetralogy alone. This suggested a by-pass to the stenosis. Dr Taussig discussed the point with Alfred Blalock, director of the department of surgery at the Johns Hopkins. On 29 November 1944 Blalock first performed his operation, known as systemic-pulmonary artery anastomosis, in the case of a girl of just over one year old. The anastomosis was made between the pulmonary artery and the subclavian vein, part of the systemic or body circulation. Although not itself an 'operation on the heart', the Blalock-Taussig operation may be regarded as the true starting point of modern cardiac surgery. In the words of Lord Brock 'it showed that cyanotic congenital heart disease, previously incurable and always fatal, could be cured by surgery. This inspired and stimulated the enormous advance in cardiac surgery that followed with almost breathless rapidity within a very short time.'[45]

Blalock's work is the beginning of modern heart surgery, but there can be no doubt that experience of battle casualties in the Second World War, as exemplified by Harken's record, gave the necessary confidence that the heart might be opened without undue risk. In 1947 Brock started to inspect the pulmonary valve by means of a specially designed cardioscope passed through the left pulmonary artery. This was not the first time that cardioscopy had been attempted, for in 1922 Duff Allen and Evarts Graham had tried to do the same by passing an instrument through the auricular appendage. Although successful in dogs, they failed in the human subject. Brock's first three patients died, but the experience gained led him to believe that direct attack upon the stenosed valve was feasible. His original idea had been to use a knife fitted to the cardioscope so that the valve could be cut under direct vision, but in the end he decided on a blind operation with a specially devised valvulotome – an instrument to cut the stenosed valve. With this he successfully cut a stenosed pulmonary valve on 16 February 1948. The patient, a girl of eighteen suffering from Fallot's tetralogy, was so ill that the anaesthetist considered a Blalock operation contraindicated. After a stormy convalescence she was allowed home on 18 March and was much improved in health when seen three weeks later.[46]

Here is another example of the remarkable fact that a new idea often occurs to more than one mind at the same time. Brock's three successful pulmonary valvotomies, of which the above was the first, must be allowed precedence of publication, but T. Holmes Sellors of the Middlesex Hospital can claim priority of operation, for he performed a manoeuvre similar to Brock's on 4 December 1947. The only difference was in the instrument used to cut the valve; Holmes Sellors used a long tenotomy knife.[47]

The work of Brock and Holmes Sellors was immediately followed by a general 'blind' attack upon the mitral valve. Harken of Boston and C. P. Bailey of Philadelphia operated through the auricular appendage in the manner of Souttar and either split the valve with a finger or cut it with a valvulotome, but the mortality was high, as many as seven dying out of Bailey's first ten patients. Results improved quickly as experience grew. By 1950 Bailey was able to report thirty mitral valvotomies with twenty-four survivals; in the same year Brock published an account of nine cases with two deaths. Brock split the valve with his finger in six of these cases and used a cutting valvulotome in two;[48] it is interesting that his technique was essentially the same as that practised by Souttar a quarter of a century before. In 1953 Holmes Sellors, using a method similar to that of Brock, reported an immediate operative mortality of only 2·7 per cent (four cases) in a series of one hundred and fifty patients. Four other patients died a month or more after operation.[49]

Until 1952 all surgery upon the interior of the heart was blind surgery. In 1951 Gross had devised a well or bag of plastic material which could be sutured to the right auricle; this gave a better approach but did not allow inspection of the operation site. It was not until the introduction of low temperature methods (hypothermia) and of the heart-lung machine or extracorporeal circulation that a dry heart could be obtained and operations performed under direct vision.

The fact that hypothermia is capable of producing relative freedom from pain has been recognized at least since Larrey noticed that frost-bitten soldiers did not appear to feel the pain of amputation; freezing by an ether spray or ice applied to the skin has been used as a means of allaying the pain of minor operations for many years. In 1940 Temple Fay and Laurence Smith of Philadelphia reported that cooling the whole body to a temperature of 27°C produced a kind of 'frozen sleep' which reduced the need for pain-allaying drugs in inoperable cancers, although it had no effect upon the cancer itself as they had hoped. This was the first attempt to produce a state of hibernation in the human; a hibernating animal such as a hedgehog has a very slow circulation, a lowered temperature, and a low metabolic rate; this means that the animal's tissues, particularly the sensitive brain, can survive unharmed without food and with little oxygen.

In 1950 W. G. Bigelow and others in Toronto investigated the effects of cooling upon animals; they came to the conclusion that cooling might be applied to the human patient and might prove a safe method of producing a bloodless heart. The first use of hypothermia in surgery seems to have been by B. A. Cookson, working with C. P. Bailey at Philadelphia, but the patient died. In September 1952 three workers Lewis, Taufic and Varco cooled a five-year-old girl to 27°C and successfully repaired a congenital defect of the heart with survival of the child.

Cooling in these early operations was done by the obvious method of immersing the whole body in a bath of iced water, or by the application of ice packs. Ite Boerema of Amsterdam cooled animals to a temperature of below 20°C by passing the blood from an artery through a refrigeration chamber and back into a vein. In 1952 E. J. Delorme, working in the department of surgery at Edinburgh, also cooled the blood directly by diverting it from an artery through a double coil condenser containing iced water and returning it to a vein. Animal experiments by Radoslav Andjus, first of Belgrade and later of Mill Hill, showed that revival is possible from temperatures far below those that had already been employed.

It is true that hypothermia could cause a fall in metabolic rate and therefore reduce the body's need for a constant, rapid circulation of oxygenated blood, so that operation upon the dry heart became possible. But it soon transpired that recovery did not always occur, usually because the brain had been damaged. Further, if the method was to be a safe one, hypothermia imposed a time limit upon the surgeon. Using a method of hypothermia alone, the permissible time for operation upon the heart at a temperature of 28°C was about six minutes, with ten minutes as the absolute maximum.

The attractive idea of an extracorporeal circulation, cutting the heart out of the circuit and pumping the oxygenated blood round the body by a mechanical device, is by no means a new one, having been thought-aloud by a visionary in 1812. Although at first sight the obvious means of producing a dry heart, in practice the difficulties of preventing breakdown of the blood corpuscles and of oxygenating the blood required much work before a solution could be found. In 1926 Brukhonenko and Tchetchilin of Russia designed a primitive heart-lung machine with which they managed to sustain life in animals. About 1935 John Gibbon of Philadelphia started to investigate the problem; in 1937 he produced the first experimental machine and stated that his object was 'to allow the surgeon to cpen the heart without losing blood and to operate in the empty inside chambers'. His machine depended on a mesh screen over which the blood was pumped and saturated with oxygen; in 1952 it was more or less perfected and in use upon animals. In 1953 John Gibbon applied his idea to the human, a baby of fifteen months. By what seems to have been pure mischance this child and two out of his next three patients died.

Another apparently simple scheme is to employ the heart of a second person as the pumping and oxygenating machine for the patient. The credit for suggesting a human donor goes to Anthony Andreason and Frank Watson, working at the Buckston Browne Experimental Farm of the Royal College of Surgeons in 1953. C. W. Lillihei and R. L. Varco of Minneapolis used this method of cross-circulation for the first time on 26 March 1954. Their patient was a one-year-old boy suffering from a severe congenital heart defect, a deficient wall between the two ventricles. The father acted as donor; the right ventricle was open for thirty minutes and the defect successfully repaired. Although the child recovered from operation, he died of pneumonia on the eleventh day. Lillihei's next two patients, both suffering from interventricular defects, recovered. In the following two years he applied the technique to Fallot's tetralogy and was able to do a more extensive repair operation. By 1956 Lillehei had recorded forty-six successes.

The method appeared a good one but, unfortunately, it was not without risk to the donor; further, the position could easily arise wherein a parent might, for very good reasons, be placed in the intolerable position of having to refuse his help in saving the life of his child. Lillehei dropped the method, not because it was unsuccessful, but on ethical grounds, and returned to the heart-lung machine, a type of bubble-oxygenator which he had devised with the help of R. A. de Wall in 1954.

The Gibbon principle of oxygenation is by a mesh screen and the Lillehei by bubbling oxygen through the given blood, but it must incorporate a de-bubbling device or the free oxygen will produce an 'air' embolus in the veins. In 1948 V. O. Björk and Clarence Crafoord had invented a pump-oxygenator on the principle of rotating discs, dipping into a trough of blood, which picked up a film and exposed it to oxygen. Denis Melrose of the Royal Post-Graduate Medical School, Hammersmith, modified and improved the Björk pump and, in 1953, applied it to animal experiment. The first use of the Melrose pump in man took place on 9 December 1953 when W. P. Cleland of Hammersmith dilated a stenosed aortic valve by open operation through the left ventricle. The patient recovered consciousness within two hours of the operation and was sufficiently clear minded to know where she was and to ask the time within five minutes of waking. Before operation she had been bedridden; by June 1954 she could climb forty-eight steps without undue difficulty.[50]

In reporting this case Melrose stated that interest in pump oxygenation was steadily growing but mortality had been so high that even a single survival must be worth recording. The position had arisen in which advocates of the pump and advocates of hypothermia pointed to the dangers of the opposing method; but in 1954 neither method could be considered safe and neither gave ideal operating conditions. Hypothermia imposed a time limit; the pump did not give a motionless heart. In order to overcome the latter difficulty, Melrose tried injecting solutions of potassium citrate or chloride into the coronary circulation which supplies the heart. He first used this method of 'elective cardiac arrest' on animals in 1955; by 1958 potassium salts had been used for arrest of the human heart on thirty-six occasions at the Stanford University Hospital, San Francisco. Although successful for its purpose, potassium proved to be dangerous. Ite Boerema tried to overcome the danger of brain damage by combining hypothermia with oxygen under high pressure in 1956. His method required a special operating chamber. Cardiac arrest could be safely extended for forty-five minutes, but the cramped operating conditions and the necessity for decompression of staff when emerging from the high-pressure 'theatre' were, to say the least, inconvenient.

A combination of the two methods, hypothermia and the heart-lung machine, provided the answer. In 1959 C. E. Drew and others at the Westminster Hospital tried the effect of combining profound hypothermia, as suggested by the Andjus experiments, with a technique which replaced the heart by a pump yet allowed the patient's own lungs to oxygenate the pumped blood. They found that at a temperature of 15°C complete circulatory arrest could be tolerated for forty-five minutes. The first of their patients, a child of twelve months, died; the next two children, operated on for ventricular defects, recovered uneventfully. Drew at the same time reported operations upon four more patients of whom three recovered and one, an infant weighing only eight pounds, died.[51] The Drew method or the Melrose pump, fitted with a cooling coil to produce hypothermia, are now in common use; cardiac arrest has been maintained for as long as two hours at a temperature of 12°–13°C.

With these techniques open surgery of the heart under direct vision became possible. In describing the development of hypothermia and the 'pump', we have already mentioned the repair of congenital defects in the wall between the right and left ventricles; repair of these septal defects, and of the atrial defect in the wall of the auricles, would have been impossible without a dry heart. Once the dry heart had been obtained, surgeons began to consider a more delicate repair of valvular defects in place of the older methods of cutting or dilatation. In 1949 G. Murray of Toronto succeeded in replacing one of the cusps of a mitral valve with a new cusp made out of a piece of vein; he first experimented on dogs and later applied his technique to the human. Hufnagel of the Peter Bent Brigham Hospital made a kind of artificial ball-valve and placed this in the aorta to take over the function of an incompetent valve in 1954. In 1962 D. N. Ross of Guy's Hospital refashioned a defective aortic valve in the human, and at about the same time B. G. Barratt-Boyes started to perform a similar operation. In 1964 Barratt-Boyes reported the results of forty-four cases, treated with plastic repair of the valves or by the insertion of a ball-valve prosthesis; forty-one of these patients survived operation. We shall have a little more to say about this type of surgery in a later chapter.

It may have been noted that modern cardiac surgery started, not with operations upon the heart itself, but with operations upon the great blood vessels which arise directly from the heart. We will therefore retrace our steps and end this chapter with a short note on the surgery of blood vessels – vascular surgery – which may be said to date from 1897 when J. B. Murphy showed that severed arteries and veins can be reunited by end to end anastomosis. In 1902 Alexis Carrel introduced the method of suture which is today used in the anastomosis of blood vessels; he also transplanted vessels from one animal to another in 1908.

In 1912 G. C. Guthrie made the important suggestion that a length of excised artery can be replaced by a length of vein. Guthrie's idea was applied to the treatment of aneurysms by Lexer of Jena in 1912 and by the military surgeon Subbovitch in 1914, who replaced lengths of damaged artery by vein in soldiers wounded during the Balkan War. The first examples in Britain were by J. Hogarth Pringle of Glasgow in 1913. He treated two patients, one for an aneurysm and the other for an injury. His second patient, a lad of nineteen, had been badly cut in the arm by a piece of metal. Pringle excised six centimetres of the damaged brachial artery and replaced it with eight centimetres of a large vein from the leg. The patient was able to work at his trade of blacksmith two months after operation.[52]

It is surprising that no progress was made in arterial grafting during the two world wars. The surgeon contented himself with ligaturing the bleeding vessel or, very occasionally, with anastomosing the two cut ends together. Partly this is due to trouble experienced by clotting, the cause of failure in the majority of early repair operations. The blood clotted in the grafted length of vessel, the lumen became obliterated by the clot, and the clot often became infected, leaving the patient worse off than before. In 1916 W. H. Howell discovered heparin which prevents clotting of the blood, but heparin was not introduced into surgical practice until 1939, when George Murray of Toronto excised an aneurysm and repaired the defect with a length of vein.[53]

Not until April 1952, during the Korean War, did grafting of the wounded artery assume any importance, and the good results then attained suggested the possibility of treating arteries that had become occluded by disease. The cause of occlusion is a thrombus, a clot, which may occur in any artery. If the clot forms in the pulmonary artery, the blood cannot be oxygenated by the lungs and death will very rapidly ensue. An unsuccessful attempt to remove the clot from the pulmonary artery was made by the German surgeon Trendelenberg in 1908 and, by a miracle, was successfully done by another German, Martin Kirschner, in 1924. But these were desperate, life-saving measures; the gangrene resulting from a clot forming in the main artery of a limb could be more safely treated by amputation.

In 1947 J. C. Dos Santos of Portugal suggested that it might be possible to remove the thrombus occluding an artery of a limb, but some experimental work done at Harvard in 1949 diverted attention from his idea. The Harvard team, Gross, Bill, and Pierce, had been experimenting with 'bridges', tubes of various materials which might be used to bridge a gap between the excised ends of a blood vessel. Glass, aluminium, gold-plate, and silver, lined with paraffin, all led to thrombosis. Lucite, a plastic material, gave more promising results. From these inorganic substances they turned to organic tissues and found that an artery removed from one dog and grafted into another (homografts) would function. From dogs they turned to the human. Arteries were taken from victims of street accidents, quickly frozen, and stored at a very low temperature. These arterial homografts were used to repair excised lengths of artery in Fallot's tetralogy and coarctation of the aorta; of nine patients so treated, three died and in one the artery failed to 'take'. In a later series of six cases, all the grafted arteries were patent three to nine months after operation.[54]

The success experienced in the Korean War led to a renewed interest in this form of surgery. 'Banks' for the storage of arterial grafts at low temperatures were set up in certain centres – the first in England was at St Mary's Hospital, Paddington. Two plastics, teflon and dacron, were tried in place of the earlier tubes of glass, metal, or lucite, and found to give good results. Replacement of a length of artery by a piece of vein or, more often, the formation of a by-pass to the block in an artery was quite commonly practised. Surgeons started to investigate the actual removal of a clot from the artery – the operation of thromboendarterectomy – first suggested by Dos Santos.

In 1963 two surgeons at St Thomas' Hospital reported their experience of nine years; a short summary of their paper may serve to describe the progress that has been made. In the first five years they used stored arterial homografts, lengths of the patient's own vein, and, later, tubes of teflon or dacron. The initial results were not very good. Out of twelve end-to-end arterial grafts, only one remained patent for more than a year. Of twenty-nine by-passes, using a length of grafted artery to by-pass the clot in the patient's own artery, eleven remained patent for two years or more. In 1959 and 1960 they did twelve by-passes with a length of teflon tube; only two of these – in the right and left leg of the same patient – remained patent for over two years. From 1956 they tended to do more thromboendarterectomies (which they less scientifically but more pleasingly and correctly described as 'rebores') and by the end of 1959 had treated thirty-three patients by this method with seven primary failures; in 1962 sixteen of these patients still had patent arteries from two and a half to five years after removal of the thrombus. From 1959 they used an improved technique of 'total rebore', a more extensive examination and cleaning-out of the artery; out of fifty-four cases with seven primary failures, forty-six still had patent arteries at the time of writing, ten months to two and a half years after operation.[55]

CHAPTER II

Ears and Eyes

The last very long chapter dealt with specialities which have come to the fore in recent years. In the present – and much shorter – chapter we shall describe the development of two of the oldest surgical specialities which, broadly speaking, have never become part of general surgery. Tumours of the brain, diseases of the chest, malformations, fractures, acute appendicitis, all these were surgically treated in the first instance by men who did not confine themselves solely or even largely to a particular type of operation or region of the body. But there has always been a tendency to regard disease of the eye and of the ear as separate from the rest of surgery. The rule was by no means absolute; William Bowman, for instance, was a general surgeon who had a marked interest in the eye, and we find occasional notes that William Watson Cheyne operated on the ear.

Surgery of the ear[1,2] is linked to surgery of the brain by the 'acute mastoid', infection of the cellular bone immediately behind the ear. For centuries deafness, pain, and discharge from the ear were thought to be signs of an abscess in the brain. One of the more interesting cases in the history of medicine is that of the seventeen-year-old King Francis II of France, who suffered from severe headache, delirium, and a discharging ear. The court surgeon, Ambroise Paré, advised that the skull should be trephined in order to drain away the pus which he suspected to be present in the brain. The queen, Mary Queen of Scots, agreed to operation but the king's mother, the formidable Catherine de' Medici, overruled her. Francis died on 5 December 1560; Paré was afterwards accused of having put poison in his ear by command of Catherine. The unfortunate boy was undoubtedly suffering from an acute mastoid; had Paré been allowed to trephine over the mastoid cells, thus allowing free drainage, he might possibly have recovered. This raises an interesting point. Mary's second marriage with her cousin Henry Stewart united the kingdoms of England and Scotland under their son James the Sixth and First. Who would have inherited the throne had Francis lived to father a child? Here is an example of the effect of disease of the individual upon world history.

The infection of the king's mastoid may have already spread to form a brain abscess, for this can occur when the disease is untreated. Trephining could still have saved his life by draining away the pus, although no successful operation is known until nearly a century later when, in 1752, S. F. Morand of France trephined a fifty-one-year-old monk who was suffering from a brain abscess which had almost certainly arisen from the infected mastoid. In 1893 William Macewen reported that he had drained nineteen brain abscesses with only one death.[3] A brain abscess is very dangerous and drainage is by no means always successful. Macewen's astonishing record has never been surpassed and, as the brain abscess usually responds well to treatment with antibiotic drugs, it is now unlikely that it ever will be.

In 1761 Giovanni Battista Morgagni of Padua published a five-volume work on the causes of disease as revealed by posmortem examination. He stated, among other equally important findings, that a brain abscess is more often the result of acute inflammation of the ear, rather than that the pain, deafness, and discharge are secondary to a brain abscess. 'On the contrary,' he wrote, 'abscess of the brain results from suppression of discharge of the ear.' In 1736 the French surgeon Jean Petit drained an infected mastoid, with survival of his patient but an account of this case was not published until 1774, twenty-four years after Petit's death. Two years later in 1776 the operation was performed by the Prussian military surgeon Jasser, also with success.

There now occurred one of those tragic events which sometimes delay progress. Baron Bergen, physician to the king of Denmark, suffered from deafness and the type of singing in the ears known as tinnitus; having heard of Jasser's success he persuaded a colleague to attempt the operation upon himself, but he died twelve days later *from a brain abscess*. Morgagni's finding seemed to have been disproved; contemporary medical men thought that the deafness and tinnitus from which Bergen suffered must have resulted from an abscess of the brain. For nearly a century no attempt was made by the medical profession to treat infection of the ear as anything but a symptom of more deeply seated trouble.

For this reason the surgeons lost interest in aural surgery, which passed into the hands of unqualified practitioners. Some of these did important work. The Eustachian catheter, an instrument commonly used today, was invented by an aural 'surgeon' named Guyot who was, in fact, a posting-house keeper of Versailles. Another unqualified man, John Harrison Curtis, founded in 1816 a special institution for the treatment of ear diseases, now known as the Royal Ear Hospital. The first qualified doctor to practise otology in London was James Yearsley, who founded the Metropolitan Ear, Nose, and Throat Hospital in 1838.

About the year 1860 another qualified practitioner named Joseph Toynbee resurrected Morgagni's idea that a brain abscess may be secondary to infection of the ear. He proved that infection could extend to the brain by way of the internal ear, or labyrinth; he suggested that treatment of the ear infection should take the form of a drainage operation, or mastoidectomy. He never performed mastoidectomy himself, but his assistant, James Hinton, did it for the first time in 1868. Toynbee was appointed aural surgeon to St Mary's Hospital in 1851, the first general hospital to have a special department for diseases of the ear. It is of some interest that William Wilde of Dublin, the father of Oscar, treated a mastoid abscess by making an incision behind the ear in 1853; he did not open the bone to allow drainage of the pus, and advised against it, so he cannot be credited with the first mastoidectomy.

In 1873 H. H. Schwartze of Halle described a method of opening and draining the acutely infected mastoid cavity. This is the 'simple' or 'Schwartze' operation which is still quite often done. Although satisfactory in acute infection, it is of little value in the chronic type of disease, which requires a more radical clearance of diseased bone. This fact was first pointed out by

A. F. von Tröltsch in 1873; in 1889 another German, E. Küster, devised a suitable operation, which was given the name of 'radical mastoidectomy' by von Bergmann. The radical operation, although good for its purpose, is a very destructive one, for it is necessary to remove the bony wall of the external auditory meatus, the passage leading from the external air to the tympanic membrane, and also the chain of small bones, incus, malleus, and stapes, which conduct the sound waves from the tympanic membrane through a tissue-covered oval window into the internal ear and so to the brain. Thus the patient is left with a deaf ear.

In these early days of ear surgery, the surgeon was primarily concerned with the treatment of infection; his operations were life-saving and the preservation of hearing was of secondary importance. The surgery of deafness itself started to develop alongside the surgery of infection, but it made little headway until knowledge of the mechanism of hearing increased and until the surgeon became less obsessed with the risk of brain abscess. The old-time surgeon put first emphasis upon extirpation of infected tissue. The modern surgeon, armed with antibiotics and an operating microscope, is able to pay more attention to preservation of the ear's function; today the surgery of deafness has attained predominance.

But successful attempts to preserve the hearing of a chronically infected ear had been made long before the introduction of sulphonamides or of penicillin. In 1899 O. Korner suggested that it should be possible to perform a 'radical' operation without removing the tympanic membrane and the ossicles – incus, malleus, and stapes. The first description of this 'modified radical operation' was published in 1906 by Christopher Heath of University College Hospital[4] and, independently, by W. S. Bryant in America, but three years later the American surgeon S. J. Kopetsky pointed out that the Heath and Bryant operation did not remove all disease. G. Bondy of Germany overcame this objection in 1910 by slightly extending the amount of bone removed yet retaining the tympanic membrane and ossicles. His modified radical mastoidectomy did not attain any great popularity until 1938 when surgeons were becoming increasingly interested in the preservation and the improvement of hearing.

Sound waves, carried through the air, impinge upon the tympanic membrane which, in turn, transmits them as vibrations through the chain of ossicles to the brain. The tympanic membrane may become perforated by a disease process or by injury, and the patient's hearing will be impaired. The first attempts to cure deafness were directed to the filling of such defects in the tympanic membrane. Marius Banzer used a disc of pig's bladder to cover the hole as early as 1640; James Yearsley in 1841 occluded the perforation with a ball of moist cotton wool, a simple device which still finds a place today. J. Toynbee invented a thin rubber disc on a silver stem (1853) and C. J. Blake of America suggested a small paper patch in 1887.

All of these had disadvantages in that they were foreign bodies, needed careful apposition and frequent renewal, and sometimes proved ineffective. The next step was an attempt to cause healing of the perforation. Thus D. B. Moosa of America cauterized the edges of the defect with silver nitrate in 1876 and W. N. Okuneff used trichloracetic acid in 1895. Then came plastic repair. In 1878 E. Berthold removed the outer epithelial layer of the damaged tympanic membrane with repeated applications of court plaster, and grafted the raw area with skin. He was successful in two cases and suggested the term 'myringoplasty' for his operation. Much the same method was revived by two Americans, Schulhof and Valdez, in 1944 and is sometimes used today. But an infective process commonly causes more extensive damage than a simple perforation, and that infection must be controlled if operation is to be successful. Hence the modern operation aims at reconstruction of the damaged hearing mechanism and control of infection; this is known as tympanoplasty and was developed by another American, H. Wullstein, in 1952.

From the tympanic membrane we pass to the chain of ossicles of which, for our purpose, the stapes is the most important. The stapes, as its name implies, is shaped exactly like a stirrup and the footplate of the stirrup is connected by a tiny ligament to the margins of the fenestra ovalis, the oval window which opens into the vestibule of the organ of hearing and balance, the three semicircular canals. The sound waves, carried through the air, impinge on the tympanic membrane and cause it to vibrate; these vibrations are passed to the first ossicle, the malleus or hammer, with which the membrane is in contact, and from the malleus to the incus or anvil. The incus has a long, thin projection which connects with the head of the stapes. So the malleus hammers on the incus which moves the stapes backwards and forwards and, since the footplate of the stapes is attached by a ligament to the oval window, causes the footplate of the stapes to oscillate the membrane covering the oval window and so to transmit impulses to the liquid contained in the semicircular canals.

These impulses will be transmitted only so long as the stapes is mobile. In 1735 A. M. Valsalva observed that the stapes may become fixed to the margin of the oval window by bony changes in the connecting ligament (bony ankylosis or otosclerosis). This was confirmed by Toynbee who found, in the course of over fifteen hundred dissections of dead bodies, that 'osseous ankylosis of the stapes to the fenestra ovalis is one of the common causes of deafness'. Adam Politzer of Vienna, having examined sixteen cases of stapes fixation during life, in 1893 gave it as his opinion that this form of deafness was due, not to some disorder of the stapes, but to a disease process of the labyrinth, that is, of the vestibule and its semicircular canals. Politzer was before his time; his findings did not receive general acceptance until the nineteen forties.

The problem was how to make use of this knowledge. The chain of ossicles is not absolutely necessary; sound can, to a certain degree, be conducted through bone, but it must be changed into waves or impulses in the liquid contents of the semicircular canals before the brain can perceive it. If the stapes is fixed firmly to the oval window, the membrane covering the oval window cannot vibrate and so the liquid cannot 'judder'. The first attempt to deal with the problem was by removing the stapes entirely; this was done for the first time by J. Kessel as early as 1876. The operation was quite an extensive one, and he abandoned it because of the risk of sepsis.[5]

Two years later, in 1878, Kessel tried a different method. He made an incision through the tympanic membrane, found the stapes, and attempted to mobilize it by making pressure on the bony head which connects with the incus. This was not nearly so severe an operation and it became fairly popular for a time;

the French surgeon Boucheron operated on sixty patients and another Frenchman, C. Miot, on over two hundred. Possibly encouraged by the French work, two Americans named C. J. Blake and F. L. Black returned to Kessel's original operation of removing the stapes in 1892 and 1893. Both methods met with a fair degree of success although hearing could never be as good as with a normal ear, but infection was common. It was dread of infection which caused more conservative surgeons to condemn this type of operation which fell into general disrepute during the eighteen nineties and was not practised again for nearly half a century.

In 1897 a man named Passow suggested that it might perhaps be simpler and equally effective to leave the stapes and the fenestra ovalis untouched but to drill an entirely new opening through the bony wall of the labyrinth. Two years later B. Floderus described a theoretical operation in which a portion of the labyrinthine wall was resected and the opening covered with a Thiersch graft, which would act in the same way as the membrane covering the fenestra ovalis. In 1910 R. Bárány of Vienna performed this operation for the first time, but he seems to have failed to restore hearing. Three years later, in 1913, G. J. Jenkins of King's College Hospital made an opening into the lateral semicircular canal of the labyrinth and covered the new fenestra or window with a Thiersch graft. He operated on only two patients; in both there was a dramatic improvement of hearing within a few hours. This improvement was not maintained; hearing gradually became worse over the next weeks, although it remained slightly better than before operation.

In 1916 G. Holmgren of Stockholm began his long and patient struggle against the more conservative school of surgeons who thought that surgical interference with the deaf ear was not justified because of the risk of infection. By 1923 Holmgren had performed a quite large series of operations upon the labyrinth. The prime importance of his work is not so much in the methods which he used as in the fact that he demonstrated the safety of surgical intervention in deafness, always provided that the surgeon adhered to a rigidly aseptic technique. Holmgren's results were not satisfactory by modern standards; thus, as in Jenkins' two cases, the initial improvement of hearing was not maintained. Holmgren is, however, the father of the modern surgery of deafness, for his work led directly to that of Sourdille, his pupil.

Maurice Sourdille of Nantes started to perform a somewhat complicated operation in 1932 and described his technique in 1937. The essential of his method was to make a plastic skin flap from the external opening (meatus) of the ear and turn it in so that it formed continuity with the tympanic membrane and the new fenestra which he cut in the labyrinth, the result being that there was some conduction of sound waves by way of the tympanic membrane. He did the operation in three separate stages and, for this reason, it never became popular. In 1938 Julius Lempert of America combined Sourdille's three-stage method into a one-stage operation and reported eighteen successes in twenty-three cases. The good results of Lempert's operation served to change the opinion of otologists; from 1938 onwards surgery of the uninfected but deaf ear assumed a new importance.

One point had been overlooked; in 1893 Adam Politzer had suggested that this form of deafness is not due to disease of the stapes but of the labyrinth. The disease process resulted in new bone formation, which was why the stapes became ankylosed to the fenestra ovalis. Just as those patients, upon whom Jenkins and Holmgren had operated, became deaf again within a matter of weeks or months, so Lempert and his followers found that the improvement in their patients' hearing was not maintained. New bone formation caused the fenestra which they had made in the labyrinth to close, thus undoing the good effects of their operation.

Surgeons now started to investigate methods of stopping new bone formation. G. E. Shambaugh of New York invented special irrigating tubes to wash away all bone dust when drilling the hole, for bone dust tends to form new bone. Lempert made his fenestra much larger in an endeavour to stop the trouble, and he also fitted shaped plugs of cartilage (1945) and rubbed lead around the rim of his new fenestra (1951). But the fenestration operation suffered from other disadvantages; the patient often experienced really severe and unpleasant giddiness during convalescence because of interference with the balancing mechanism, and in some 25 per cent of cases there was chronic discharge from the ear, because the operation was done through the extensive radical mastoidectomy approach, and the cavity became secondarily infected. For these reasons surgeons began to reinvestigate the simpler, less traumatic, method of removing the stapes, first practised by Kessel in 1876.

In 1946 Terence Cawthorne of King's College Hospital returned to Kessel's stapedectomy operation but, in a series of fourteen patients, he obtained improvement of hearing in only two cases; three years later he achieved the more hopeful result of better hearing in five out of eight. But the gain in hearing was not sufficient to warrant replacement of the Lempert fenestration.

In April 1952 S. Rosen of America started to attempt re-mobilization of the stapes by pressure upon the end of the bone, a similar method to that of Kessel in 1878 and almost the same as that of Miot; surprisingly enough, Rosen does not seem to have been aware of Miot's quite extensive work in this field. The relative simplicity of his operation was an advance but his results, although fairly successful, could only compare with those of Lempert in about half his cases.

The practical value of stapedectomy was proved in 1957 when J. J. Shea of America introduced his much improved operation. He removed the stapes, cleaned the fenestra ovalis and covered it with a graft made from a small piece of vein, and fitted a very small piece of fine polythene tubing, sharpened at one end, between the incus and the grafted fenestra. Thus he not only treated the cause of trouble, ankylosis of the stapes to the oval window, but he reestablished the normal hearing mechanism through the chain of ossicles by means of the polythene tube. In 1962 he described a modification, a tiny piston made of teflon which was anatomically better shaped for the purpose than a cut piece of tubing. In the same year Cawthorne reported that, by using the Shea technique since 1959, he had improved hearing in no less than 248 out of a series of 300 patients.

Surgery such as this, in which grafts, tubes, and pistons are measured in millimetres, would be impossible without adequate lighting and magnification. It is almost unbelievable that Kessel must have removed the tiny stapes with ordinary spectacles and by the reflected light of an oil lamp, gas, or a candle – or the sun. Sourdille and Lempert used headlamps, lit by electricity, and special magnifying spectacles known as loupes. The modern surgeon works with a high powered, electrically illuminated, microscope. The first practical instrument was invented by Nylen of Lund as long ago as 1921, but it suffered from the disadvantage of being monocular, which makes appreciation of depth uncertain. Holmgren introduced a binocular instrument in 1923 and used this in his series of operations, but most surgeons remained content with loupes until Shambaugh brought an improved operating microscope into general use in 1940.

The story of the efforts to cure deafness has entailed a great deal of explanation and may appear a dull one for that reason. It would be nice to tell it as a romantic, exciting tale, full of incident, something in the nature of a James Bond fantasy. This cannot be done; it must be left to the reader to glimpse the triumphant endeavour that lies behind the uninteresting façade. For here we have one of the major victories of surgery; every day the deaf are being made to hear again by operations which are not dramatic, in which indeed very little can be seen by an onlooker, but which are now part of routine practice.

Linked with the ear is surgery of the throat and of the nose; the modern surgeon sometimes calls himself an otorhinolaryngologist and the part of the hospital in which he works is usually called the ENT Department. One of the more important and commonly performed operations is that for tonsils and adenoids. Tonsillectomy or, to be exact, partial tonsillectomy is of ancient origin, for Celsus advised that the tonsil should be removed with a scalpel when all other methods of treatment had failed. The German Heister described three methods of dealing with the tonsil in 1798; these were corrosion, which meant treatment by corrosives such as silver nitrate, excision, and ligature. Ligature was used by Cheselden, who pierced the tonsil with a needle bearing a double thread and tied off the two halves, leaving them to slough off.

Excision of the tonsil with a sharp scalpel was not only very difficult in the conscious patient but also could result in dangerous bleeding. A method that came into use nearly a hundred and fifty years ago and persisted until almost the present day is guillotining, the catching of the tonsil between a metal loop and a blade and its removal partly by cutting and partly by pressure; this has the effect of sealing the open ends of blood vessels. The first guillotine was invented by Philip Syng Physick of Philadelphia in 1828; it consisted of two metal plates ending in rings; a sharpened blade, carried between the two plates, could be advanced so as to cut the tonsil caught in the rings. This is essentially the same principle as the modern guillotine, although Physick's instrument has been modified and remodified. Coxeter, a well-known London instrument maker, made a very similar one to the design of Robert Liston; another incorporated a fork to hold the tonsil and prevent it sliding from between the rings. The best of these early instruments was one designed by Morell Mackenzie; save in small details it is the same as that used today.

Some surgeons would never use a guillotine. Syme of Edinburgh preferred to hold the tonsil in a pair of forceps and dissect it out with a blunt-ended knife. This may be called the 'Edinburgh method' for it was followed by Lister and his successors. Other surgeons destroyed the tonsil with the cautery; the chief advocate of this method, Krishaber, submitted the patient to repeated operations, puncturing the tonsil with a cautery point five or six times at each sitting. A technique approaching the dissection of today was introduced by an Italian surgeon, Borelli, in 1861; he enucleated the tonsil with his finger. But guillotining was the most popular method; an annotation of 1882 in the *British Medical Journal* stated that removal by the finger, the ligature, caustics, or the cautery had all fallen into disuse and that guillotining was the only method employed, an assumption that evoked angry protest from Edinburgh.[6]

In 1910 S. S. Whillis and F. C. Pybus of America revolutionized tonsillectomy by what is known as the 'reverse' method of guillotining. Until this date the guillotine had simply been slipped over the tonsil and the blade pressed home; part of the tonsil, the pedicle, was almost invariably left to provide a focus for renewed infection. In the reverse method a finger is pressed behind the tonsil and pushes it outwards into the ring of the guillotine. This is one of the simple little manoeuvres that makes for successful surgery. Whillis and Pybus claimed to have removed the complete tonsil in 74 per cent of cases, and Greenfield Sluder of St Louis, using the same method, credited himself in 1912 with a success rate of 99·6 per cent. The average guillotinist could not approach this figure. In 1909 G. E. Waugh of Great Ormond Street published his method of 'blunt dissection'; he did not use a finger, as had Borelli, but dissected out the tonsil with a pair of forceps. Then he slipped a wire snare around the pedicle and removed the tonsil with firm pressure and a twisting motion. Nearly all surgeons would regard the method of blunt dissection, in one of its innumerable modifications, as the method of choice today.

The existence of adenoids was not recognized until 1852 when Köllicker described the presence of tissue similar to the tonsil in the space where the back of the nose joins the throat, the nasopharynx. In 1868 Hans Wilhelm Meyer of Copenhagen published a paper on adenoids which was translated into several languages.[7] Meyer had first observed the presence of adenoids when examining a deaf child; he found them to be present in 102 patients during the next eighteen months. Correctly believing that adenoids might be a cause of deafness, Meyer started to remove them, with good results. Again, this is one of the small operations which has added so greatly to the usefulness of surgery, and it is nice to know that the Danes appreciated Meyer's work; there is a statue to his memory in Copenhagen. Meyer removed adenoids with a ring knife, fitted over the finger; other surgeons used a specially sharpened finger nail. Gottstein invented a curette in 1885, and this is the prototype of the instrument used today. The adverse effect of adenoids upon mental and physical development, due to obstructed breathing particularly during sleep, was first described by A. Guye of Amsterdam in 1884.

Accurate examination of the throat demands special instruments, of which the most important is the laryngoscope, briefly mentioned in the last chapter. The early history of the laryngoscope is bound up with that of the cystoscope, for the instruments of Desormeaux and Nitze were devised to gain a view of body canals in general. Benjamin Guy Babington of Guy's Hospital invented a combined tongue depressor and mirror in 1829, but no practical instrument was evolved until Manuel Garcia hit on the idea of reflecting an image of the vocal cords upon a mirror by means of a second mirror held against the back of the throat.

Garcia was not medically qualified. Born in Spain in 1805, he became professor of singing at the Paris Conservatoire, and fled to England during the revolution of 1848. He had a professional interest in the mechanism of the human voice and found himself frustrated by being unable to obtain a clear view of the movements of the vocal cords. According to Garcia's own account he returned to Paris on holiday and, while idly strolling in the gardens of the Palais Royal on a sunny day in September 1854, casually observed the sun reflecting itself from one window to another. He immediately conceived his scheme of twin mirrors. By means of his mirrors, Garcia was able to describe the action of the vocal cords during inspiration, expiration, and speech in a paper communicated to the Royal Society in 1855. After Garcia's publication, Ludwig Türck of Vienna and J. N. Czermak of Budapest claimed priority for the invention of the laryngoscope and a wordy battle developed, which nearly resulted in a legal action between Czermak and Türck. There is no need to revive this ancient squabble; all three men did much to develop the science of laryngoscopy. Garcia lived to a hundred and one and to be recognized as the father of modern laryngology. There is a pleasing little tale that a grand reception was organized on Garcia's hundredth birthday at which the father of laryngology was presented with medals, orders, and his portrait painted by Sargent. The delightful old gentleman, still remarkably alert, 'wondered what all the fuss was about; he had never meant to become the founder of a new medical speciality – and the mirrors had only cost him six francs'.[8]

Garcia's method only permitted the image of the larynx to be seen on a mirror; the larynx was first seen by direct vision in 1894 when Kirstein of Berlin invented his 'autoscope', a flat spatula and prismatic incandescent lamp. By then laryngoscopy had become a routine method of examination and had extended itself into examination of the bronchi of the lungs, and of the oesophagus. All the early instruments, most of which have already been described under cystoscopy and gastroscopy, depended upon reflected light and the image was observed in an attached mirror. The first direct vision instrument, the parent of the present oesophagoscope and bronchoscope, was introduced by Mikulicz-Radecki in 1881. This was a straight metal tube with a slanting distal end, illuminated by incandescent platinum. Rosenheim of Berlin lit the tube with an electric bulb in 1895. In 1896 Gustav Killian of Freiburg began to study methods of endoscopy. He adopted Mikulicz's principle for his instruments, but he enlarged the 'tubes'. Killian was the first to remove a foreign body by an endoscopic method. A six-year-old girl had inhaled a metal collar-stud which had become lodged in the larnyx. Using Kirstein's autoscope, Killian successfully extracted the stud. He also introduced the important method of 'suspension laryngoscopy', in which the instrument is affixed to the ceiling or is supported by a jack, thus allowing the surgeon to use both hands for operating. This was in 1912. Killian's work was taken up in Britain by Logan Turner of Edinburgh and by E. B. Waggett of London. In 1904 Chevalier Jackson of Philadelphia much improved endoscopy instruments, established the largest and most famous clinic in the world, and transformed bronchoscopy and oesophagoscopy into a routine method of examination. In more recent years (1932) the Jackson instruments have been modified by Victor Negus of King's College Hospital, another world-famous laryngologist. Many ingenious devices have been invented, particularly for the removal of foreign bodies. For instance an open safety pin is sometimes swallowed and lodges with the open, sharp end uppermost; it cannot be removed in this state because the point would tear the oesophageal or bronchial wall. A special forceps has been devised by which the pin can be turned and closed.

If Manuel Garcia is the father of the science of laryngology, Morell Mackenzie of the London Hospital is undoubtedly the father of practical laryngeal surgery. When only twenty-six years old he founded the Metropolitan Free Dispensary for Diseases of the Throat and Loss of Voice, which became the Throat Hospital, Golden Square, the first hospital in the world devoted solely to diseases of the throat. He published a book *Use of the Laryngoscope* in 1865 and another *Growths of the Larynx* in 1871. His greatest work, called by the world-famous St Clair Thomson 'the laryngologist's bible', was *Diseases of the Throat and Nose* in two volumes, published 1880 and 1884. Mackenzie's very real importance in medical history has been overshadowed by his notorious and much-discussed failure to diagnose a cancer of the throat in the case of Frederick III of Germany. The most fantastic stories of political intrigue have been woven around this incident; whatever the true facts may be, Mackenzie's error cannot have affected the fatal outcome. Here is another instance of the impact of disease upon world history; had the liberal Frederick survived to the age of ninety-two as did his father, instead of dying of cancer at the age of fifty-seven, that singularly idiotic autocrat, Kaiser Wilhelm II, would not have occupied the throne of Germany in 1914 and the nations might have been spared much suffering.

Mackenzie could only have excised the projecting portion of the cancer in Frederick's throat, which would have been useless. It was left to his successor, Felix Semon, to devise an effective operation. Felix Semon, a German, came to England in 1875 with a letter of introduction to Morell Mackenzie, who appointed him to the staff of his Golden Square hospital. In 1882 Semon took charge of the throat department at St Thomas' Hospital. He carried on Mackenzie's work, translated his *Diseases of the Throat and Nose* into German, was one of the first to treat tuberculosis of the larynx by completely resting the voice, and was largely responsible for developing the operation of laryngofissure for cancer.

Laryngofissure, splitting of the larynx and removal of the affected vocal cord, was established as an operative technique by St Clair Thomson of King's College Hospital, one of the greatest of laryngologists, who particularly interested himself in surgery of cancer and of syphilis. It is of some interest that this well-skilled ENT surgeon had taken his MD London in 1888 without ever seeing the vocal cords or the living eardrum. He had a hard struggle to establish himself in what was then an unrecognized speciality. He developed tuberculosis in 1902 and was probably the first patient in Britain to be ordered complete silence, the treatment suggested by Semon. Thomson's *Diseases of the Nose and Throat*, published in 1911, is now in its sixth edition and is the standard text book on the subject. The operation of laryngofissure, which he did so much to perfect, is still done but not commonly for cancer. A more extensive procedure, removal of the whole larynx, or radiotherapy gives better results.

From otorhinolaryngology we pass to surgery of the eye, which has in its early stages a somewhat similar history to surgery of the ear. Until the nineteenth century treatment of the eye lay almost entirely in the hands of quacks. An unqualified practitioner, rather than a quack, was Richard Banister of Stamford, who died in 1626 having published a quite important series of treatises upon eye diseases. Another publication, probably but not certainly by Banister or his son, throws light upon the doings of less reputable colleagues. Here are mentioned Luke of Erith who charged from twenty to sixty pounds for couching a cataract – from two to six hundred pounds in our depreciated currency – and who rarely succeeded in improving the patient's sight; Surphlete of King's Lynn 'a man of excellent diet and crusty fashion of body' who had as apprentice a barber 'of weak understanding and given to drink'; Henry Blackbourne, like Banister an itinerant practitioner, who 'could do good in these cures yet he was so wickedly given that he would cozen and deceive men of great sums of money by taking incurable diseases in hand. He was lusty amorously, given to several women so that his cozening made him fearfully to flee from place to place and often change his name and habits.'

Practice was equally bad in the eighteenth century. Notable among the real charlatans is 'The Chevalier' Taylor, oculist to George III, whose son and grandson also became royal retainers. To be just, Taylor was often ahead of his time, but he pretended to a knowledge and a skill which he most certainly did not possess. He travelled about the countryside calling himself 'Ophthalmiator Pontifical, Imperial, and Royal'. Another charlatan named William Read, a tailor by trade, not only acted as court oculist but acquired a knighthood from Queen Anne. He published a *Treatise for the Eyes* which is nothing but a reprint of parts of Banister's works enlivened by fulsome advertisements of his own skill. Read cannot have written the book himself, for he was entirely illiterate.

A few qualified practitioners attempted to treat disorders of the eye; among these were the sixteenth-century Daubigney Turbeville of Salisbury, possibly the first medical ophthalmologist, William Cheselden, and Cheselden's pupil Samuel Sharp of Guy's. The first ophthalmologist worthy of the name was

Thomas Young, physician to St George's Hospital, who was elected FRS at the early age of twenty-one for his work on the ciliary muscles, which cause the eye to accommodate itself to changed conditions of light. John Cunningham Saunders, an apprenticed but unqualified surgeon who also practised otology, founded the Dispensary for Curing Diseases of the Eye and Ears in 1805; two years later this became a specialized hospital for diseases of the eye, the first of its kind in the world. The success of 'Moorfields', now the Royal London Ophthalmic, stimulated the foundation of similar institutions; the West of England Eye Infirmary in 1808, and the Royal Westminster Ophthalmic founded by George James Guthrie (whom we have met before) in 1816. The first systematic teaching of ophthalmology started at the Royal Westminster when Guthrie began a regular course of lectures in 1817.

The majority of early nineteenth-century ophthalmologists were physicians. Among the first surgeons to turn their attention to the subject may be mentioned George Critchett and William Bowman. Both had rather similar careers. Critchett of the London Hospital was elected to the staff of Moorfields in 1843 and resigned from the London in 1863 in order to devote more of his time to ophthalmology. In 1877, at the age of sixty, he was appointed ophthalmic surgeon to the Middlesex Hospital. Bowman, notable for his work upon the kidney as well as for his researches into the structure and physiology of the eye, was appointed surgeon to Moorfields in 1846. He remained a general surgeon at King's College Hospital until 1863, when he resigned to devote all his time to ophthalmology. Bowman and Critchett left Moorfields in the same year, 1877.

Of all the many operations performed upon the eye, that for cataract has the longest history and is one of the oldest in surgery. The lens of the eye is exactly the same as the lens of a camera or microscope; it transmits the image of a thing seen to the back of the eye or retina, from which there is the pathway, the optic nerve, to the brain; but the lens of the eye, unlike the lens of a camera, can accommodate itself to near or far-off objects. If the lens of a camera is dirty, the photograph will be fogged and the same thing happens with the lens of the eye; when the opacity known as a cataract develops in the lens, vision will first be blurred and, if the cataract is not treated, will fail. The

268

lens of the eye can be 'replaced' by the lens of a pair of glasses.

The term 'cataract' is probably, but not certainly, derived from the Greek word for a waterfall, which also had the meaning of a sluice-gate, something which could be dropped down to cut off the flow of water; how the term came to be applied to the opaque lens is a mystery which has exercised the ingenuity of many a curious mind. Celsus, who treated cataracts by operation, used the word 'suffusio'. Ambroise Paré spoke of 'cataracte en coulisse'; the meaning of 'coulisse' is 'portcullis' and, in 1611, was applied to 'a web in the eye', so Paré, unless guilty of tautology, must have had some different meaning of the word 'cataracte' in mind.

For a long time cataract was supposed to be a collection of corrupted humour, the liquid contained in the anterior chamber of the eye between the cornea or pupil and the lens; it was also thought that the lens was the essential organ of vision, the importance of the retina not being understood. For this reason early cataract operations consisted of pushing the lens away from the supposed cataract, backwards or downwards into the posterior chamber of the eye, the vitreous body. The operation was known as depression or reclination, and this latter term gave the common expression 'couching for cataract', from the French 'se coucher' to lay oneself down. Couching was carried out with a pointed, awl-like needle and it has been reckoned that at least 60 per cent of patients lost their sight owing to infection, haemorrhage, or the increase in intraocular pressure now known as glaucoma. In many cases the operation was also quite useless because the cataract, that is, the opaque lens, simply returned to its original place.

The knowledge that the lens is not the essential organ of sight, that it is a thick, rounded 'lens-like' body and not a thin membrane, that a cataract is an opaque lens and not an opacity between lens and cornea, all resulted from the work of a French physician, Michel Brisseau, at the beginning of the eighteenth century, although the age-old concept had been suspect for nearly fifty years. Brisseau's revolutionary views aroused much opposition, but he was supported by the great physician Boerhaave of Leyden and by such men as Cheselden, Morgagni, and Valsalva. It was, however, not until 1748, five years after

Brisseau's death, that Jacques Daviel started to put his theories into practice.

Some years before this date, J. L. Petit had removed particles of a broken-up lens which had floated into the anterior chamber after couching; in 1722 Charles St Yves, another Frenchman, extracted a whole lens which had become displaced into the anterior chamber during a similar operation. Daviel was faced with a like emergency, and he extracted the lens through a slit in the cornea; it proved so successful that, in a second case, he deliberately made an incision through the cornea and removed the lens piecemeal. Next came a failure to couch a cataract and Daviel decided 'to open the lower portion of the cornea in order to get my needle the more effectively into the posterior chamber. Then for a long time I held the cornea by a small forceps and brought forth the lens'.

Daviel first published his method in 1748, nearly a year after this operation, but only in a private letter to another surgeon; he had not yet decided whether extraction was preferable to couching. He soon made up his mind and he became famous for his excellent results, travelling over Europe to treat his patients; in 1750 he was called to extract a cataract from the Princess Palatine of Mannheim. In 1752 he was sufficiently sure of his operation to describe it at a meeting of the surgical section of the Royal Academy in Paris. Daviel made his incision at the lower edge of the cornea, for the interesting reason that an unanaesthetized patient always tends to roll his eye upwards. He devised special instruments for his operation, cut through the capsule of the lens with a sharp needle, and expressed the lens from its capsule by pressure from below and counter-pressure from above – squeezed it out, in fact. Daviel's spoon or spatula is still in use in eye surgery.

At first the new operation was taken up enthusiastically, but a reaction in favour of the old-fashioned couching soon developed. Arnold Sorsby, in his *Short History of Ophthalmology*,[9] states that Daviel's operation was on trial for a century. During this time many modifications were introduced, mainly in the type of instruments. In 1753 Samuel Sharp simplified the rather complicated incision of Daviel, who used three cutting instruments, into a single incision needing only a knife; this resulted in the invention of no less than sixty-nine different patterns of cataract knife between 1753 and 1821. The knife commonly used today is over a century old, having been devised by the German ophthalmologist Albrecht von Graefe in 1865. For the rest, Daviel's principle of operation is similar to the modern method. But here is an interesting point; the modern operation is a *return* to Daviel's technique.

Daviel extracted the lens from its surrounding capsule. Both Daviel and Sharp contemplated removal of the lens complete within its capsule, but apparently never attempted the operation. Alexander Pagenstecher, a German, first performed this 'extracapsular extraction' in 1866 but the technique, although favoured by William Bowman, remained practically unknown until Pagenstecher's brother Hermann described it in his *Atlas of the Eye* in 1875. Colonel Mulroney of the Indian Medical Service began to extract all cataracts by the extracapsular operation in 1895. Mulroney's method was adopted by Major Henry Smith of Jullundur (the IMS was a fertile breeding ground of distinguished ophthalmologists because of the very high incidence of eye diseases in India) and was so perfected by him that it became known as the Smith Indian operation and was the method of choice until only a very short time ago.

Extracapsular extraction is an excellent operation but is really only suitable for mature, hard cataracts. It therefore became the practice in the early years of the twentieth century to allow cataracts to 'ripen' before operation; the opacity is soft at first but hardens with time. Cataracts are much more common in elderly people. These two facts bring us to an example of how change in social habits can influence surgical technique. The majority of people of the poorer class who were in their seventies during the first two decades of the twentieth century had never known compulsory education and were unable to read or write; so long as the majority of the elderly poor were illiterate, little hardship resulted from delaying operation until the cataract matured. Compulsory education has produced a greater dependence on the printed word; the elderly in particular find life intolerably dull if deprived of books and newspapers or, in more recent times, of television. For this reason there has been a tendency to return to the intracapsular operation, more suitable for soft cataracts, and the method, with modifications, remains essentially that which Daviel introduced two hundred and more years ago.

To the ancients, cataract was a form of blindness that might be curable; glaucoma, a word derived from the dull greyish green or blue colour of opacity of the blind pupil (cornea), implied blindness that could not be cured. Thus 'glaucoma' was not a clinical entity; the modern glaucoma, increase in intraocular pressure which will lead to blindness if untreated, is a disability which has been attached to an old name. From opacity of the lens, attention turned to opacities of the cornea. In 1795 the great Erasmus Darwin of Derby, notable physician, eccentric poet, and grandfather of Charles Darwin, suggested the possibility of trephining out small areas of the opaque cornea, so that the patient could see through it again. Vision would be limited because only a small area could be safely cleared, but at least the patient would not be blind. Darwin's idea met with no success, but his suggestion stimulated surgeons to try whether the opaque cornea could not be replaced. Nussbaum of Germany cut away part of the opacity and inserted a small, thin, piece of glass; his attempt failed because the glass simply acted as an irritant foreign body in the eye.

In the early years of the nineteenth century a certain amount of experimental work was done on the actual transplantation of the cornea; these important experiments proved successful in rabbits and some other animals but failed in man. Memory of the successful animal experiments lingered on to tantalize the surgeon. In 1878 the German Sellerbeck had to enucleate the damaged eye of a 2½-year-old child; he trephined out an area of corneal opacity from another patient and grafted in part of the child's clear cornea. The graft was not rejected but soon became opaque itself. Von Hippel in 1886 transplanted a graft from the cornea of a rabbit into the cornea of a young woman and designed a special clockwork trephine for the purpose. In 1901 Ernst Fuchs transplanted part of a cornea taken from a corpse a few hours after death.

These are the small beginnings of one of the greatest advances in surgery. The continuing history of corneal transplantation or grafting starts on 7 December 1905 when Eduard Konrad Zirm of Olomouc or Olmutz in Czechoslovakia, removed the right eye, injured by a piece of iron, from an eleven-year-old boy named Karl Brauer. He placed the eye in normal saline solution at body temperature and, using von Hippel's trephine, removed areas from the opaque corneae of both eyes of a forty-five year old labourer named Alois Glogar. Zirm formed discs, of exactly the same size as his trephine holes, from the donated cornea, and he fixed them in place in both Glogar's eyes. The right one he tucked under a bridge of conjunctiva, the tissue covering that part of the eye around the cornea, and he attached the left by simple suture. Both grafts 'took' but, after a week, the right graft gave trouble and had to be removed. The left graft remained clear until Glogar died three years later.[10]

A. Magitot used the cornea of a still-born child in 1912 and, with another surgeon named Morax, he was in the same year successful with a cornea taken from the enucleated eye of a living subject, preserved in the donor's blood at a temperature of $-6°C$ for eight days. This is the first 'stored' graft. The first successful transplant in Britain was by J. W. Tudor Thomas on 15 November 1930. The patient, a man of twenty-two, had opacities of both corneae, and he was so blind that he could only count fingers held up close to the eyes. Tudor Thomas grafted the left eye with cornea taken from a man aged forty-two, of the same blood group, who had sustained a severe injury requiring enucleation. Four months after operation the patient could count fingers at a distance of two feet; two years later, at a distance of thirty-three inches.[11]

In 1937 V. P. Filatov of Odessa stated that successful transplants from enucleated eyes had been recorded on about seventy occasions since 1905. But Filatov himself used the eyes of dead subjects; he had started doing so in 1932 and had operated on 95 patients in the years 1932–6; of these 18 had retained a transparent cornea, 17 a half transparent cornea, and in the remainder transplantation had failed.[12]

The work of Tudor Thomas and of Filatov stimulated a renewed interest in corneal grafting. Tudor Thomas organized the collection and registration of grafting material from freshly enucleated eyes. In Britain the law did not permit removal of eyes from the dead body, even though the relatives expressed no objection. Many public-spirited people desired to bequeath their eyes but this, too, was contrary to law. After the Second World War, when new techniques and lessened risk of infection showed that corneal grafting could give excellent results, a nation-wide campaign was launched through the public press and the BBC. This well-run campaign, which received the strong support of the Royal College of Surgeons, presented the facts clearly without pandering to mass-hysteria or sensationalism. As a result, the Corneal Grafting Act became law on 24 September 1952. The Ministry of Health established eye banks throughout the country, where cadaveric eyes, removed within ten hours of death, could be preserved for up to ten days in liquid paraffin at a temperature of 4°C.

There are, of course, many other eye operations done today which are of interest and importance; those for squint and for a detached retina are examples. Space does not permit an account of their history, but one technique, the magnetic removal of foreign bodies from the eye, must be shortly mentioned because so few people realize what an old operation it is. Wilhelm Fabry first used a magnet to extract a metallic object from the eye as long ago as 1627. Powerful magnets were used by James Dixon in 1859 and by W. A. McKeown in 1874. The modern electromagnet was introduced for this purpose in 1875 by Julius Hirschberg.

We will end this chapter with a type of surgery that fits into no speciality; the only reason for placing it here is that the thyroid gland lies in front of the throat, although it is not usually treated by a throat surgeon. The thyroid is an endocrine gland, that is, an internally secreting or ductless gland which delivers its product into the circulation and not on to the skin or mucosal surface as do sweat or salivary glands. Disorders of the endocrine glands can result in too much or too little of their secretion entering the blood stream, with consequent ill effects upon the patient. Deficiency of thyroid secretion will produce myxoedema, slowing of the mental processes, lethargy, coarsening of the skin and loss of hair. Too much thyroid secretion, spoken of as thyrotoxicosis, exophthalmic goitre, or Graves' disease, renders the patient abnormally excitable and nervous, with a very rapid pulse, loss of weight, and protruding eyes. There is also simple enlargement of the gland, a simple goitre, which causes much less general disturbance but is unsightly, uncomfortable, and may produce respiratory obstruction by pressure on the trachea.

Attempts to remove the abnormal thyroid were made from time to time by the ancients but it was not until the last years of the eighteenth and opening years of the nineteenth centuries that the operation was done with any frequency. Syme and Liston removed part of the gland, but both condemned the procedure in their text books of surgery. 'Extirpation of such growths has been frequently attempted,' wrote Liston, 'but the patients, almost without exception, have perished from haemorrhage under the hands of the knivesmen.' Surgery of the thyroid went out of fashion for thirty years, but during this time a good deal of work continued on the function of the gland and on the treatment of goitre.

Richard Russell, a London physician, had made the empirical observation that drinking of sea water appeared to be 'good for goitre' in 1750. Sea water contains quite an appreciable amount of iodine; in 1820 J. F. Coindet, a physician in Switzerland, one of the home countries of simple goitre, drew attention to the value of treatment with iodine; nine years later J. G. A. Lugol of Paris introduced an iodine solution, for oral administration, which is in use today. Lugol did not originally suggest his solution for the treatment of thyroid disorders, but of tuberculosis. It is of some interest that, when J. H. Green of St Thomas' Hospital tried to remove the whole gland from a woman, aged twenty-four, in 1829, he noted that the patient had been treated with iodine for some weeks and that the gland had decreased in size.[13] A French physician, G. A. Chatin, produced evidence that iodine would prevent simple goitre and have some effect upon the congenital type of thyroid deficiency, known as cretinism, in 1850. Another important date is 1869, when W. B. Cheadle of St Mary's recommended the routine use of iodine in cases of exophthalmic goitre.

Exophthalmic goitre, in those days a most dangerous condition, was described as a clinical entity by C. H. Parry, an English physician, in 1786 and by Giuseppe Flajani, an Italian, in 1802. It became commonly known as Graves' disease after Robert Graves of Dublin, a physician, published his classical and now much sought-after monograph in 1835. In

1840 K. A. von Basedow of Merseburg enunciated the three cardinal signs, goitre, protruding eyes, and a rapid pulse, which have become known as 'the Merseburg triad'. The nature of the gland was not understood until T. W. King of Guy's, sometimes called the father of endocrinology, first suggested that the thyroid is a ductless but secreting gland in 1836. But there was still no general agreement on the question of whether Graves' disease caused the enlarged gland or the enlarged gland caused Graves' disease when the first important work on the pathology and nature of secretion of the thyroid was published in 1893.

Meanwhile interest in surgery of the thyroid had been re-awakened by Patrick Heron Watson of Edinburgh. Watson was one of Lister's fellow house surgeons at the Edinburgh Royal Infirmary in 1854; despite this, he became an obstinate opponent of antisepsis. Watson operated on his first case in 1871, and the patient almost died from haemorrhage. He decided that the blood vessels must always be ligated before any attempt was made to remove the gland and, with this new technique, he performed thyroidectomy in six cases with only one death. At least one of these patients, and possibly more, suffered from an exophthalmic goitre.[6]

Six years later, in 1878, Theodor Kocher of Berne turned his attention to thyroid surgery. A brilliant pupil of Langenbeck and Billroth, Kocher held the chair of surgery at Berne from 1872 until his death in 1917 at the age of seventy-six. He was a dapper, handsome, little man with neat moustaches and a pointed beard. During his life he added much to many aspects of surgery, but he should be primarily remembered for his superb operating technique at a time when the majority of surgeons still practised the spectacular but somewhat hazardous methods of the old school. Kocher was one of the first surgeons to understand that speed has little place in surgery; his work was slow and precise, skilful and meticulously careful; he excelled in minute dissection. He adopted rigid antisepsis from the start but was one of the earliest surgeons to practise asepsis, with which he obtained remarkably successful results.

In thyroidectomy, Kocher probably introduced the 'collar' incision, which follows the natural transverse fold of the skin and leaves only a faintly perceptible scar, but Bassini may have anticipated him. Kocher performed over two thousand thyroidectomies with a mortality of only 4½ per cent, but many of these were the endemic simple goitres of Switzerland. At the beginning he removed the whole gland, with the result that thirty out of his first hundred cases developed thyroid deficiency, myxoedema; by 1883 he had recognized that part of the thyroid must be left if 'cachexia strumipriva' – as he christened post-operative myxoedema – is to be avoided. Kocher undoubtedly deserves the title 'Father of thyroid surgery'.

James Berry of the Royal Free Hospital, T. P. Dunhill of Melbourne and later of St Bartholomew's, Charles Mayo and Henry Plummer of the Mayo Clinic, and G. W. Crile of Washington were the pioneers of thyroid surgery before the First World War. Berry's book *Diseases of the Thyroid Gland* (1901) is a classic; Dunhill insisted on preliminary medical treatment with iodine until the patient had been brought to the best possible state for operation; Charles Mayo and Plummer not only introduced routine pre-operative treatment with iodine but made Rochester one of the centres of thyroid surgery; Crile devised the important technique of 'stealing' the gland in Graves' disease. The patient suffering from exophthalmic goitre is, as has been said, abnormally nervous and the thought of operation will send the pulse bounding up to a dangerously rapid rate. 'Stealing' consisted of giving the patient a daily enema at a prearranged time; on the day of operation the simple enema was replaced by a mixture of olive oil and ether (introduced by the American anaesthetist J. T. Gwathmey in 1913) which sent the patient to sleep. This became a much simpler and more effective technique after 1927, when a German chemist, Otto Butzengeiger, introduced the famous avertin, a narcotic drug which is given by rectum. The use of basal narcosis, as this form of semi-anaesthesia is called, reduced the operative mortality of thyroidectomy in Graves' disease to 1·8 per cent. The modern operation owes much to Cecil Joll of the Royal Free Hospital, who worked with James Berry and became the foremost 'thyroid surgeon' during the twenty years before his death in 1945.

In recent years operative mortality has been greatly decreased by the use of 'antithyroid' drugs, which antagonise the gland secretion. The first of these was used by E. B. Astwood of America in 1943. Antithyroid drugs are now given preoperatively in the majority of cases and have the effect of converting the dangerous Graves' disease into something similar to a simple goitre, which can be removed with much greater safety. Lugol's iodine solution is still given before operation, as the antithyroid drugs increase the tendency of the gland to bleed and iodine reduces it. Another treatment, especially for the elderly patient whose heart is badly affected, is radioactive iodine, first introduced in 1941, which has the effect of destroying the secreting power of the gland.

There is no doubt that the effect of antithyroid drugs has been beneficial. A long stay in hospital is often avoided, because out-patient treatment only is necessary before operation. It was common in the old days for a patient to stay in hospital for weeks or even months before being judged fit for surgery. The safety of operation has been so increased that thyroidectomy now carries a mortality of only 0·5 per cent from all causes, a figure that is commonly regarded as the 'irreducible mortality' of surgery. The patient suffering from Graves' disease is always treated with medication before being submitted to surgery; here is an example of the way in which the physician and the surgeon co-operate in the modern treatment of disease.

CHAPTER 12

The Surgeon and
His Operating Theatre

It is time for us to make a pilgrimage. But, before setting out for Edinburgh, we must read part of the story *His First Operation* in Conan Doyle's *Round the Red Lamp*. 'The students were pouring down the sloping street which led to the infirmary – each with his little sheaf of note-books in his hand. There were pale, frightened lads, fresh from the High Schools, and callous old chronics, whose generation had passed on and left them. They swept in an unbroken, tumultous stream from the University gate to the hospital. The figures and gait of the men were young, but there was little youth in most of their faces. Some looked as if they ate too little – a few as if they drank too much. Tall and short, tweed coated and black, round-shouldered, bespectacled and slim, they crowded with clatter of feet and rattle of sticks through the hospital gate. Now and again they thickened into two lines as the carriage of a surgeon of the staff rolled over the cobblestones between.

'They passed under an archway and down a long, stone-flagged corridor with drab-coloured doors on either side, each marked with a number. Some of them were ajar, and the novice glanced into them with tingling nerves. He was reassured to catch a glimpse of cheery fires, lines of white-counterpaned beds and a profusion of coloured texts upon the wall. The corridor opened upon a small hall with a fringe of poorly-clad people seated all round upon benches. A young man with a pair of scissors stuck, like a flower, in his button-hole, and a note-book in his hand, was passing from one to the other, whispering and writing. ... They rejoined the throng which was hurrying to the theatre of the famous surgeon.

'The tiers of horse-shoe benches, rising from the floor to the ceiling, were already packed, and the novice as he entered saw vague, curving lines of faces in front of him, and heard the deep buzz of a hundred voices and sounds of laughter from somewhere up above him. His companion spied an opening on the second bench, and they squeezed into it.

'Only a single row of heads intervened between them and the operating table. It was of unpainted deal, plain, strong and scrupulously clean. A sheet of brown waterproofing covered half of it, and beneath stood a large tin tray full of sawdust. On the further side, in front of the window, there was a board which was strewed with glittering instruments, forceps, tenacula, saws, canulas and trocars. A line of knives, with long, thin, delicate blades, lay at one side.

'A flutter of interest passed through the closely-packed bench as a woman in petticoat and bodice was led in by two nurses. A red woollen shawl was draped over her head and round her neck. The face which looked out from it was that of a woman in the prime of her years, but drawn with suffering and of a peculiar bees-wax tint. Her head drooped as she walked, and one of the nurses, with her arm round her waist, was whispering consolation in her ear. She gave a quick side glance at the instrument table as she passed, but the nurses turned her away from it.

' "What ails her?" asked the novice.

' "Cancer of the parotid. It's the devil of a case, extends right away back beyond the carotids. There's hardly a man but Archer would dare to follow it. Ah, here he is himself."

'As he spoke, a small, brisk, iron-grey man came striding into the room, rubbing his hands together as he walked. He had a clean-shaven face of the Naval officer type, with large, bright eyes, and a firm, straight mouth. Behind him came his big house surgeon with his gleaming pince-nez and a trail of dressers, who grouped themselves into the corners of the room.

' "Gentlemen," cried the surgeon in a voice as hard and brisk as his manner. "We have here an interesting case of tumour of the parotid, originally cartilaginous but now assuming malignant characteristics, and therefore requiring excision. On to the table, nurse! Thank you! Chloroform, clerk! Thank you! You can take the shawl off, nurse."

' "Adherent at one place, gentlemen," he cried "The growth

involves the carotids and jugulars, and passes behind the ramus of the jaw, whither we must be prepared to follow it. It is impossible to say how deep our dissection may carry us. Carbolic tray, thank you! Dressings of carbolic gauze, if you please! Push the chloroform, Mr Johnson. Have the small saw ready in case it is necessary to remove the jaw."

' "I propose," said he, passing his hand over the tumour in an almost caressing fashion, "to make a free incision over the posterior border and to take another forward at right angles to the lower end of it. Might I trouble you for a medium knife, Mr Johnson."

'The novice, with eyes which were dilating with horror, saw the surgeon pick up the long, gleaming knife, dip it into a tin basin and balance it in his fingers as an artist might his brush. Then he saw him pinch up the skin above the tumour with his left hand. At the sight, his nerves, which had already been tried once or twice that day, gave way utterly.'

These are the main points from Conan Doyle's story of an operation when he was a student at Edinburgh during the early eighteen eighties. Now let us make the pilgrimage. We can start, as did Conan Doyle's students, from the great gateway of Edinburgh University, cross the road, and take the short street down to the old infirmary, now the Geographical School. We pass through a pillared entrance – the doorkeeper will point out the letters WS scratched on one pillar as the monogram of Walter Scott – and enter the building. It is surprisingly small, far smaller than Conan Doyle's 'long corridor' would suggest. The corridor is still stone-flagged and the doors are painted a colour which may be described as drab, but they no longer open on glimpses of cheery fires, white counterpanes, and a profusion of coloured texts, for the wards are now offices and laboratories. We cross the little hall where outpatients once sat waiting to be seen by the outpatient clerk with his scissors worn, like a flower, in his buttonhole, and we follow a short passage to a door on the left hand side.

The old operating theatre comes as another surprise. Here is a vast room out of all proportion to the modest scale of the building; it is now the great lecture theatre of the geographical school. The curving tiers of seats, reaching to the ceiling, have gone; in their place are rows of desks and a gallery; but the wide, high windows remain, filling the whole of one side and flooding the room with light. Close to the wall at right angles to the windows and facing the rows of desks is a rostrum for the lecturer; on either side and behind the rostrum are doors leading to two smaller rooms.

The lecture theatre is empty and we can stand at the rostrum, once the site of a plain, strong, and scrupulously clean table of unpainted deal. We use that inward-turning eye of the mind which we call imagination; the gallery and the lines of desks become blurred and dissolve into nothing; once more the curving tiers rise to the ceiling, every seat occupied by a student, tweed coated or black, perhaps bespectacled, some looking as though they ate too little, a few as if they drank too much. Not all are students; in the two front rows are older men, and a French surgeon edges away from his German neighbour, for we are back in the early eighteen seventies and memories are bitter; it is only a year or two since the German Empire was proclaimed in the mirror hall of Versailles.

We cross the small amphitheatre and take our seats in the second tier of benches, hearing behind us the chatter of young voices, looking before us across only a single row of heads at the deal operating table, flanked by a desk and a chair. But Time has flowed still further back and the operating table has gone; in its place is another, more ominous, chair, upright, strong, furnished with straps. The talk behind us is hushed as the door to the surgeons' small room softly opens and the shades of those men who have worked in this place, who by their work have added so much to the fame of British surgery, come back to the theatre which they have known so well.

First Robert Liston, a magnificent figure of a man with the muscles of a blacksmith; he speaks a short sentence of rough encouragement to his patient, orders the attendants to fix the straps, turns to the audience and tells them in the fewest possible words – coarse words at that – of what he is going to do, and picks up a knife. Next, the young William Fergusson, fashionably dressed, jutting nose, long upper lip, already superb in his arrogance and self-confidence; he lectures upon the case haltingly, ineptly, in the broadest Scots, while the students yawn and fidget behind us. Silence grips the audience as the lecture ends, attention is riveted on the knife which seems to flash with the speed of light, every movement swift, controlled, and certain. Then James Syme, small, eager, pugnacious; he sits in his chair, elbow leaning on the desk, one leg carelessly thrown across the other – 'sic sedebat, sic docebat' as a student once wrote above a casual sketch of his master – and in a dry, pawky voice teaches the art of surgery as it has never been taught before nor since. He rises from his chair and takes up a knife; we see that Time has moved forward, for the patient is quiet, relaxed, breathing softly and regularly. The sickly sweetness of chloroform is in our nostrils, and a heavily built figure crosses the theatre floor. Here are the kindly, plebeian features of James Young Simpson; he exchanges a short, angry snarl with Syme, and they vanish together.

Now the audience is hushed and expectant. The Chief, as they have named him, comes through the door with his quick, athletic stride and takes his place at the table. Tall, slimly built, fresh coloured; hazel eyes, short side-whiskers, nose slightly snub; wide mouth tucked in at the corners, hair brushed across his broad forehead in a thick wave. He speaks to the silent students in his quiet, slow voice, haltingly at first and then, as the subject grips him, with greater authority but still with a little hesitation, for always at the back of his mind lies a memory of the stammer that he defeated in boyhood. The lecture over, he turns back his cuffs and plunges his hands in a basin, softly instructs the clerk whose duty it is to administer chloroform and, when he is certain that the patient is unconscious, tells the student in charge of instruments to uncover the trays that stand beneath the long windows. Then, head bowed, he stands for a moment in silence, and in that silence we hear only the hiss of the sprays as the pungent smell of carbolic acid fills the room. He takes up a knife in his hand.

What are they thinking, these shades of long-dead students who surround us on the tiered seats, as they watch Joseph Lister at his silent work in the operating theatre of the old Edinburgh Royal Infirmary? Do they understand that they are witnessing the birth of a new era? Do they instinctively know that the rare operation of today, and many more that they have never seen, will be commonplace tomorrow? They do not. Probably they will say, as they go back to the university gates, that Professor Lister seems to have a good idea, but he cannot teach nearly so well as did Professor Syme, and his operative technique is not at all exciting to watch. Here is the evidence of Sir St Clair Thomson, who was dresser to Lister in the early years at King's.

'Looking back, it is astounding that we never realized then that his principles were creating a new world of medicine. Even his favourite house surgeon, Sir Hector Cameron, said, "We little realized how great was the value of his lessons, or what was to be their unspeakable fruitfulness in the fulness of time."

'It might be asked what then did we think about it? I would answer that we were in the presence of a great and good man who taught us the foundations of physiological surgery, and who had evolved a technique of wound dressing, based on demonstrable scientific tests, which would ensure their healing by first intention and so abolish suppuration, septicaemia, pyaemia and other wound diseases.

'But we never foresaw that this would safely open up to the surgeon all the cavities of the body and, within little more than a decade, enable him to carry out as many new and undreamt-of life saving operations in one afternoon, in any operating theatre of the world, than were wont to be performed or attempted in a month when I was a student.'

They could not know, for it is given to very few people to understand fully what is taking place around them, and fewer still can make an accurate forecast of where any great discovery will end; perhaps we, too, are as ignorant of the future of Lister's work as were these students. But now it is time for us to leave them, to end this pilgrimage which we have made to the only remaining theatre in which Lister operated.

A modern operating theatre is very different; in fact, the American term 'operating room' is a better description. The old theatres were enormous because they were used for lectures and demonstrations; the surgeon gave a talk about his case before operating and usually described the stages of his operation as he worked. In more recent times, and certainly since the Second World War, fear of cross-infection has suggested that as few people as possible shall be present during an operation. Sometimes the theatre is by no means under-populated; for instance, operations on the dry heart will fill the room with cumbersome apparatus and the team of experts required to attend it; with surgeons, nurses, and technicians, the number present will be as great as in the nineteen thirties, when twenty or more students of a surgical firm watched their 'honorary' operate. There are still demonstration theatres in some centres, but the audience watches from behind glass screens or from galleries. A developing method of teaching large numbers, which shows promise, is the use of closed circuit television.

The surgeon exchanged his frock coat for a white gown, which is now more generally green; the white glossy walls of the theatre have been painted a neutral colour with a matt finish; the sterile drapes which cover trolleys and the patient are also of green; for it has been found that white is tiring to the eyes. Until the late nineteen thirties, operating theatres were kept at a very high temperature, in the mistaken belief that warmth prevented shock. A high temperature, combined with damp steam from the sterilisers, produced most unpleasant working conditions. Just before the Second World War, experiments were made with air conditioning, the then aim being to provide a hot, dry atmosphere, with a humidity as low as 20 per cent at 80°F, which, it was believed, would both prevent shock and allow staff to work in greater comfort. It had exactly the opposite effect; the patient became more shocked and the surgeon consumed vast quantities of tea, lemonade, and orange squash; in both cases the dry heat caused increased fluid loss. The modern air-conditioned theatre is kept at a comfortable temperature and a humidity of about 50 per cent.

Good lighting is a boon which the present day surgeon takes for granted. Older theatres were lit by a skylight, the operating table being placed directly beneath; this had the advantage of good downward illumination, but imposed a strain on the surgeon in hot, sunny weather. At the end of the nineteenth century, architects began to design theatres with large windows on the north side, the 'cold north light' of the artist's studio. Many such theatres remain, but some of the more modern ones have no natural lighting at all. Opinon on this subject is mixed; there is evidence that people who work long hours in windowless rooms can develop claustrophobia. But the surgeon of today never relies upon daylight; the main source of light is from a special type of lamp directly above the operating table. A system of mirrors or lenses makes this lamp almost shadowless;

thus the surgeon's hand will not obscure the site of operation. The lamp is movable and can be tilted at an angle or swung from side to side in the simpler models. The beam of more complicated lamps can be focused, and some incorporate a camera or even a television lens. A few are powered by motors and directed by remote control.

In moments of wrath we say that electricity is the most unreliable of modern amenities, the invariable cause of breakdown in the home, the motor-car, and the operating theatre. A surgeon who spends long minutes in fiddling adjustment of the lighting to his exact desire should spare a thought for the difficulties of his predecessors who had no electricity. Their only means of illuminating a body cavity was by light reflected from mirrors for, unlike us, they had no instruments incorporating a lamp. Their routine operations were performed under ordinary daylight. When daylight was not available they had to exercise ingenuity; there is a student's note in the case books which records, as a surprising item, 'operation performed by gas and candlelight'; one of Conan Doyle's stories relates that the patient, becoming excited under the influence of chloroform, knocked over the candles on a side table and plunged the theatre into darkness. An 'improved' method of illuminating the eye during operation, described in a late nineteenth century *Lancet*, consisted of rays from a paraffin lamp passed through a globe of water. The modern surgeon must surely find it remarkable that these old time practitioners managed to perform even the simplest of operations with the feeble lighting, not easily adjustable, which was all they had at their disposal.

Lister and the generation of surgeons who immediately followed him walked straight into the operating theatre from a corridor which carried a stream of people off the streets to the various parts of the hospital. This would not commend itself to a modern bacteriologist. The first advance came with the provision of surgeons' changing rooms, in which they removed their outer clothes and donned pyjamas or operating suits, an apron, and boots or plimsolls. This part of the costume was more for the protection and comfort of the surgeon than for the safety of his patient. From there he entered the theatre, 'scrubbed up' at the sink and was tied into his sterilized gown, cap, and mask, thus protecting the patient from bacterial invasion.

The next step was to divide the scrubbing-up place off from the theatre by glass screens; the surgeon, instead of entering the theatre with bare head and face, now did not come into the theatre proper until gowned, capped, and masked. More recently the theatre has been subdivided into 'dirty' 'clean' and 'sterile' zones; nothing soiled may ever go back to the 'clean' or 'sterile' zones, and no one may pass from the 'clean' to the 'sterile' zone without protective clothing; this rule applies to surgeon, nurse, anaesthetist, and patient alike. Some very modern theatres incorporate a system of 'locks' which may not be traversed by anyone unless covered with sterile clothing.

Early theatres consisted of one large room with, perhaps, two small rooms leading off, one for the surgeon and the other for storage and cleaning of instruments. The modern theatre has developed into a suite of rooms, of which the theatre proper forms only a small part. There is a separate room where the patient is anaesthetized and another for his recovery before being returned to the ward. Special cases may be sent from the recovery room to an intensive care unit, a development of the accident service, where highly trained staff cope with the various difficulties which may follow operation on the brain, the heart, and the lungs before the patient can be judged fit for routine nursing in the open ward. There is the surgeons' room and the scrubbing-up room, a section for sterilization of instruments, a place to set up instrument and dressing trolleys, often a special room for the messy application of plasters, and sometimes a separate endoscopy room where examinations with the various 'scopes' may be performed. This is not all; space is required for nurses' changing rooms, technicians' rooms, for office work, and for the bulk storage of equipment, but these various compartments do not usually form part of the actual operating suite.

Sterilization by carbolic or mercuric chloride gave place to sterilization by boiling or by steam. This had disadvantages. Boiling sterilizers filled the theatre with steam; steam treated gowns and drapes often emerged from the sterilizers wringing wet. The method of 'wet' sterilization has given place to 'dry' autoclaving, in which everything used in an operation is submitted to superheated steam under pressure. The big, complicated, autoclaves suggested a central service for the whole hospital; now the sterilizing department has been largely separated from the operating theatre; gowns, dressings, syringes, drapes, are prepacked in suitable containers, autoclaved, and sent out to the wards and theatres. Some items of equipment are bought packed and ready sterilized by irradiation with gamma rays.

The original ether gave place to chloroform which, in turn, was superseded by ether and nitrous oxide. Conan Doyle's patient walked into the theatre supported by two nurses who persuaded her to lie down on the operating table at the surgeon's command. Not until then did she start to inhale chloroform, and she was anaesthetized in full view of a hundred students while the surgeon continued with his lecture. Such treatment gives some basis of truth to Bernard Shaw's dictum that an anaesthetic only saves the patient the actual pain of operation. Of course Shaw was wrong; anaesthesia has given freedom from operative pain, diminished risk of shock and, above all, the necessary time without which advance in surgery would have been impossible. But an anaesthetic such as this must have been a most unpleasant experience and today would only be permitted in the direst emergency.

The patient is now premedicated before he leaves the ward with a morphia derivative or similar drug, and is wheeled, in a relaxed, sleepy state, to a room adjoining the operating theatre. Even the days of the mask have gone. Instead he receives an intravenous injection of a quick-acting barbiturate, such as pentothal, which sends him to sleep within fourteen seconds. Many patients describe their experience as 'Click, I was asleep – click, I was awake again'; some of them recover consciousness when the nurse is injecting a post-operative sedative and imagine that the pentothal is still being given – the author himself has had this experience.

During this lost period of time, which may be as long as five or six hours, the patient will be entirely unaware of what is happening to him. An endotracheal tube will probably be passed through his vocal cords and the anaesthetic vapour pumped into his lungs; his muscles will be relaxed and his breathing may be stopped by means of a curarizing agent; the anaesthetist will assist or take over his respiration by 'squeezing the bag' or with a mechanical respirator. His temperature may be lowered to the point where his heart ceases to beat, and the circulation maintained by means of a pump. It is possible, when the operation is finished, to have the patient almost fully conscious within five minutes. But here we are on dangerous ground, for there is much difference of opinion as to whether quick recovery is or is not the best treatment. As with so many other points in medical practice, the anaesthetist must weigh the safety against the comfort of his patient when making this decision.

Much thought has gone into the design of various parts of the theatre and, because the conscious patient can appreciate them, particularly into details of the anaesthetic room. A matt wall surface of pastel colour – beige is supposed to be best – has been found more soothing than glossy white or green. Overhead ceiling lighting glares straight down into the patient's eyes when he lies face upwards on a trolley; it has therefore been laid down that all lighting should be indirect and of low power, with a bright, adjustable lamp for the anaesthetist's use. In a modern anaesthetic room all walls are sound-proofed and lined with acoustic tiles, for noise is the one thing that the pre-medicated patient remembers. Absolute silence is impossible so long as nurses are of the female sex – especially if, by some mishap, two nurses are in the room together – but there is one anaesthetist at least who lives in hope that the golden age will dawn when everyone in the theatre will fully understand the truth of those words which Humphry Davy wrote in the year 1800 'When breathing nitrous oxide amid noise, I have sometimes found that the organs of hearing are painfully affected.' Despite all the changes in methods of anaesthesia, Davy's words are true today.

We have come a very long way from the time when a large audience tramped into a vast operating theatre direct from the street or the post-mortem room, when the chloroformist induced anaesthesia with a few breaths of the drug and the surgeon swiftly operated during the short period before complete recovery. We may have been somewhat too detailed and too long-winded in our description of a modern operating theatre, but this has been done for a purpose. Too few members of the public appreciate the immense amount of work, thought, and research which has added to the safety and the comfort of the patient during his operation. That work has been done, not by doctors and nurses only, but by architects, engineers, and designers. No detail is too insignificant for consideration; the texture of the blanket that covers the patient, relative impermeability of various types of surgeons' mask, the best kind of soap or detergent for 'scrubbing up'. About the year 1952, all 'ordinary' rubber in the theatres was changed for 'conducting' rubber, and theatre floors were ripped up to be replaced by 'conducting' surfaces. The object of this extremely costly manoeuvre was to prevent explosion of inflammable anaesthetics – now rarely used – by a static spark, which will only be dangerous in abnormally dry conditions. Even the most enthusiastic explosion 'expert' could not produce evidence that the risk was greater than one in three and a half million cases.

What of the surgeon, the man who is lord and master of this operating theatre? Let it be said in the first place, jumping ahead to modern days, that he is no longer the absolute master whose word is law. Once upon a time this was true, but now operating theatre life has become too complicated for one man to impose his will upon every detail of conduct. The bacteriologist will insist that certain things are done according to his own ideas; experts in electrical safety will require safety measures; if a new theatre is to be built, the architect will most certainly refuse to countenance some of the surgeon's pet schemes; even the anaesthetist has raised a timid voice to suggest that swinging doors are a danger to the unconscious patient and that sliding doors are safer.

Let us go right back to the beginning and briefly trace the development of the surgeon rather than of surgery. At the start of the first chapter he was, with a few honourable exceptions, an ill-educated man, trained by apprenticeship, only differing from the bone setter or the quack by possession of a qualification. He was the lowest member of the medical order, less considered than the physician and apothecary, often content to act as a specialized technician who skilfully performed his operation when instructed by the physician that operation was desirable. He, in turn, passed on his skills to apprentices, and his teaching was all too often coarse and obscene, by no means of the type to add to the dignity of his profession. An early nineteenth-century apologist declared this to be no bad thing, for it hardened the callow apprentice to the sights and sounds which would confront him.

From 1840 onwards there came a change which developed rapidly. In part this change was due to the more humane approach made possible by anaesthesia and of which anaesthesia was also an outward sign. But the alteration in the method of medical education did still more to effect a change. The apprentice, often indentured at twelve or thirteen years of age, had no cultural background; the medical student, schooled in the classics until seventeen or eighteen, was able to speak on terms of equality with 'the educated classes'. Thus the surgeon, no longer a harbinger of intolerable agony and now a man of some pretension to learning, began to achieve a status on a par with that of the cultured physician. It was not until some years later that the two branches of the profession met upon an entirely equal footing; the physician still tended to be a graduate of one of the ancient universities while the surgeon, with rare exceptions, was trained only at the medical school and hospital. But, by 1847, a man of the stamp of Lister, with a family background, education, and temperament that would suggest a physician's career, had decided upon the life of a surgeon.

The surgeon's outlook and the scope of his ordinary work had broadened by the time that Lister qualified. A generation of surgeons trained in general medicine, rather than in surgery alone, no longer depended upon the physician for diagnosis, but diagnosed their own cases before operating. Lister taught them that the after-treatment of a wound is just as important as is infliction of a wound; as time went on the surgeon accepted full responsibility for the care of his patient from the moment that he first saw him until cure was complete, although he might delegate some of the responsibility to others. Increasing interest in diagnosis and after-care introduced him to skills which were not part of surgery in the narrow meaning of the word; Pasteur's germ theory heralded the science of bacteriology; Virchow's work on cellular structure made it essential that the surgeon should have a knowledge of histology and pathology. For some years, until the coming of specialized bacteriologists and pathologists, he could only depend upon himself.

Thus there came into being the typical scientific surgeon of the eighteen eighties, learned, comfortably off, of a higher social status than his predecessors. In that secure, settled age of the rich man in his castle and the poor man at his gate, the surgeon, like everyone else, was expected to conform to a certain and definite pattern of living, behaviour, even of appearance. It is more instructive to consider one who did not so conform than to describe an exemplar of the type. Robert Lawson Tait of Birmingham would today be classed as 'anti-Establishment'. At a time when the importance of scientific advance in surgery had become fully recognized, Tait preached that apprenticeship is better than scientific training, that the budding surgeon should spend part of his time at the metal worker's lathe, the carpenter's bench, and the blacksmith's forge in order to learn the practical handling of tools, rather than that he should waste his short training in the laboratory or in the acquisition of theoretical knowledge. Tait practised antisepsis until the method was fully accepted, then became an opponent;[1] he preached the truth of the germ theory, but held that bacteria could cause changes only in tissues already dead. His character is a mass of contradictions; in his insistence that surgery is a trade and not a profession, yet depends upon a knowledge of the classics; in his determinedly plebeian behaviour and appearance, combined with a genuine cultured passion for beautiful things; in his puritan cleanliness of speech coupled with the revolting lechery that finally broke him. As a surgeon, he was undoubtedly the most brilliant operator and advanced thinker in England during the latter half of the nineteenth century; we can now understand that he was the British counterpart of Billroth and should have been honoured as such in his time. But he had little or no influence on his generation, for he would not conform; his obstinate heterodoxy made him suspect. Tait's failure gives us a measure of the rigid pattern of society in which the Victorian surgeon – and not the surgeon only – was expected to take his proper place.

X-rays, radium, radiotherapy entailed a wide extension of the surgeon's learning. At first he translated X-ray appearances himself; when the speciality grew into a separate department he still had, and has, to possess sufficient knowledge to discuss a questionable diagnosis. Radiotherapy cannot be handed over entirely to the expert; the surgeon must know what kinds of tumour respond best to irradiation and be prepared to argue the pros and cons of operative treatment in consultation with the radiotherapist. Then came the modern treatment of shock, problems of blood transfusion, the bacteristatic and antibiotic drugs; more recently biochemistry, alteration of the normal chemical constituents of the body fluids in disease, has assumed a most important place in surgery: the surgeon must have at least a working familiarity with all these allied sciences. It is a far cry from the days when he needed to rely solely upon a knowledge of anatomy and his own technical skill.

Often they had a hard road to travel, for many surgeons rose to the heights of their profession from very humble beginnings. Bartimeus, in one of his 1914 war stories, makes a character point to an island somewhere near Scapa Flow with the remark that a famous Harley Street surgeon was 'born in one of those crofts'. Bartimeus probably had in mind Sir William Watson Cheyne, consulting surgeon to the Royal Navy, who is often said to have been a native of Fetlar. In fact the true story of his birth is more interesting, for he was born in a storm at sea off the coast of Australia. Cheyne's father, skipper and part owner of a small trading schooner, died soon after the event and Cheyne was brought up by a maternal uncle, the minister of Fetlar. Men such as this somehow educated themselves; there were few scholarships and no state grants for medical students in those days. They lived in squalid lodgings, were often insufficiently fed, and had no money at all for amusements. Sir St Clair Thomson worked as a clerk in the evenings to earn his keep, and many others did the same.

Life was no less difficult for the intending specialist after he qualified. The ambitious man must serve as house surgeon before he could expect a staff appointment – not necessarily at the same hospital. House surgeons were rarely paid; a few hospitals offered an honorarium of £50 a year; some not only paid nothing at all but made a charge for board and lodging. Then came years of waiting until a suitable appointment offered. During this period many promising young men found it impossible to carry on; they could not scrape a sufficient income by coaching, assisting established surgeons, acting as curators of medical school museums, or by medical journalism; they became disheartened by the struggle and joined one of the services – usually the IMS – or went into general practice. Such wastage, although disappointing to the individual, was not altogether against public interest; a steady stream of brilliant young men, particularly interested in a speciality, ensured a very high standard of work in the 'general practitioner' hospitals. We face a similar problem today; part of the younger man's dissatisfaction with the National Health Service stems from the fact that he spends seven or eight years in postgraduate training, only to find that consultant posts are in short supply and that, because he is a highly qualified specialist, he is not suited to general practice. The solution lies in a return to the old-fashioned 'general practice' of three or four men, all well qualified and interested in a different speciality. Given adequate rewards and access to hospitals, such a change would do much to make the GP's life a more interesting one, to improve the standard of general practice, and to ease the burden on the hospital service.

This is wishful thinking for the future, and we must return to the surgeon of the past. The successful candidate for a hospital post still had a period of difficulty ahead of him. He was an 'honorary', receiving no payment at all for his work at the hospital and only rarely being granted a small honorarium for teaching the students. He had embarked upon a Robin Hood career, treating the sick poor in the hospitals free of charge and relying upon the rich for his livelihood. Just as a barrister can only receive his brief from a solicitor, so the honorary surgeon was debarred from touting for patients; he depended upon his contacts with the general practitioner. Almost without exception the successful surgeon made his name – and his fortune – by the excellence of his unpaid hospital work; the general practitioner sent his poorer patients to the surgeon's out-patient clinic, and the good results encouraged him to send his more wealthy patients to the same surgeon in Harley Street. Unlike the general practitioner, the specialist surgeon or physician did not buy a share in an established practice, and his own practice was not a saleable asset. Every specialist was a 'squatter' waiting, often waiting long years, for the paying patients to come. Such a life entailed hardship, all the greater because there must be an outward appearance of prosperity. Joyce Dennis in her *Mrs Dose the Doctor's Wife* delightfully tells the early struggles of Sir Joshua Tonsil; his party dinners in Harley Street were admirably cooked by a hired chef and deftly served by a hired butler, but it was Joshua and Mrs Joshua who washed up afterwards – and Mrs Joshua donned a wig and spectacles when she scrubbed the front door steps and polished the brass plate every morning. There is more than a grain of truth in this fable; many surgeons and their wives were forced to bitter economy in private, but the rent of the Harley Street room must be paid, a smart car maintained, and the surgeon be immaculately dressed.

The young surgeon without private means had a hard struggle before the Second World War. In 1948 the National Health Service gave him an assured income and, for all the disappointments and frustrations which the registrar must be prepared to face before becoming a consultant, the road to specialization is smoother and less hazardous than in the past. When the doctor tried to obtain higher pay and better working conditions by negotiation and even by threat of strike action – fortunately never yet implemented – the public image of the profession was tarnished. Those who are so quick to criticize should bear in mind that the doctor is now a state employee and must make the best bargain with his employer that he can. A greater though perhaps inevitable loss is the long tradition of voluntary service.

Because the young surgeon had a hard struggle in the years before 1948, he found it necessary to resort to various little stratagems. Good, hard work was often not enough to make his fame; debarred from open advertising by the ethical code of his profession, he had to develop a distinctive personality for himself by other means. Quite a long essay could be written on the peculiarities of surgeons' names, their love for the double-barrelled and the unusual. Bland Sutton, Webb Johnson, Tudor Edwards are random examples of the hyphen or assumed hyphen; so common did the habit become that Wells is generally spoken of as Spencer Wells, Tait as Lawson Tait, and Cheyne as Watson Cheyne. Berkeley Moynihan, St Clair Thomson, and D'Arcy Power are examples of the unusual Christian name.

Trivial though this seems, it is symptomatic; an 'ordinary' name such as Sutton or Edwards was not sufficiently distinctive.

Some surgeons gloried in the fact that they had risen from the lower ranks. John Bland Sutton, a baronet and President of the Royal College of Surgeons, cultivated an exaggerated Cockney accent, to which he had little right for he was the son of a grazier-butcher of Enfield. Bland Sutton was once called to operate on a duchess at the family seat. After the operation was over, the ducal butler suggested that he might like a little refreshment; Bland Sutton gratefully accepted and was given his lunch in the housekeeper's room. Relating this terrible indignity, Bland Sutton added: 'Little did 'Is Grice know that this piece of hinfernal himpertinence cost 'Is Grice an extra 'undred guineas.' But others hated the memory of their grim struggle. Berkeley, Lord Moynihan of Leeds, orphan of a penniless soldier who won the Victoria Cross and was awarded a commission, could never bear mention of the fact that he had been educated at Christ's Hospital. It is true that he was bitterly unhappy there, as many boys have been before and since his time, but his biographer is probably correct in his opinion that Moynihan angrily resented that he had never had the advantages of a more fashionable school.

Surgeons have to be quick thinkers and it is for this reason that many have become famed for their wit; indeed, a London newspaper for a short time recorded the sayings of a living surgeon under the heading 'Dicksoniana'. Many good stories have been fathered on to Wifred Trotter of University College Hospital; there seems no doubt that he did once say 'Mr Anaesthetist, if the patient can keep awake I see no reason why you should not do the same.' Philip Mitchener of St Thomas' is credited with many swift repartees; unfortunately most of these are somewhat broad, but there is one gem that can be reproduced here. He swore at a nurse in the theatre and was summoned before the formidable matron of St Thomas'. 'Mr. Mitchener,' she said. 'I understand that you told one of my nurses to go to the devil.' 'Quite right, matron,' answered Mitchener cheerfully. 'I never thought she'd do it.'

And now we must embark upon the most dangerous thing that a historian can do, take the lessons of the past and apply them to a forecast of the future. Where is surgery leading? This brings us to some work that has not yet been mentioned, the replacement of a diseased organ by one which is healthy, or the insertion of an inert prosthesis which will assume the function of the natural structure. An example of the latter is the 'artificial heart' made of plastic called silastic, which was inserted into the chest of a calf by suture to the great blood vessels in 1965.[2] In 1966 De Bakey of Houston, Texas, applied the idea to the human and succeeded at the third trial. This is not true replacement of an organ, because the artificial heart, worked by a pump, is only designed to tide the patient over a period of failure, but the insertion of plastic valves is a true replacement technique.

The answer probably does not lie in the use of synthetic organs; despite all the problems that remain to be solved, a 'Henry Ford scrap-and-replace' technique will, in the end, depend upon a steady and readily available supply of human material.

The attractive idea of killing off a valueless but healthy member of the lower classes and transferring some part of his anatomy to a diseased social superior is a very old one, but alleged successes must be regarded with a certain suspicion. In more modern times O. M. Lannelongue of France is said to have successfully transplanted a sheep's thyroid into the human for the cure of myxoedema in 1890, and Victor Horsley among others transplanted human thyroid for the same purpose.[3] Alexis Carrel published his *Results of the Transplantation of Blood Vessels, Organs, and Limbs* in 1908 and, as we have seen, attempts have been made from time to time to graft one individual with skin, cartilage, or bone from another.

At present the most hopeful work is that in connection with the kidney. Although C. S. Williamson performed a number of animal experiments in 1923–6, the idea could not be applied to the human because there was no means of tiding the patient over the inevitable period of renal failure before the graft became functional. The first artificial kidney or dialyser was built by W. J. Kolff in 1944. It must have been a miracle of ingenuity for Kolff was working in a provincial Dutch hospital under the German occupation and had only elementary appliances and materials at his command. The modern 'artificial kidney' is descended from the Kolff machine and is in routine use when patients suffer from kidney failure. The first attempt to graft a kidney in the human seems to have been by E. Landsteiner and C. Hufnagel at the Peter Bent Brigham Hospital in 1945, but the first well-documented case is that of Lawlor and others in Chicago. The patient, a woman of forty-four, suffered from a cystic disease of the kidneys; they functioned but with reduced efficiency. The operation was therefore not replacement of a kidney, but addition of a third in the hope that this would relieve her symptoms. On 17 June 1950 Lawlor transplanted a kidney from a woman of forty-nine who had just died from cirrhosis of the liver – not, one would have thought, the best possible type of donor. After a fairly uneventful recovery the patient was on 26 August 'able to take a 300-mile automobile trip to attend a convention of a week's duration. During her attendance at the convention she freely participated in the banquets, dancing and other convention activities.'[4] But the operation was not successful; in 1951 Lawlor reported that the transplanted kidney, although still living, was much diminished in size and not doing its work of secreting urine.

In 1951 Servelle of France tried the experiment on a twenty-four-year-old female who suffered from congenital absence of the right kidney and ureter. Servelle used the kidney of an executed criminal; his patient died on the nineteenth day after operation. At about the same time C. Dubost of Paris reported two transplants. In 1952–5 D. M. Hume performed kidney transplants upon nine patients; only four of the transplanted kidneys functioned for more than thirty-seven days, and none for more than just under six months. All these grafts had been taken from unrelated donors; in 1953 L. Michon transplanted a kidney from a mother to the son, but the graft failed within three weeks.

The surgeons had encountered a difficulty which had been foreseen but which, it was hoped, would not materialize. Just as the skin of one person will often refuse to 'take' when grafted on to another, so the body mechanism of the recipient refused to accept the kidney of a donor. The transplanted kidney simply acted as a foreign body and was rejected. Until 1956 no kidney transplants met with more than temporary success, save for one experimental operation performed on *identical twin* calves.

In 1954 John P. Merrill, Joseph E. Murray and others at the Peter Bent Brigham Hospital had under their care a twenty-four-year-old man who suffered from a disease which caused atrophy of both kidneys, a high blood pressure, and the type of poisoning by retained products which is known as uraemia. It happened that this youth was one of a pair of identical twins, and the brother was healthy. Merrill and his co-workers, having knowledge of the calf experiment, started to investigate the possibility of grafting one kidney from the healthy twin into the sick brother. First of all they took a piece of skin from the potential donor and grafted it on to the patient and vice versa. This was done to make certain that the twins were, in fact, identical and that tissue rejection would not be sure to occur when the kidney was transplanted. At the end of thirty-one days the grafts on both twins appeared to have survived as normal skin.

On 23 December 1954 the left kidney was removed from the healthy twin and transplanted to the patient. The donor twin recovered uneventfully; he left hospital on the fourteenth day after operation. The recipient also recovered quite well; nine days after transplantation, tests showed that the grafted kidney was secreting urine satisfactorily and that the patient's own diseased kidneys were not secreting at all – he would have been dead by this time if left untreated. He was discharged from hospital on the thirty-eighth day; later he had to return for treatment of a mild urinary infection but otherwise he remained in good health. However, his blood pressure was still high and the surgeons thought that removal of the diseased kidneys might have a good effect; the first was removed three months after the original operation, the second two and a half months later – and the blood pressure fell to a normal level. Eleven months after the last operation an account of the case was published in the *Journal of the American Medical Association;* at this time, 1956, the patient appeared in excellent health with a fully functioning kidney, and there could be no doubt that grafting had been successful.[5] He married one of the nurses who looked after him, fathered a child, and was working as a television engineer three and a half years after transplantation.

Perhaps the most remarkable part of this story is the fact that there were found a sufficient number of pairs of identical twins, one suffering from severe kidney disease and the other healthy, to make up a worth-while series of cases. In 1958 – only four years after their original operation – Murray and Merrill reported on the results of transplantation between seven pairs, including that already described. In one case the kidney failed to function and the recipient died on the twelfth day from renal failure; one patient died after four months because the disease from which he suffered spread to the transplanted kidney; one had signs of active disease in the transplant at the time of publication. The remaining four patients were living in good health. By 1963 some twenty-five transplants had been made between identical twins, with considerable success.

These hopeful results stimulated work on the problem of tissue rejection. It may here be said that such work is by no means yet complete but sufficient progress has been made to render possible the transplantation of kidneys from an un-related human to another with some hope of success. The 'immune' or 'rejection' response of the body is suppressed ('immunosuppression') by irradiation of the whole body and by the use of drugs, of which prednisone and azathioprine are examples. Further, the artificial kidney enables the patient to be cleared of toxic products which his own kidneys or the graft cannot expel during periods of diminished function.

The first successful kidney transplant from one individual to another (for identical twins can be looked upon as a single individual) was by J. Hamburger of Paris in 1959; he operated on twins, but non-identical twins, and the grafted kidney was functional four years later. In the same year Merrill used the kidney of an unrelated donor in the case of a twenty-four-year-old man who had suffered from renal disease since the age of seven. Merrill made preliminary cross skin grafts, but these were rejected. However tests showed that the two individuals were very similar, and the recipient was submitted to whole body irradiation. A week after transplant he became severely ill but, after removal of both his own kidneys, he recovered with the help of prednisone and further whole body irradiation. In the end he was able to resume his studies at college.

By 1963 renal transplantation had been performed success-fully in America, Canada, France, and Great Britain, but always using living donors. That year F. M. Parsons, F. R.

Raper and others in Britain reported that they had used kidneys taken from dead persons in two cases.[6] At the end of 1965 J. R. Kenyon, W. S. Peart and others at St Mary's Hospital, London, reported a series of twenty patients, suffering from hopeless renal failure, who had been treated by transplantation of cadaveric kidneys between October 1963 and April 1965. The only 'matching' test between the donor and the recipient was to see that they were of the same blood group. Eight out of these twenty patients were alive and well, with functioning transplants, at three to twenty months after operation.[7]

Work still goes on and work will go on until the various problems are solved. We shall then find that the surgeon will proceed from the kidney to the stomach, the lungs, the heart and other body organs. Here is the surgery of the future; instead of cobbling-up a diseased organ, the surgeon will replace it with a healthy one. But this 'scrap-and-replace' technique will demand that the new structure is taken from a dead body. We have already seen that Lillihei gave up his cross-circulation method in heart surgery partly because of risk to the donor and partly because of the criticism that might fall upon a parent who refused his aid. No healthy individual should ever be put at risk for the sake of a diseased one. This is common sense; not only is the donor of a kidney risking his life, however small that risk may be, but he has no warranty that his remaining – and now essential – kidney will not become diseased. If this is true of the kidneys, one of which can be spared, it is certainly true of a single organ such as the heart. Therefore the future will require a free supply of cadaveric material and suitable methods of storage. Again, we have seen that a similar problem has been solved in the case of corneal grafts; the far more complex problem of other parts of the body is equally capable of solution. And this will entail a more logical, less emotional approach to the disposal of a corpse.

Transplantation of organs and tissues implies a widening of the surgeon's present field, but there is little doubt that an important part of his work will be taken over by the physician or biochemist in the foreseeable future. Operative surgery of infection – the acute mastoid and osteomyelitis are examples – has receded in importance during the last twenty-five years because antibiotic drugs have proved so effective in the treatment of these disorders. Tuberculosis, the reason for nearly a quarter of all operations in the nineteenth century, has been brought under control by establishing the cause, by preventive treatment, and by streptomycin. Cancer has taken the place of tuberculosis as a surgical disease. Research into the cause of various types of cancer is being carried out in a number of centres, and the day will come when that cause is found. Once the cause has been discovered, a means of treatment will soon follow, and it is unlikely that such treatment will involve operative surgery. It is, of course, useless to forecast the nature of the treatment but one might, perhaps, be permitted to hazard a guess that the development of a cancer may prove to depend upon deficiency or excess of some internal secretion and that the cure will take the form of injecting a stimulating or inhibiting substance.

We, or our children, will very probably witness the simplification of present surgical methods. Antisepsis gave way to asepsis, but the introduction of bacteristatic and antibiotic drugs has not affected aseptic technique as much as might be expected. Part of the reason for this is that the antibiotics have proved unsatisfactory, almost dangerous, in one respect; bacteria can and do develop a resistance and can breed a strain which will not be destroyed by the antibiotic. This is why antibiosis, useful though it is, does not provide the complete answer to the problem of infection. On the other hand, there is no known strain of bacteria which has developed resistance to an efficient antiseptic. An antiseptic kills at once, just as a man dies at once when shot through the heart, but an antibiotic kills more slowly by interfering with the organism's nutrition. If the organism develops a resistance to this interference, its progeny will also be resistant because it reproduces itself by division. Thus a resistant strain will emerge.

In this one respect the antiseptics are better drugs than the antibiotics and it is therefore probable that, within less than a century, penicillin will be as outdated as is carbolic acid today. But the change will be a larger one than this. Asepsis works – and gives very good results – but, in order to maintain those good results, it has been found necessary to erect an immense structure of safeguards, requiring cumbersome, costly apparatus and innumerable man-hours to support it. Nor is that structure a safe one. The aseptic system has been likened to a leaking dam; the efforts of bacteriologists, nursing staff, technicians, and surgeons are harnessed to patch up the leaks and, as soon as one leak is stopped, another breaks through. Thus the whole system, although it works, is outworn and potentially dangerous. Even a vintage Rolls-Royce can be wrecked by the snapping of a rusted split pin.

Again, it is useless to attempt an accurate forecast of the method that will take the place of asepsis. Not antibiotics, certainly, for the reason given above. It will possibly be a return to some kind of antisepsis, not necessarily by chemical agents, for gamma rays have already proved effective in the sterilization of certain articles, or perhaps something in the nature of a selective weed-killer will be developed. We must hope that, whatever the means evolved, the technique will be a simple one. That is the great drawback of 'modern' asepsis; it lacks the simplicity in which Lister so firmly believed and which he rightly stated to be the outstanding advantage of his own method. But the principle of preventing invasion of the wound by bacteria will remain; for that principle, first taught by Joseph Lister, is the eternal rock upon which the whole practice of surgery is founded.

REFERENCES

CHAPTER 1

1 *Lancet*, 1830, i, 112.
2 Cope, Sir Zachary, *The Royal College of Surgeons of England*, 1959, 64.
3 ibid, 75.
4 Lonsdale, Henry, *Robert Knox*, 1870, 131.
5 Taylor, Shephard T., *The Diary of a Medical Student during the Mid Victorian Period*, 1927, 98, 151, 170.
6 *Lancet*, 1832–3, ii, 321.
7 Cartwright, F. F., *The English Pioneers of Anaesthesia*, 1952, 11.
8 *Lancet*, 1830–1, ii, 86ff.
9 *Lancet*, 1870, i, 387.
10 *Lancet*, 1824, ii, 291.
11 *Lancet*, 1833–4, i, 99.
12 New Sydenham Society. *Year Book of Medicine and Surgery*, 1864, 194.

CHAPTER 2

1 *Med-Chir. Transactions*, 1819, x, 153.
2 *Gentlemen's Magazine*, 1825, xcv, 628 *Lancet*, 1825–6, ix, 646.
3 Beddoes, T., *Notice of Some Observations Made at the Medical Pneumatic Institution*, 1799.
4 Sykes, W. Stanley, *Essays on the First Hundred Years of Anaesthesia*, 1960, i, 50.
5 *Lancet*, 1848, i, 70, 119, etc.
6 *Lancet*, 1858, i, 604.
7 *Lancet*, 1858, ii, 603.
8 *Lancet*, 1858, ii, 350.
9 *British Medical Journal*, 1880, i, 933.

CHAPTER 3

1 *King's College Hospital Gazette* 1937 (supplement) p. xxvi.

304

CHAPTER 3

2 *Lancet*, 1865, i, 651.
3 Sykes, W. Stanley, *Essays on the First Hundred Years of Anaesthesia*, 1960, i, 71.
4 *Med-Chir. Transactions*, 1859, xlii, 67.
5 *British Medical Journal* 1864, i, 264.
6 Nisbet, W. *The Clinical Guide*, 1801, ii, 377.
7 Simpson, Sir James Y., *Acupressure, a New Method of Arresting Surgical Haemorrhage and of Accelerating the Healing of Wounds*, 1864.
8 Simpson, Sir James Y., *Edinburgh Medical Journal*, 1869–70.
9 Nightingale, F., *Notes on Hospitals*, 3rd Edn, 1863, 56.
10 *Punch*, 1858, xxxiv, 26/6, 255.
11 Cheyne, W. W., *Lister and His Achievement*, 1925, 44.
12 *Lancet*, 1870, i, 40.
13 *Lancet*, 1867, i, 327.
14 Guthrie, Douglas, *Lord Lister*, 1949, 59.
15 *Lancet*, 1867, ii, 353.

CHAPTER 4

1 *Lancet*, 1868, ii, 695.
2 *British Medical Journal*, 1871, ii, 228.
3 *Lancet*, 1870, i, 155.
4 *Lancet*, 1875, ii, 597.
5 *Lancet*, 1879, i, 577.
6 *Lancet*, 1882, i, 1088.
7 *British Medical Journal*, 1879, ii, 210.
8 *Lancet*, 1868, ii, 634 et seq.
9 Taylor, Shephard T., *Diary of a Medical Student during the Mid-Victorian Period*, 1927, 24.
10 *Lancet*, 1875, i, 511 et seq.
11 *Lancet*, 1870, i, 91.
12 *Lancet*, 1870, i, 175.
13 *British Medical Journal*, 1870, ii, 243.
14 *Lancet*, 1870, ii, 908.
15 *Lancet*, 1870, ii, 871.
16 *British Medical Journal*, 1870, ii, 317.
17 *Lancet*, 1879, i, 337.
18 *Lancet*, 1879, i, 575.
19 *Lancet*, 1879, i, 336.
20 *Lancet*, 1879, ii, 731.
21 *British Medical Journal*, 1871, ii, 227.

CHAPTER 5

1 Power, Sir D'Arcy, *British Masters of Medicine*, 1936, 134.
2 Bleich, A. R., *The Story of X-rays*, 1960, 4.

CHAPTER 5

3 *Nature*, 23/1/1896, 274.
4 *Lancet*, 1896, i, 257.
5 *Lancet*, 1896, i, 477.
6 Lister, Lord, *Collected Papers*, 1909, ii, 491.
7 *Lancet*, 1903, ii, 271.
8 *Lancet*, 1903, ii, 1388, 1904, i, 1046.
9 *Lancet*, 1890, ii, 1158.
10 *British Journal of Surgery*, 1939, xxvii, 436.

CHAPTER 6

1 *Lancet*, 1876, ii, 553.
2 *Lancet*, 1900, i, 1485.
3 *Lancet*, 1899, ii, 441.
4 *Lancet*, 1905, i, 820.
5 *J. Bone and Joint Surg.*, 1950, 32B, 666.
6 *Lancet*, 1915, ii, 213, 1009, 1063.
7 *The Medical Annual*, 1911, 14.
8 *Lancet*, 1936, i, 1279, 1286.
9 *Lancet*, 1938, i, 1210.
10 Lister, Lord, *Collected Papers*, 1909, i, 280.
11 *Brit. J. Experimental Pathology*, 1929, x. 226.
12 *Biochemical Journal*, 1932, xxvi, 1907.
13 *J. of Bacteriology*, 1935, xxix, 215.
14 *Lancet*, 1940, ii, 226.
15 *Lancet*, 1941, ii, 177.
16 *Med-Chir. Transactions*, 1819, x, 296.
17 *Lancet*, 1824, ii, 295.
18 *Lancet*, 1825, vi, 14.
19 Keynes, Geoffrey, *The History of Blood Transfusion, Brit. J. of Surgery*, 1943, xxi.
20 *Lancet*, 1831–2, ii, 274.
21 *Lancet*, 1935, i, 977.
22 *Lancet*, 1937, ii, 361.
23 Massy, John, 1959, *King's College Hospital Gazette.* 38, ii, 101.
24 Edwards, Harold C., ibid, 66.

CHAPTER 7

1 Power, Sir D'Arcy, *Cutting for the Stone, British Journal of Surgery*, 1930, xviii, 541.
2 ibid, 1.
3 ibid, 185.
4 ibid, 24.
5 Power, Sir D'Arcy, *Lithotrity, British Journal of Surgery*, 1931, xix, 1.

CHAPTER 7

6 Fergusson, Sir W., *System of Practical Surgery*, 1846, 2nd Edn, 627.
7 *Lancet*, 1878, ii, 624.
8 *Lancet*, 1870, i, 1.
9 *Lancet*, 1888, i, 215.
10 *Lancet*, 1930, i, 1163.
11 *British Medical Journal*, 1901, ii, 125
12 *Lancet*, 1904, ii, 197.
13 *British Journal of Surgery*, 1920, vii, 525.
14 *Lancet*, 1945, ii, 693.
15 *Med-Chir. Transactions*, 1880, lxiv, 181.
16 *Med-Chir. Transactions*, 1879, lxxiii, 421.
17 *J. of Bone and Joint Surgery*, 1950, 32B, 620.
  (for section on the orthopaedic service)

CHAPTER 8

1 Taylor, Shephard T., *Diary of a Medical Student in the Mid-Victorian Period*, 1927, 188.
2 *Lancet*, 1871, i, 685.
3 *Trans. Clinical Soc. Lond.*, 1871, iv, 49.
4 *British Medical Journal*, 1875, ii, 360.
5 Hey Groves, E. W., *Methods and Results of Transplantation of Bone*, Brit. Jour. of Surgery, 1917, v, 185.
6 *British Medical Journal*, 1879, i, 656.
7 *Jour. of Bone and Joint Surgery*, 1952, 34B, 126.
8 Warren Woodroffe, H. L., *The Reparation of Cranial Defects by Means of Cartilaginous Grafts*, Brit. J. Surg., 1917, v, 42.
9 ibid.
10 *Plastic Surgery at the Queen's Hospital, Sidcup*, Brit. J. of Surgery, 1921, ix, 87.
11 *Lancet*, 1894, i, 1008.
12 Edwards, Harold, *Inguinal Hernia*, Brit. J. of Surgery, 1943, xxxi, 172.
13 *Med-Chir. Transactions*, 1860, xliii, 71.

CHAPTER 9

1 Dinnick, T., *The Origins and Evolution of Colostomy*, Brit. J. of Surgery, 1934, xxii, 142.
2 *British Journal of Surgery*, 1914, ii, 292.
3 *British Medical Journal*, 1897, i, 341.
4 *Med-Chir. Trans*, 1844, xxvii, 468.
5 *British Journal of Surgery*, 1927, xiv, 385.
6 *British Medical Journal*, 1864, ii, 384.
7 *British Medical Journal*, 1879, ii, 911.
8 *British Medical Journal*, 1880, i, 931.

CHAPTER 9

9 *British Medical Journal*, 1879, i, 926.
10 Moynihan, Berkeley, *Surgery of the Spleen. Brit. J. of Surgery*, 1920, viii, 307.
11 *Med-Chir. Transactions*, 1880, lxiii, 17.
12 *British Journal of Surgery*, 1934, xxii, 274.
13 Ogilvie, Sir Heneage, *A Hundred Years of Gastric Surgery. Ann. Roy. Coll. Surg. Eng.*, 1947, i, 37.
14 Gordon Taylor, Sir Gordon et al., *The Remote Results of Gastrectomy. Brit. J. of Surgery*, 1928, xvi, 641.
15 Hurwitz and Degensheim. *Milestones in Modern Surgery*, 1958, 276.
16 *Lancet*, 1885, i, 903.
17 *British Medical Journal*, 1888, i, 719.
18 Ogilvie, Sir Heneage, *op. cit.*
19 ibid.
20 ibid.
21 Taylor, Herman, *Gastroscopy. Brit. J. of Surg.*, 1936, xxiv, 469.
22 *British Journal of Surgery*, 1919, vii, 404.
23 Taylor, Herman, *op. cit.*
24 *Lancet*, 1848, ii, 380.
25 Bockus, H. L. et al., *Gastroenterology*, 1964, ii, 1091.
26 Rendle Short, A., *The Causation of Appendicitis. Brit. J. of Surgery*, 1920, viii, 171.
27 Power, Sir D'Arcy, *Treves' First Appendix Operation. Brit. J. of Surgery*, 1935, xxiii, 89.
28 *British Medical Journal*, 1939, ii, 56.

CHAPTER 10

1 Ballance, Sir Charles, *A Glimpse into the History of the Surgery of the Brain. Lancet*, 1922, i, 111, 165.
2 *British Medical Journal*, 1877, ii, 75.
3 *Med-Chir. Transactions*, 1880, lxiii, 21.
4 *British Medical Journal*, 1877, ii, 75.
5 *Med-Chir. Transactions*, 1880, lxiii, 17.
6 *British Medical Journal*, 1922, ii, 157.
7 *Lancet*, 1922, i, 170, *British Medical Journal*, 1922, ii, 157.
8 *Lancet*, 1884, ii, 1090.
9 *British Medical Journal*, 1886, ii, 670; 1887, i, 863.
10 *British Medical Journal*, 1865, i, 357.
11 *Lancet*, 1888, ii, 260.
12 Bailey, Hamilton, & Love, R. S. McNeill, *A Short Practice of Surgery*, 1932, ii, 800.
13 *Lancet*, 1890, ii, 914, 925.
14 *British Medical Journal*, 1923, ii, 796.
15 *British Journal of Surgery*, 1922, x, 165.
16 *Lancet*, 1947, i, 265.

CHAPTER 10

17 *Lancet*, 1885, i, 894.
18 *Lancet*, 1911, ii, 150.
19 *Lancet*, 1880, i, 810.
20 Thomas, Sir C. Price, *Pulmonary Tuberculosis in Retrospect and prospect.*
   Ann. Roy. Coll. Surg. Eng., 1964, xxxv, 67.
21 *British Medical Journal*, 1893, i, 1152.
22 *British Medical Journal*, 1906, ii, 6.
23 *British Journal of Surgery*, 1926, xiv, 100.
24 *British Medical Journal*, 1880, ii, 122.
25 *British Medical Journal*, 1880, ii, 163.
26 *British Medical Journal*, 1881, ii, 523.
27 *International Abstracts of Surgery*, 1922, xxxv, 12.
28 *British Journal of Surgery*, 1934, xxii, 310.
29 *British Medical Journal*, 1939, i, 809.
30 *Ann. Roy. Coll. Surg. Eng.*, 1947, i, 248.
31 *Med-Chir. Transactions*, 1873, lvi, 203.
32 Ballance, Sir C., *The Surgery of the Heart. Lancet*, 1920, i, 1.
33 *British Medical Journal*, 1896, i, Epitome 82.
34 Ballance, Sir C., *Lancet*, 1920, i, 1.
35 ibid.
36 *Lancet*, 1920, i, 77.
37 *Surgery, Gynaecology & Obstetrics*, 1946, lxxxiii, 117.
38 *Lancet*, 1902, i, 619.
39 *Lancet*, 1898, i, 927.
40 *Lancet*, 1902, i, 352.
41 *British Medical Journal*, 1923, ii, 530.
42 *British Medical Journal*, 1925, ii, 603.
43 *Jour. of the American Med. Assoc.*, 1939, cxii, 729.
44 *British Journal of Surgery*, 1944, xxxii, 1.
45 *Ann. Roy. Coll. Surg. Eng.*, 1965, xxxvi, 64.
46 *British Medical Journal*, 1948, i, 1121.
47 *Lancet*, 1948, i, 988.
48 *British Medical Journal*, 1950, i, 1283.
49 *British Medical Journal*, 1953, ii, 1059.
50 *British Medical Journal*, 1954, i, 1284.
51 *Lancet*, 1959, i, 748.
52 *Lancet*, 1913, i, 1795.
53 *British Journal of Surgery*, 1939, xxvii, 567.
54 *Surgery, Gynaecology & Obstetrics*, 1949, lxxxviii, 689.
55 *British Medical Journal*, 1963, i, 353.

CHAPTER 11

1 Mawson, Stuart R., *Diseases of the Ear*, 1963, *passim.*
2 Shambaugh, George E. Jr., *Surgery of the Ear*, 1959, *passim.*

3 Macewen, W., *Pyogenic Infectious Diseases of the Brain and Spinal Cord*, 1893, 332.
4 *Lancet*, 1906, ii, 353.
5 *Journ. of Laryngology and Otology*, 1962, lxxvi, 87.
6 *British Medical Journal*, 1882, i, 130, 265.
7 *Med-Chir. Transactions*, 1870, liii, 191.
8 Stevenson, R. Scott & Guthrie D. *A Short History of Otolaryngology.* 1949, 103.
9 Sorsby, Arnold, *A Short History of Ophthalmology*, 1933, 47.
10 *Archives of Ophthalmology.* 1965, lxxiv, 871.
11 *Proc. Roy. Soc. Med.*, 1933, xxvi, 597.
12 *Lancet*, 1937, i, 1395.
13 *Lancet*, 1828–9, ii, 351.
14 *British Medical Journal*, 1875, ii, 386.

CHAPTER 12

1 *Med-Chir. Transactions*, 1880, lxiii, 22.
2 *Annals of Surgery*, 1965, clxi, 365.
3 *British Medical Journal*, 1892, i, 215, 265.
4 *Jour. of the American Medical Association*, 1950, cxliv, 844.
5 *Jour. of the American Medical Association*, 1956, clx, 277.
6 *British Medical Journal*, 1963, i, 930.
7 *British Medical Journal*, 1965, ii, 1387.

BIBLIOGRAPHY

Annals of the Royal College of Surgeons of England.
Annals of Surgery.
Brain.
British Journal of Experimental Pathology.
British Journal of Ophthalmology.
British Journal of Radiology.
British Journal of Surgery.
British Journal of Urology.
British Medical Journal.
Guy's Hospital Reports.
International Abstracts of Surgery.
Journal of the American Medical Association.
Journal of Bone and Joint Surgery (British and American).
Journal of Laryngology and Otology.
Journal of Urology.
King's College Hospital Gazette.
Lancet.
Medical Annual.
Medico-Chirurgical Transactions.
Proceedings of the Royal Society of Medicine.
St Bartholomew's Hospital Reports.
Surgery, Gynaecology and Obstetrics.
Transactions of the Medical Society of London.

Allen, J. G. et al., *Surgery* (Pitman Med. Pub. Co., London, 1957).
Atkins, Hedley, *The Surgeon's Craft* (Manchester University Press, Manchester, 1965).
Bateman, D., *Berkeley Moynihan* (Macmillan, London, 1940).
Bett, W. R., *Sir John Bland Sutton* (Livingstone, Edinburgh, 1956).
Bick, Edgar M., *Source Book of Orthopaedics* (Williams & Wilkens, Baltimore, 1948).
Bleich, A., *The Story of X-rays* (Dover Publications Inc., New York, 1960).
Bockus, H. L., *Gastro-enterology* (Saunders, Philadelphia, 1946).
Brock, R. C., *The Life and Work of Astley Cooper* (Livingstone, Edinburgh, 1952).
Cartwright, F. F., *The English Pioneers of Anaesthesia* (John Wright, Bristol, 1952).
Cartwright, F. F., *Joseph Lister* (Weidenfeld & Nicolson [Educational], London, 1963).
Castiglione, A., *A History of Medicine* (Alfred A. Knopf, New York, 1947).
Cheyne, W. Watson, *Antiseptic Surgery* (Smith, Elder & Co., London, 1882).

Cheyne, W. Watson, *Lister and His Achievement* (Longmans, London, 1925).

Cope, Z., *The Royal College of Surgeons of England* (Anthony Blond, London, 1959).

Cope, Z., *Some Famous General Practitioners* (Pitman Med. Pub. Co., London, 1961).

Curie, Eve, *Madame Curie* (W. Heinemann, London, 1947).

Fergusson, W., *A System of Practical Surgery* (John Churchill, London, 1842).

Fulton, J. F., *Harvey Cushing* (Charles C Thomas, Springfield, Illinois, 1946).

Garrison, F. H., *An Introduction to the History of Medicine* (Saunders, Philadelphia, 1929).

Gask, George, *Essays in the History of Medicine* (Butterworth's Med. Pub. Ltd., London, 1950).

Godlee, Rickman J., *Lord Lister* (Macmillan, London, 1917).

Gordon Taylor, Gordon, and Wells, E. W., *Sir Charles Bell* (Livingstone, Edinburgh, 1958).

Grey Turner, G., (Ed) *Modern Operative Surgery* (Cassell & Co. Ltd., London, 1955).

Guthrie, Douglas, *A History of Medicine* (Nelson, Edinburgh, 1949).

Guthrie, Douglas, *Lord Lister* (Livingstone, Edinburgh, 1949).

Harding Rains, A. J. & Melville Capper, W., (Eds.) *Bailey and Love's Short Practice of Surgery* (Lewis, London, 1965).

Hilton, John, *Rest and Pain* (Ed. E. W. Walls et al.) (G. Bell & Sons Ltd., London, 1950).

Holmes, T., *Sir Benjamin Collins Brodie* (T. Fisher Unwin, London, 1898).

Keith, Arthur, *Menders of the Maimed* (Oxford Med. Publ., London, 1919).

Laing Gordon, H., *Sir James Young Simpson* (T. Fisher Unwin, London, 1897).

Layton, T. B., *Sir William Arbuthnot Lane* (Livingstone, London, 1956).

Leeson, J. R., *Lister as I Knew him* (Baillière, Tindall & Cox, London, 1928).

Le Vay, D., *The Life of Hugh Owen Thomas* (Livingstone, Edinburgh, 1956).

Lister, Joseph, Baron, *The Collected Papers of* (Clarendon Press, Oxford, 1909).

Lonsdale, H., *Life of Robert Knox* (MacMillan, London, 1870).

Maingot, R., (Ed.) *Post-Graduate Surgery* (Med. Pub. Ltd., London, 1936).

Major, R. H., *A History of Medicine* (Blackwell Sc. Pub., Oxford, 1954).

Mawson, Stuart R., *Diseases of the Ear* (Edward Arnold, London, 1963).

Mettler, C. C., *History of Medicine* (The Blakiston Co., Philadelphia, 1947).

Moynihan, Berkeley, *Addresses on Surgical Subjects* (Saunders, Philadelphia, 1928).

Ogilvie, W. Heneage, *Surgery Orthodox and Heterodox* (Blackwell Sc. Pub., Oxford, 1948).

Power, D'Arcy, (Ed.) *Plarr's Lives of the Fellows of the Royal College of Surgeons of England* (John Wright, Bristol, 1930).

Power, D'Arcy, & LeFanu, W. R., *Lives of the Fellows of the Royal College of Surgeons of England 1930–51* (Roy. Coll. Surg. Eng., London, 1953).

Power, D'Arcy, (Ed.) *British Masters of Medicine* (Med. Press & Circular, London, 1936).

Poynter, F. N. L., (Ed.) *The Evolution of Medical Practice in Britain* (Pitman Med. Pub. Co., London, 1961).

Richardson, R. R., *The Surgeon's Tale* (Charles Scribner's Sons, New York, 1958).

Rock Carling, E., & Paterson Ross, J., *British Surgical Practice* (Butterworth Med. Pub., London, 1947–61).

Shambaugh, George E., Jr., *Surgery of the Ear* (Saunders, Philadelphia, 1959).

Sigerist, H. E., *Great Doctors* (George Allen & Unwin, London, 1935).

Sigerist, H. E., *A History of Medicine* (Oxford University Press, Oxford, 1951).

Singer, C., & Underwood, E. A., *A Short History of Medicine* (Clarendon Press, Oxford, 1962).

Sorsby, A., *A Short History of Ophthalmology* (John Bale, Sons & Dannielson., London, 1933).

Stevenson, R. Scott, & Guthrie, D., *A History of Otolaryngology* (Livingstone, Edinburgh, 1949).

Welch, H., & Marti-Ibanez, F., *The Antibiotic Saga* (Medical Encyclopaedia Inc., New York, 1960).

Index of Subjects

Index of Names

Macewen, Sir William
(1848–1924), 167–8, 181,
213, 214, 215, 224, 225,
226–7, 253
McIndoe, Sir Archibald
(1900–60), 173, 177, 179
Mackenzie, Sir Morell
(1837–92), 262, 265–6
Matas, Rudolph (1860–1957),
125, 227
Mayo, Charles Horace
(1865–1939), 102–5, 177,
277
Mayo, William James
(1861–1939),102–5, 195,
200
Mêlier, François (1798–1865),
204, 205
Melrose, Denis Graham, 247
Metchnikoff, Elie Ilya Ilyich
(1845–1916), 79, 114
Merrill, John Putnam, 299–300
Meyer, Hans Wilhelm
(1825–95), 263
Mikulicz-Radecki, Johann
von (1850–1905), 72, 81,
199, 201, 205, 265
Millin, Terence, 140, 143
Miot, Camille (1838–1904),
258, 260
Moynihan, Berkeley, Lord
(1865–1936), 81, 113, 195,
199, 200, 295
Murphy, John Benjamin
(1857–1916), 125, 198,
206, 222, 249

Nissen, Rudolph, 232
Nitze, Max (1848–1906), 138,
201, 263
Nussbaum, Johann von
(1829–90), 72, 192

Ochsner, A. J. (1858–1925),
207
Odelberg, A., 199
Oliver, Percy Lane, 126–7
Ollier, Louis (1825–1901), 74,
164, 165, 167
Ombrédanne, L., 177, 178
Orr, Hiram Winnett
(1877–1956), 112, 115

Paget, Sir James (1814–99),
38–9, 87–9
Paré, Ambroise (1510–90), 173,
194, 252–3
Pasteur, Louis (1822–95),
50–1, 57, 74, 89, 118, 193
Péan, Jules (1830–98), 74, 194,
197
Physick, Philip Syng
(1768–1837), 7, 262
Pirogoff, Nikolai Ivanovitch
(1810–81), 33, 37
Platt, Sir Harry, 157
Pólya, Eugene (1876–1944), 200
Pott, Percivall (1744–88), 6, 210,
211

Rehn, Ludwig (1849–1930),
237
Reverdin, Jacques Louis
(1842–1929), 163, 164
Röntgen, Wilhelm Konrad
(1845–1922), 92–4
Rokitansky, Carl (1804–78),
85, 206
Rose, William (1847–1910),
63, 175, 216
Ryle, John Alfred
(1889–1950), 129

Sauerbruch, Ernst Ferdinand
(1875–1951), 175, 222,
228, 232

541   A 74 2ʲ